Handbook of Experimental Pharmacology

Volume 100

Targeted Drug Delivery

Contributors

K.L. Audus, N. Bodor, R.T. Borchardt, M.E. Brewster, Y.W. Chien
G. Degols, R.L. Juliano, A.S. Kearney, J. Kopeček, N.L. Krinick
B. Lebleu, J.-P. Leonetti, F.R. Maxfield, T.E. McGraw, G.L. Scherphof
V.J. Stella

Editor

Rudolph L. Juliano

With 112 Figures

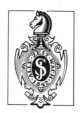

Springer-Verlag
Berlin Heidelberg New York
London Paris Tokyo
Hong Kong Barcelona
Budapest

Rudolph L. Juliano, Prof., Ph.D.
Professor and Chairman
Department of Pharmacology
University of North Carolina
School of Medicine
CB#7365, Faculty Laboratory Office Building
Chapel Hill, NC 27599-7365
USA

ISBN 3-540-52843-1 Springer-Verlag Berlin Heidelberg New York
ISBN 0-387-52843-1 Springer-Verlag New York Berlin Heidelberg

Library of Congress Cataloging-in-Publication Data. Targeted drug delivery / contributors, K.L. Audus . . . [et al.]; editor, R.L. Juliano. p. cm.—(Handbook of experimental pharmacology; v. 100) Includes bibliographical references and index. ISBN 3-540-52843-1 (alk. paper).—ISBN 0-387-52843-1 (alk. paper) 1. Drug targeting. I. Audus, Kenneth L. II. Juliano, R.L. III. Series. [DNLM: 1. Drug Administration Routes. 2. Drug Carriers. 3. Drugs—adminstration & dosage. W1 HA51L v. 100 / QV 748 T 185] QP905.H3 vol. 100 [RM301.63] 615'.1 s—dc20 [615.5'8] DNLM/DLC for Library of Congress.

© Springer-Verlag Berlin Heidelberg 1991
Printed in Germany

Typesetting: Best-set Typesetter Ltd., Hong Kong
27/3130-543210 – Printed on acid-free paper

Preface

The chapters in this volume describe a powerful emerging approach for the therapy of disease. Targeted drug delivery, that is control of the kinetic behavior, tissue distribution, and subcellular localization of pharmacologically active agents, offers an important means for improving the efficacy of a wide variety of drug therapies. This is particularly true for therapeutic approaches based on newer agents which are the products of recombinant DNA research. These agents, be they peptides, proteins, or oligonucleotides, tend to be larger, more complex, and less stable than traditional drugs. Thus they stand to benefit most from drug delivery systems which can protect them from premature degradation and which can carry them to critical target sites in the body.

This volume examines several important aspects of the current state of drug delivery research; it also attempts to project future directions for this field. Successful approaches to drug targeting are based, first of all, on a sophisticated understanding of the biological barriers encountered by the drug-carrier complex as it moves from the portal of administration to the ultimate target site. A second aspect of successful drug delivery is appropriate matching of the disease entity with the pharmacologically active substance and with the delivery system. Thus it is important to be aware of the variety of delivery technologies which currently exist and to be sensitive to their strengths and limitations. Finally, successful application of drug targeting approaches to therapeutics will require a continued evolution of new technologies as our understanding of cellular function and disease processes increases. Each of these aspects of targeted drug delivery are well represented in this volume through chapters from leading investigators in the field.

I hope that this volume will serve both to provide an overview of drug targeting research as it currently exists, and to stimulate new contributions to this exciting and rapidly developing field.

I would like to thank the chapter authors for their fine contributions, the patient staff of Springer-Verlag for their support, and Mrs. Branda Rosen for secretarial and organizational assistance.

R. L. JULIANO

List of Contributors

AUDUS, K.L., Department of Pharmaceutical Chemistry, The University of Kansas, School of Pharmacy, 3006 Malott Hall, Lawrence, KS 66045-2504, USA

BODOR, N., Center for Drug Discovery, Box J-497 JHMHC, Gainesville, FL 32610, USA

BORCHARDT, R.T., Department of Pharmaceutical Chemistry, The University of Kansas, School of Pharmacy, 3006 Malott Hall, Lawrence, KS 66045-2504, USA

BREWSTER, M.E., Research Department, Pharmatec, Inc., P.O. Box 730, Alachua, FL 32615, USA

CHIEN, Y.W., Controlled Drug-Delivery Research Center, Rutgers-State University of New Jersey, College of Pharmacy, Busch Campus, P.O. Box 789, Piscataway, NJ 08855-0789, USA

DEGOLS, G., Université de Montpellier II, Laboratoire de Biochimie des Protéines, UA CNRS 1191 "Genetique Moleculaire", Place E. Bataillon CP 012, F-34095 Montpellier Cedex 5, France

JULIANO, R.L., Department of Pharmacology, University of North Carolina, School of Medicine, CB 7365, Faculty Laboratory Office Building, Chapel Hill, NC 27599-7365, USA

KEARNEY, A.S., 11 Alpine Drive, Randolph, NJ 07869, USA

KOPEČEK, J., Department of Bioengineering, 2480 MEB, University of Utah, Salt Lake City, UT 84112, USA

KRINICK, N.L., Department of Bioengineering, 2480 MEB, University of Utah, Salt Lake City, UT 84112, USA

LEBLEU, B., Université de Montpellier II, Laboratoire de Biochimie des Protéines, UA CNRS 1119 "Genetique Moleculaire", Place E. Bataillon, F-34095 Montpellier Cedex 5, France

LEONETTI, J.-P., Université de Montpellier II, Laboratoire de Biochimie des Protéines, UA CNRS 1119 "Genetique Moleculaire", Place E. Bataillon, F-34095 Montpellier Cedex 5, France

MAXFIELD, F.R., Department of Pathology, Columbia University College of Physicans and Surgeons, 630 W. 168th Street, New York, NY 10032, USA

McGRAW, T.E., Department of Pathology, Columbia University College of Physicans and Surgeons, 630 W. 168th Street, New York, NY 10032, USA

SCHERPHOF, G.L., Laboratory of Physiological Chemistry, Faculty of Medicine, State University Groningen, Bloemsingel 10, NL-9712 KZ Groningen, The Netherlands

STELLA, V.J., Department of Pharmaceutical Chemistry, University of Kansas, Malott Hall, Lawrence, KS 66045-2504, USA
Present address: Center for Drug Delivery Research, Victorian College of Pharmacy, School of Pharmaceutics, 381 Royal Parade, Parkville, Victoria, Australia 3052

Contents

CHAPTER 3

Transport of Macromolecules Across the Capillary Endothelium
K.L. AUDUS and R.T. BORCHARDT. With 3 Figures 43

CHAPTER 6

Systemic Delivery of Pharmacologically Active Molecules Across the Skin

CHAPTER 1

A New Perspective for Drug Delivery Research

R.L. Juliano

A. Promises Realized:
A Recent History of Controlled Drug Delivery

As one of the old warhorses of drug delivery research, probably I am entitled to look backward and to take some satisfaction from the enormous progress which has been made since the time, some 15 years ago, when I first became involved with this field. Many things which were merely ephemeral dreams or vague concepts at that point have advanced to clinical application and commercial success. On the other hand, especially in the realm of targeted delivery, many of the problems anticipated in the 1970s remain unsolved. The goal of radically improving the cellular specificity of a drug (and consequently its therapeutic index) through targeted delivery persists as the unrealized Holy Grail of drug delivery research. We move incrementally toward the goal of specific targeting, but formidable chemical and biological barriers remain. However, new hope for specific targeting comes with fundamental new insights into how cells work, and with the technological mastery provided by molecular biology.

This prefatory chapter will examine selected examples of recent successes in drug delivery research and its applications. It will also point out some of the remaining problem areas and discuss ways of solving or getting around those problems. This is an enormous undertaking, and I can be concise only at the risk of slighting some of the many fine investigators who have contributed so effectively to the field of controlled and targeted drug delivery. With apologies, then, to many of my esteemed colleagues, let me begin a biased and very personalized analysis of the field.

I. Sustained Delivery Systems: A Clinical and Commercial Success

Typically, applied research and product development build on basic research done 20 or more years previously. This has certainly been true of drug delivery research. The drug delivery systems now enjoying widespread clinical utilization and considerable commercial success are, for the most part, sustained release systems whose goal is to provide constant blood levels of a drug over a protracted period of time. These systems depend very heavily on polymer chemistries developed in the period after World

War II. Using either rate-limiting polymer membranes or various types of polymer matrix release strategies, investigators working on sustained delivery preparations have honed and refined their technology over the past 20 years. Issues that needed to be addressed included the choice of drugs and therapeutic indications which were amenable to sustained delivery, the optimization of release kinetics, questions of biocompatibility and safety of the delivery system, questions of convenience and patient compliance, problems of scale-up and efficient manufacturing, and, finally, multiple factors relating to cost, market share, and the overall economics of a new pharmaceutical entity. I dwell on these considerations because other technologies in the drug delivery arena are just beginning to address some of the issues which have already been solved for sustained delivery preparations.

1. Implantable Systems

Implantable delivery systems have enjoyed their greatest use in connection with contraception (LEONG and LANGER 1987; LANGER 1990) but may have many other applications. The Norplant system, approved for use in 15 countries, including recent approval in the USA, consists of a progestin in a set of Silastic membrane-coated rods which are implanted under the skin. This system can provide effective contraception with minimal need for patient compliance and complete reversibility for a period of 5 years. This system would seem to have many advantages for fertility control in a variety of populations in both developed and developing nations. Another promising system uses a biodegradable matrix composed of copolymers of lactic and glycolic acids whose degradation products are natural metabolites. Devices of this type do not require surgical removal at the end of the treatment period. An implantable lactic-glycolic copolymer system containing a gonadotropin releasing hormone analog has recently become the first FDA-approved system for controlled release of a peptide (LANGER 1990).

2. Transdermal Systems

Perhaps the most widespread advance in the practical application of controlled delivery technology has occurred in the area of transdermal systems (CHIEN, this volume; CHIEN et al. 1987). Patch-like devices with rate-limiting membranes or rate-controlling microreservoirs are affixed to the skin with drug-compatible, hypoallergenic adhesives. These can provide sustained and controlled blood levels of drug for periods of hours to days. The attractiveness of transdermal delivery has led to rapid progress both in the design of devices for that purpose and also in our understanding of the biology and transport characteristics of the skin. There are several transdermal products currently available for the delivery of nitroglycerin for control of angina; sales of this type of product amount to approximately 500 million dollars per year (CHIEN, this volume). Transdermal systems for controlled delivery of scopolamine (for motion sickness), clonidine (for hypertension), and estradiol (for post-menopausal symptoms) are also on the market. An intriguing new development is the possible use of iontophoresis to promote transdermal delivery of polypeptides (CHIEN et al. 1987); as discussed below, effective means for the delivery of peptides and proteins is a major issue for the practical application of recombinant DNA technology.

II. Microparticulate Delivery Systems

The basic science underlying microparticulate delivery systems such as liposomes, protein microparticles, and emulsions is of more recent vintage than that which supports polymeric sustained delivery systems. Liposomes were first rigorously described in the late 1960s, and the basic physical characteristics of lipid bilayer membranes were worked out in the 1970s. Likewise, our understanding of the biology of the two organ systems which most affect the *in vivo* behavior of microparticulates, the vascular endothelial lining and the mononuclear phagocytic cells, dates from the 1970s and 1980s. While the story of microparticulate delivery systems has been replete with biological misconceptions, over-expectations, and dashed hopes, nonetheless there has also been steady progress both scientifically and technologically.

1. Solving Old Problems

In years past, critics of microparticulate delivery systems have insisted that they were "pharmaceutically unacceptable", that is, their constituents were too costly, their preparation quite complex and unsuited to scale-up, their stability questionable, and their polydispersity a potential regulatory problem. At this juncture, the critics will hopefully begin to fall silent, as most of their objections have been met and overcome.

In the case of liposomes, for example, the creation of an industrial scale market for ultra-pure lipids has led to the development of clever synthetic and preparative technologies, and to a precipitous decline in the price of pure bulk phospholipids (WEINER 1989). As to scale-up, commercial pilot plants are now generating liposomes in hundred-liter quantities, thus providing the ability to generate hundreds to thousands of doses weekly of liposome-incorporated drugs (CROSSLEY 1990; Press Release, July 1990). The problem of liposome stability has been approached in several ways. A simple expedient is to focus on use of lipid-soluble drugs, thereby eliminating much of the concern about stability (JULIANO et al. 1987). Another approach is remote loading, that is, use of a strategy which allows the liposomes to be loaded with drug at the time the sample is used in the clinic. This approach has been exploited very effectively in connection with a liposomal form of the anti-cancer drug doxorubicin (CULLIS et al. 1987). The liposomes are prepared in low-pH buffer and, at the time of use, are exposed to doxorubicin in a buffer of physiological pH; since doxorubicin has a titratable amino group, the pH gradient results in the accumulation of most of the doxorubicin in the vesicles. The liposomes, buffer, and drug are provided as a kit, and the preparation can be done at the bedside. Thus it is clear that tremendous progress has been made in overcoming many of the scale-up and pharmaceutical manufacturing problems previously believed to be barriers to the clinical application of liposomes.

2. Clinical Evaluation

An exciting aspect of progress in the microparticulate delivery system area has been the movement of several of the most advanced liposomal drug candidates into phase I and phase II clinical trials. Thus considerable clinical experience has accrued with various preparations of "liposomal" amphotericin B in connection with treatment of systemic fungal infections. Some of these preparations are actually drug-lipid complexes with a non-bilayer structure, rather than "classical" liposomes. In the USA, phase I trials (MARTIN 1990; JANOFF 1990) have been completed for two liposomal amphotericin B preparations, and phase II trials have begun for one of these (JANOFF 1990). In Europe, a third formulation of liposomal amphotericin B has been approved for clinical use and sale in at least one nation and is being considered for approval in several others (CROSSLEY 1990). Several liposomal antitumor drug candidates have also reached the stage of phase I and phase II clinical trials. Thus, at least two groups are currently conducting phase II trials in the USA of liposomal doxorubicin in breast cancer (RAHMAN 1990), and in non-lymphocytic leukemia (CREAVEN 1990a). Phase I trials have also been done on a liposomal platinum drug (PEREZ-SOLAR 1990) and on liposomal muramyl tripeptide, an immunomodulator (CREAVEN 1990b). It is also evident that regulatory agencies are beginning to look more favorably on the use of microparticulate carriers. This is borne out by the fact that approval has been granted for numerous clinical trials in the USA and Europe and by the fact that a liposomal preparation of gentamicin rapidly received approval as an orphan drug for treatment of *Mycobacterium avium intracellulare*, an opportunistic pathogen in AIDS patients (Press Release, October 1990). Thus, approximately 15 years after the first experiments with liposomal anti-tumor and anti-infectious drugs, significant clinical trials with these agents are now underway in many centers. It seems reasonable to expect that the next few years will see the appearance on the market of several liposomal drug formulations for therapy of cancer and serious infections. Experience with other microparticulate carriers lags behind that with liposomes by several years. However, some good results in animal experimentation have been observed with anti-tumor drugs in other carrier systems, including emulsions and solid microparticles (COUVREUR et al. 1990), suggesting that clinical trials may eventually be pursued.

B. The Opening Door:
Molecular Biology Generates New Opportunities and Challenges for Drug Delivery Research

I. Using the Body's Own Pharmaceuticals

One of the most exciting challenges in modern drug delivery research concerns optimizing the formulation and delivery of the products of recombinant DNA technology. We are now at the point where it seems feasible to clone, and to express in large quantities, virtually any peptide or protein found in the human body. This awesome technology gives rise to the opportunity to use the body's own regulatory and defense factors in the treatment of disease. Thus hormones, growth factors, lymphokines, monoclonal antibodies, and enzymes are now all part of the therapeutic armamentarium. The use of endogenous proteins and peptides in medicine constitutes both an enormous opportunity and an equally enormous challenge. We now have the chance to develop therapies that are more effective and more precise than those employed previously. However, we are faced with the prospect of using, as therapeutic agents, molecules which are much more complex, unstable, and difficult to analyze than traditional drugs. The multiple problems involved in efficient production, analysis, purification, and stabilization of protein/peptide-based drugs has been reviewed recently (SHARMA 1989; CARR 1989; MOZHAEV and MATINEK 1990). It seems clear that delivery systems of various types will play major roles in protein/peptide-based therapeutics. At this point, however, we are learning to match disease states and therapeutic entities with the most appropriate delivery systems. No clear "winner" seems appropriate for all problems in protein/peptide therapeutics, and delivery via the skin, the respiratory tract, and the gastrointestinal tract (at least for short peptides) are contending with intravascular delivery for therapeutic use.

II. Endocrine Vs Paracrine: A Drug Targeting Problem

A very interesting problem has emerged in connection with use of some of the peptide factors produced by recombinant DNA techniques this problem should provide a fertile field for controlled drug delivery approaches. Until recently, most of our experience with peptides as therapeutic agents has been with hormones such as insulin, products of the endocrine system. The basic physiology of endocrine control implies that a peptide hormone is designed by nature to be released at one site in the body, traverse the bloodstream, and then regulate cellular activities at distant sites. By contrast, many of the recombinant DNA products coming into use currently are not involved in *endocrine* regulation, but rather are involved in *paracrine* or *autocrine* regulation; that is, their physiology involves local production and local action (BAGBY and SEGAL 1991). Thus, molecules such as the various lymphokines, interferons, tumor necrosis factors, and colony-stimulating factors are, under normal physiological conditions, primarily involved in local regulation of cells which are in close proximity to the cells which secrete these factors. In general, these molecules have rather short lifetimes in the circulation and are rapidly degraded and/or excreted. Thus, in order to attain therapeutic levels of autocrine or paracrine factors at tissue sites, it has usually been the practice to inject enormous quantities of these materials into the systemic circulation. Quite predictably, this has led to the appearance of severe undesirable side effects, such as those observed in early therapeutic studies of interferons and of interleukin-2 (QUESADA et al. 1986; Parkinson 1988). The challenge to drug delivery experts, then, is to find ways of stabilizing these peptide factors, thus increasing their circulation lifetime, and, perhaps even more importantly, to find ways of delivering them selectively to their ultimate targets.

C. An Overview of this Volume:
Building on the Past and Looking Toward the Future

The purpose of this volume is both to analyze some of the current developments in the drug delivery arena and to anticipate the future evolution of the field. I am firmly convinced that progress in controlled and targeted drug delivery will be contingent upon an increasingly sophisticated understanding of the pathogenesis of disease processes at the molecular level, as well as on an understanding of the biological barriers to successful targeting. With this in mind, the volume stresses the biological and conceptual underpinnings of the field rather than attempting a comprehensive recapitulation of developments to date. A major bias in the volume is that it emphasizes delivery of macromolecules, including proteins, peptides and oligonucleotides, rather than delivery of more traditional drugs.

   The first part of the volume is comprised of two chapters on the transport of macromolecules by McGraw and Maxfield and by Audus and Borchardt. These chapters provide the groundwork for an understanding of how cells transport and process proteins, and how proteins and other macromolecules are transported across a multicellular barrier, the capillary endothelium. These chapters emphasize that we must first have insight into physiological processes for macromolecular transport before we can find effective means for modifying and controlling such transport. A chapter by Stella and Kearney examines the problem of targeted drug delivery in pharmacokinetic terms and thus provides a quantitative basis for the design of delivery systems. These first three chapters thus supply basic background information which impinges on the subsequent chapters.

The chapter by Krinick and Kopecek on the development of synthetic polymer carriers, gives insight into recent biological and chemical technologies for the design of macromolecular delivery systems. This chapter illustrates the ingenuity and flexibility of currently available approaches. The authors also discuss in general terms the stability, clearance behavior, and metabolic processing of exogenous macromolecules. The next three chapters provide insight into exciting current areas of drug delivery research. Chien discusses the important problem of transdermal delivery, emphasizing the delivery of peptides by iontophoretic mechanisms. Bodor and Brewster deal with the pro-drug concept and its application to targeted drug delivery. Scherphof reviews the basic characteristics and current applications of liposomal drug delivery as a timely example of microparticulate systems. These three chapters ably summarize recent development in three of the major branches of contemporary research on targeted delivery of therapeutic agents. The final chapter by Degols, Lebleu, and Leonetti turns to the future to consider a form of targeting at the molecular level. Their discussion of antisense oligonucleotide technology illustrates the exciting potential of this approach for gene-specific targeting.

These eight chapters, while heterogeneous and covering multiple aspects of research will, I hope, give the reader both a broad perspective and keen insights into the current state and future aspirations of the the field of targeted drug delivery.

D. Drug Targeting Research
in the Twenty-First Century: A New Perspective

The developments of the past decade indicate that significant progress has been made in several areas of targeted and controlled drug delivery. What, then, are the prospects for the future? Gazing into crystal balls can be hazardous, at least to one's professional reputation. Let me take the risk, however, and offer a few prognostications. First, I would venture that drug delivery research will become less of an autonomous field and, at least in major pharmaceutical companies, will be integrated with the overall process of drug development. Investigators will spend less time exploring the characteristics of delivery systems studied in splendid isolation and more time on evaluating specific match-ups of delivery technology with therapeutic moieties. Thus, considerations of potential for sustained or targeted delivery will be implicit in drug development programs and not just an afterthought.

Second, I believe we will see a continuation and expansion of concern about the delivery properties of macromolecular drugs, including polypeptides and oligonucleotides. In addition to work aimed at improving the stability and transport behavior of peptides, there will be concern about improving the verisimilitude of their use. Thus, we will try to find ways to deliver autocrine and paracrine polypeptides locally so as to mimic their normal biology; we will also see more emphasis on the chronobiology of peptides, using pulsatile delivery systems to couple into the body's physiological rhythms.

Third, advances in protein engineering and in the design and synthesis of polynucleotides will permit the merging of therapeutic moiety with targeting moiety. Thus, we may be able to design peptides which not only interact with the appropriate receptor, but which also have built into their structure features which enhance their transport and delivery. In line with this, I believe that delivery systems of the future will be miniaturized and be on a molecular scale. Thus, rather than coupling a therapeutic moiety to a large and often cumbersome delivery vehicle such as a liposome, polymer, or antibody, protein engineering (and nucleic acid engineering) will permit the design of relatively compact molecules incorporating both therapeutic and targeting features.

More than 10 years ago, in reviewing the field of controlled drug delivery as it existed at that point, I wrote, "The practitioners of drug delivery research find themselves in the interesting but difficult position of being at a nexus between an ever growing stream of information about drugs and about biological systems, and an ever-expanding reservoir of demand for more sophisticated therapeutic agents" (JULIANO 1980). This statement is probably one of the few things that has remained true about the field. Therapeutics has gotten more complex and more demanding with the challenges of AIDS, transplantation medicine, and new approaches to cancer. Our ability to respond to these challenges, however, has increased extraordinarily with the progress of molecular and cellular biology, and is now limited only by the scope of our imaginations.

References

Bagby GC, Segal GM (1991) Growth factors and the control of hematopoiesis. In: Hoffman R, et al. (eds) Hematology: basic principles and practice. Livingstone, New York, pp 97–121

Carr SA (1989) Recent advances in the analysis of peptides and proteins by mass spectrometry. Adv Drug Delivery Rev 4:112–148

Chien YW, Siddiqui O, Sun Y, Shi WM, Liu JC (1987) Transdermal iontophoretic delivery of therapeutic peptides/proteins. Ann NY Acad Sci 507:32–51

Couvreur P, et al. (1990) Nanoparticles as microcarriers for anticancer drugs. Adv Drug Delivery Rev 5:209–230

Creaven P (1990a) Conference Abstract. Liposomes in Drug Delivery: 21 Years On. London

Creaven P (1990b) Conference Abstract. Liposomes in Drug Delivery: 21 Years On. London

Crossley RJ (1990) Conference Abstract. Liposomes in Drug Delivery: 21 Years On. London

Cullis P, et al. (1987) Liposomes as pharmaceuticals. In: Ostro MJ (ed) Liposomes: from biophysics to therapeutics. Dekker, New York, pp 39–72

Janoff A (1990) Lecture. Liposomes in Drug Delivery: 21 Years On. London

Juliano RL (1980) Drug delivery systems: characteristics and biomedical applications. Oxford University Press, New York

Juliano RL, Daoud S, Krause HJ, Grant CWM (1987) Membrane to membrane transfer of lipophilic drugs used against cancer or infectious disease. Ann NY Acad Sci 507:89–103

Langer R (1990) New methods of drug delivery. Science 249:1527–1533

Leong KW, Langer R (1987) Polymeric controlled drug delivery. Adv Drug Delivery Rev 1:199–233

Martin F (1990) Conference Abstract. Liposomes in Drug Delivery: 21 Years On. London

Mozhaev VV, Matinek K (1990) Structure stability relationships in proteins: a guide to stabilizing enzymes. Adv Drug Delivery Rev 5:359–386

Parkinson DR (1988) Interleukin-2 in cancer therapy. Semin Oncol [Suppl 6] 15: 10–26

Perez-Soler R (1990) Conference Abstract. Liposomes in Drug Delivery: 21 Years On. London

Press Release, The Liposome Co., Princeton NJ, July 18, 1990

Press Release, The Liposome Co., Princeton NJ, October 1990

Quesada JR, Gutterman JU, Hersh EM (1986) Treatment of hairy cell leukemia with alpha interferons. Cancer 57:1678

Rahman A (1990) Conference Abstract. Liposomes in Drug Delivery: 21 Years On. London

Sharma SK (1989) Key issues in the purification and characterization of recombinant proteins for therapeutic use. Adv Drug Delivery Rev 4:87–112

Weiner AL (1989) Liposomes as carriers for polypeptides. Adv Drug Delivery Rev 3:307–341

CHAPTER 2

Internalization and Sorting of Macromolecules: Endocytosis

T.E. McGraw and F.R. Maxfield

A. Introduction

Endocytosis is a process used by cells to internalize a variety of macro-molecules, supramolecular complexes, and organisms. This large variety of molecules that enter cells by endocytosis illustrates the general physiological importance of this pathway. An understanding of endocytosis will provide insight into the methods available for a cell to sense and respond to its environment as well as a potential means for targeted drug delivery.

As illustrated in Fig. 1, several types of endocytic processes have been characterized in mammalian cells. Each of these processes involves the formation of a sealed vesicle formed from the plasma membrane which encloses part of the extracellular medium. The best characterized of these processes is receptor-mediated endocytosis via the clathrin-coated pit pathway. This mechanism is used for the internalization of many proteins, hormones, growth factors, viruses, and toxins. Clathrin-coated pits are used for receptor-mediated endocytosis in all nucleated mammalian cells examined to date. In addition to this well studied pathway, several ligands are internalized by non-clathrin-coated pit pathways. These endocytic pathways are not as well characterized at present, but they appear to be used for the uptake of some toxins, hormones, and nutrients.

Phagocytosis is used mainly by specialized cells such as macrophages and neutrophils for the engulfment of large particles, cells, and micro-organisms (Silverstein et al. 1977). However, nonspecialized cells such as fibroblasts also take up large particles adsorbed to their surface by a phagocytic mechanism (Okada et al. 1981).

In addition to the adsorbed molecules, extracellular fluid is also trapped in the endocytic vesicles by each of these processes (Silverstein et al. 1977). This uptake is described as fluid phase pinocytosis, and it can be largely accounted for by the endocytic processes used for internalizing adsorbed molecules or particles. However, additional processes can contribute to fluid phase pinocytosis. For example, under certain circumstances cultured cells form ruffles which collapse back onto the cell surface and trap extracellular fluid in large vesicles called macropinosomes (Willingham and Yamada 1978; Haigler et al. 1979).

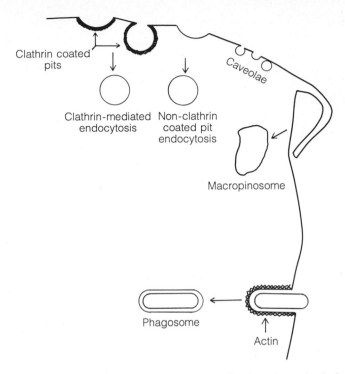

Fig. 1. Endocytic internalization pathways. Internalization through clathrin-coated pits is the best characterized of the endocytic pathways. Clathrin-coated pits are regions of the plasma membrane, of varying degrees of curvature, with a bristle-like-protein coat comprised of clathrin and clathrin associated proteins. Non-clathrin-coated pit internalization can occur through smooth invaginations, through smaller caveolae, or by a folding back of a plasma membrane ruffle to form a macropinosome. Internalization of some parasites into phagosomes by phagocytosis represents a more specialized form of internalization. All of these pathways result in the internalization of a portion of the plasma membrane and some of the extracellular milieu

There are also very specialized types of endocytosis. Malarial parasites enter red blood cells in a vacuole formed from the host cell's membrane. The bacterium *Legionella pneumophila* causes the membrane of human monocytes to wrap around it, forming a specialized type of phagosome in which the bacteria proliferate (Horwitz 1983). Other intracellular parasites use additional specialized mechanisms for entry.

The molecules or particles brought into cells by these endocytic processes have a variety of different fates. Many are delivered to lysosomes and degraded. However, the majority of receptors and some ligands are returned to the cell surface and can be reutilized. In polarized cells molecules can be transported vectorially from one side of the cell to the other, providing a mechanism for selective delivery of molecules across endothelial or epithelial layers. Some endocytosed molecules escape from the sealed vesicles and enter the cytoplasm; this process has been characterized for certain toxins and viruses. In some cases, the endocytic routes are not well understood. For example, the fate of molecules brought into the cell by non-clathrin-coated pit endocytosis is only partially characterized.

Given this rather impressive feat of delivering an array of receptors and ligands to their various destinations, cells must utilize complex sorting mechanisms along endocytic pathways. In this chapter we will describe the cellular and molecular mechanisms used to carry out the sorting of endocytosed molecules.

B. Pathways of Endocytosis in Nonpolarized Cells

The organelles involved in endocytosis have been studied in great detail in cultured fibroblast cell lines. Receptor-mediated endocytosis is initiated by the occupancy of a cell surface receptor. The distribution of unoccupied receptors on the cell surface is variable. The low density lipoprotein (LDL) receptor tends to cluster over clathrin-coated pits even in the absence of ligand (ANDERSON et al. 1982). For other receptors, such as the epidermal growth factor (EGF) or α_2-macroglobulin (α_2m) receptors, ligand occupancy is required to initiate clustering over coated pits (WILLINGHAM et al. 1979; SCHLESSINGER et al. 1983). Occupied receptors diffuse in the plasma membrane with diffusion coefficients of approximately 10^{-10} cm^2/s (WEBB et al. 1982). This diffusion is rapid enough to allow random collisions with a coated pit within a few seconds. Thus, a specific mechanisms is not required for movement of receptors to clathrin-coated pits. It should be noted that fluorescence photobleaching recovery experiments generally reveal a significant percentage of receptors that are immobile or slowly mobile. This immobile fraction, which can be as high as 50%, is thought to result from interactions with cytoskeleton (WEBB et al. 1982), but the basis for restricted mobility is poorly characterized at present.

In order to directly demonstrate that endocytosis occurs via clathrin-coated pits, electron microscopic studies must be performed. For the LDL receptor as many as 50%–70% of cell surface receptors are localized over clathrin-coated pits, which occupy approximately 2% of the plasma membrane. Thus, it is clear that the vast majority of LDL receptors enter cells via clathrin-coated pits. For many other receptors, it is difficult to see such a high percentage of receptors over coated pits. This is because the unoccupied receptors are not concentrated over coated pits, and the pits rapidly pinch off so that occupied receptors do not accumulate there. Nevertheless, it has been shown that a variety of ligands including α_2m, (WILLINGHAM et al. 1979) transferrin (WILLINGHAM et al. 1984; HARDING et al. 1983), EGF (SCHLESSINGER et al. 1983), asialoglycoproteins (WALL et al. 1980), diphtheria toxin (MORRIS et al. 1985), and Semliki forest virus (MARSH 1984) enter cells by clathrin-coated pits. This list is not meant to be comprehensive,

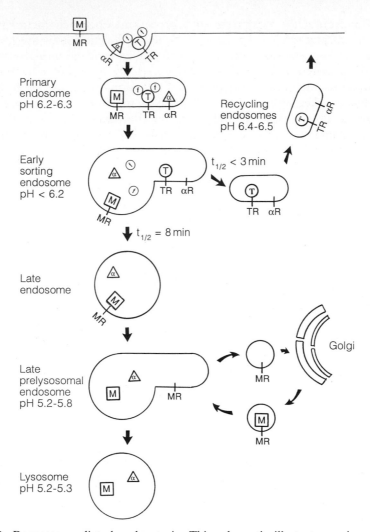

Fig. 2. Receptor-mediated endocytosis. This schematic illustrates various fates of internalized molecules. α_2-Macroglobulin (α) is released from its receptor in the acidic milieu of early endosomes. The α_2-macroglobulin receptor (αR) is sorted from the free ligand and recycled back to the cell surface. Internalized α_2-macroglobulin is eventually delivered to lysosomes. Diferric transferrin ($^f T^f$) releases its bound iron in an early endosomal compartment. Apo-transferrin, at the acidic pH of endosomes, remains associated with its receptor (TR) and is recycled back to the plasma membrane. This sorting of recycled from non-recycled molecules takes place in an early tubulovesicular endosomal compartment referred to as an early sorting endosome. Different recycled molecules, for example, the transferrin receptor and the α_2-macroglobulin receptor, are trafficked back to the plasma membrane by the same membrane-enclosed compartments. Endocytosed mannose-6-phosphate bearing proteins (M) are released from the receptor (MR) in a late prelysosomal endosome. this is the compartment to which newly synthesized mannose-6-phosphate bearing proteins are delivered from the trans-Golgi network. The mannose-6-phosphate

but rather to indicate the variety of ligand types that use the coated pit pathway.

The rate of internalization of ligand-receptor complexes has been measured in several cell types. At 37°C, half-times for internalization are approximately 1–10 min (CIECHANOVER et al. 1983; KLAUSNER et al. 1983b; WILEY 1985; McGRAW and MAXFIELD 1990). A method for measuring internalization without shifting temperature has been described (WILEY 1985). This is advantageous since temperature shifts (for example, binding on ice to prevent internalization and then rapidly shifting to 37°C) can affect the distribution of receptors (WEIGEL and OKA 1983).

At present it is unclear how coated pits pinch off from the membrane. Each clathrin-coated pit on the surface is approximately 150 nm in diameter, and the vesicle that forms from the pits rapidly loses its clathrin. These small uncoated vesicles fuse with larger compartments within minutes of formation.

I. Endosomes

These larger vesicles are part of a class of organelles called endosomes. While there has been much progress in understanding the role of endosomes over the past 10 years, many of their fundamental properties are only partially characterized. Unfortunately, this has led to a variety of names for these compartments, usually based on different sets of operational definitions depending on the property being examined. The names used in this chapter are shown in a schematic diagram (Fig. 2). We will use these names in this chapter but will try to make appropriate references to other systems of nomenclature.

The endosomes carry out several of the important processes associated with endocytosis. These include sorting and transport of internalized molecules and receptors to specific intracellular destinations as well as partial hydrolysis of some ligands. Several specialized functions have been shown to occur in endosomes. These include release of iron from transferrin, the entry of some enveloped viruses and toxins into the cytoplasm, and some critical steps in antigen processing by antigen presenting cells.

At least three types of endosomes can be distinguished. The early sorting endosome is the organelle that clathrin-coated pit-derived vesicles fuse with

---

receptors are retrieved and recycled back to the trans-Golgi. The hydrolases are eventually delivered to lysosomes. This late prelysosomal endosome is a second sorting compartment in the endosomal pathway. The late endosomal compartment (that is, post early sorting endosome) is depicted as both a late endosome and late prelysosome. The late endosome represents a compartment containing endocytosed molecules destined for the lysosomes that do not contain recycling molecules or newly synthesized lysosomal enzymes. Presently, there is no experimental evidence for this intermediate compartment. For specific details of this pathway the reader is referred to the text

almost immediately after pinching off from the cell surface. Delivery of newly internalized ligands to the early sorting endosome can be seen within 2 min (YAMASHIRO et al. 1984; DUNN et al. 1989). These endosomes are approximately 200–300 nm in diameter, and they tend to be near the cell surface. The early sorting endosome is responsible for sorting most recycling receptors from their lysosomally directed ligands. For example, LDL receptors are separated from LDL in this compartment.

The recycling endosomes carry recycling molecules back to the cell surface. Not much is known about these recycling endosomes. In Chinese hamster ovary fibroblast (CHO) cells, they are composed of small vesicles and narrow (diameter ~60 nm) tubules which accumulate in the vicinity of the Golgi apparatus but do not mix with the Golgi elements (YAMASHIRO et al. 1984). In most other cell types these recycling endosomes are dispersed throughout the cell. There is no evidence that any sorting activities are carried out by the recycling endosomes. Their main function seems to be transporting recycling molecules back to the cell surface.

The third type of endosome is the late endosome or prelysosome. The compartment contains lysosomally destined molecules like LDL, but it is essentially devoid of recycling molecules such as transferrin or the LDL receptor. This endosome is also approximately 300 nm in diameter, and in the electron microscope it often appears to contain other vesicles and has been called a multivesicular endosome. This endosome is the main site for delivery of newly synthesized lysosomal enzymes from the trans-Golgi network (KORNFELD and MELLMAN 1989; GRIFFITHS and SIMONS 1986). In Fig. 2 the late endosomal compartment is subdivided, depicted as a late endosome and a late prelysosomal endosome. The late endosome in Fig. 2 represents an intermediate stage that contains neither recycling molecules nor newly synthesized lysosomal enzymes. In the discussion that follows late endosome is synonymous with late prelysosmal endosome.

At later times internalized ligands are completely broken down by the action of lysosomal hydrolases. This process is classically described as occurring in lysosomes. However, with our current understanding, the distinction between late endosomes and lysosomes has become blurred. Newly synthesized lysosomal enzymes are delivered to late endosomes from the trans-Golgi network (GRIFFITHS and SIMONS 1986). These enzymes are routed to the endosomes by binding in the Golgi apparatus to selective receptors for mannose-6-phosphate, which is added selectively to lysosomal enzymes. Transport vesicles containing enzymes bound to the mannose-6-phosphate receptors bud off from the trans-Golgi, and these vesicles fuse with late endosomes. The lysosomal acid hydrolases are retained in the endosomes, and the receptors are recycled to the trans-Golgi network. In one categorization, organelles containing recycling mannose-6-phosphate receptors are defined as late endosomes, while the term lysosomes is reserved for organelles that are no longer acquiring newly synthesized enzymes and therefore lack the mannose-6-phosphate receptors (KORNFELD and MELLMAN 1989). This distinction is convenient for immunochemical identification of organelles, but it must be understood that many protein ligands are broken down to amino acids before entry into this compartment which lacks mannose-6-phosphate receptors. A more functional definition would be to say that late endosomes increasingly acquire lysosomal characteristics (i.e., the presence of high levels of acid hydrolases in an acidic organelle).

II. Properties of Endosomes

The mechanisms by which endosomes carry out their sorting functions are only partly understood. However, many of the important aspects of sorting can be explained at least partially from the known properties of the different types of endosomes.

1. Acidification

One of the most significant properties of endosomes is their acidic internal pH (MAXFIELD 1985). Since the spectroscopic properties of fluorescein fluorescence are strongly pH dependent, fluorescein labeled ligands can be used to measure the pH of various endocytic compartments (OHKUMA and POOLE 1978; MAXFIELD 1989). It has been found that different types of endosomes are acidified to different pH values, between pH 5.0 and pH 6.5 (TYCKO and MAXFIELD 1982; TYCKO et al. 1983; VAN RENSWOUDE et al. 1982; YAMASHIRO et al. 1984; YAMASHIRO and MAXFIELD 1987b; Roederer et al. 1987; SIPE and MURPHY 1987). The most thorough studies of endosome acidification have been carried out in cultured fibroblasts. Using a variety of fluorescein labeled ligands and different incubating protocols, the pH of the endosomal compartments in CHO cells have been determined, as summarized in Fig. 2 (YAMASHIRO et al. 1984; YAMASHIRO and MAXFIELD 1987a,b). Within 2 min, endocytosed molecules are found in organelles with an average pH of 6.2. The average pH drops over the next several minutes as molecules enter the early sorting endosomes and then the late endosomes. These later endosomal compartments maintain pH values between 5.0 and 6.0. The pH of lysosomes in these cells is between pH 5.0 and 5.5. The pH of the recycling endosomes has been measured using fluorescein-transferrin, taking advantage of the fact that transferrin remains receptor-associated as it recycles back to the cell surface (YAMASHIRO et al. 1984). The pH of the recycling endosomes in CHO cells is approximately 6.5. These pH values, which have been obtained by quantitative fluorescence microscopy and digital image analysis, are in general agreement with the pH values found in other cell types, including other fibroblast lines (TYCKO and MAXFIELD 1982), cultured human hepatoma cells (TYCKO et al. 1983), and erythroleukemia cells (VAN RENSWOUDE et al. 1982). The kinetics of acidification determined in single cells by fluorescence microscopy are also in agreement with studies on large numbers of cells by flow cytometry (SIPE and MURPHY 1987; ROEDERER et al. 1987).

The low pH is caused by the presence of an ATP-dependent proton pump in the membranes (YAMASHIRO et al. 1983). These vacuolar pumps are electrogenic (i.e., they are not directly coupled to transport of another ion to retain electroneutrality) and are part of a family of multi-subunit proton pumps which includes the pumps on chromaffin granules and on plant vacuoles (AL-AWQATI 1986). The mechanism for maintaining the pH at different values in different types of endosomes is not known, but it is probably dependent on the presence of other ion transporters in the endosome membranes. Since the pump is electrogenic, its activity will lead to an inside positive membrane potential which will increase the free energy required for proton transport. Other ion transporters (for example, chloride channels) will dissipate the electrical potential and facilitate acidification (AL-AWQATI 1986; NELSON 1987). Thus, the regulation of pH in different types of endosomes may be governed by the levels of other transporters which affect the membrane potential.

The acidification of endosomes has several important consequences. Many of the ligands that enter the cell by receptor-mediated endocytosis dissociate from their receptors at the acidic pH found in endosomes, and this is obviously a prerequisite for sorting the ligand and receptors to separate destinations. It has been shown that exposure to pH 5.5 causes conformational changes in the epidermal growth factor receptor and in the hepatocyte receptor for asilaloglycoproteins (DIPAOLA and MAXFIELD 1984). These conformational changes are presumably responsible for the loss of binding activity at low pH. The dissociation of ligands from their receptors in cells can be measured using differential precipitation methods (HARFORD et al. 1983a). It has been shown that the dissociation of several ligands including asialoglycoproteins, insulin, and lysosomal enzymes occurs as a result of endosome acidification (HARFORD et al. 1983a; TYCKO et al. 1983; BORDEN et al. 1990). When cells are treated with ionophores such as monensin that prevent endosome acidification, the dissociation of these ligands from their receptors is inhibited (HARFORD et al. 1983b).

Mutations in receptors confirm the importance of pH-induced conformational changes in receptors for the release of ligands. A variant in the human insulin receptor has been described which does not release insulin efficiently at low pH (TAYLOR and LEVENTHAL 1983). This altered receptor was found in a patient with severe insulin-resistant diabetes, and it is possible that the disease may have been related to an inability to properly recycle insulin receptors. Mutations have been introduced into the LDL receptor which alter the pH dependence of binding (DAVIS et al. 1987a).

Several of the ligands that enter cells by receptor-mediated endocytosis also undergo pH-dependent conformational changes. The iron carrier transferrin releases its two tightly bound iron atoms at low pH. The apo-transferrin remains receptor-associated at the low pH found in endosomes, but it rapidly dissociates from its receptor when it is recycled to the cell surface and is exposed to pH 7.4 (DAUTRY-VARSAT et al. 1983; KLAUSNER et al. 1983a). The apo-transferrin binds iron in the plasma, and the diferric transferrin binds again to cell surface receptors. Thus, both transferrin and its receptor are reutilized, and the pH changes are a key part of the cycle for releasing iron from transferrin within the cell.

Some toxins, such as diphtheria toxin, also undergo conformational changes at low pH (BLEWITT et al. 1983). In the case of diphtheria toxin, exposure to pH 5.0 exposes a hydrophobic surface which is thought to be important for insertion of the toxin into the membrane (DRAPER and SIMON 1980). Exposure to low pH is a requirement for entry of endocytosed diphtheria toxin into the cytoplasm. If the acidification of endosomes is blocked by ionophores or weak bases, endocytosed toxin will not enter the cytoplasm. The role of low pH has also been established by binding diphtheria toxin to the surface of cells at 4°C and forcing toxin entry from the surface by brief exposure to pH 5.0 at 37°C (SANDVIG and OLSNES 1980).

Several enveloped viruses also take advantage of the low pH in endosomes to gain entry into the cytosol. Influenza virus and Semliki forest virus have been shown to have coat proteins that undergo conformational changes at the acidic pH values found in endosomes (WHITE et al. 1983; WHITE and WILSON 1987; KIELIAN and HELENIUS 1985). These conformational changes are essential for facilitating the fusion of the viral membrane with the membrane of the target cell, allowing entry of the viral nucleocapsid into the cytosol (MARSH 1984; MARSH et al. 1983).

The hydrolytic enzymes found in late endosomes and lysosomes generally have acidic pH optima (BARRETT 1972), so development of their full activity requires acidification to approximately pH 5. Thus, lysosomal proteolysis requires acidic organelles; inhibition of intracellular hydrolysis by weak bases such as chloroquine, which raises lysosomal and endosomal pH, is often used as suggestive evidence that degradation occurs in lysosomes. One must be cautious in this interpretation since chlorquine and other lysosomotropic agents have effects in addition to those in lysosomes.

Recent evidence suggests that the cell uses the different pH values within endosomes to carry out processes in an ordered way within specific types of endosomes. The pH dependence for ligand dissociation varies with different ligand-receptor compelxes. Many ligands (e.g., insulin, EGF, and α_2m) are quite sensitive to pH, and these ligands show almost complete loss of binding at pH 6.2. Thus, these ligands will begin dissociating in the earliest endosomes. The kinetics for pH-dependent dissociation of insulin in CHO cells confirm that this occurs with a half-time of less than 5 min. In contrast, lysosomal enzyme binding to the mannose-6-phosphate receptor requires a much lower pH for dissociation. Little dissociation is found until the pH is dropped below 6.0, but the binding falls off sharply around pH 5.8 (BORDEN et al. 1990). Approximately 10% of lysosomal enzyme receptors are found on the surface of cells (KORNFELD and MELLMAN 1989), and these internalize extracellular enzymes via clathrin-coated pits (WILLINGHAM et al. 1981). Based on the measured pH values in CHO cells, dissociation of internalized lysosomal enzymes should not occur until entry into late endosomes. The dissociation of internalized mannose-6-phosphate bearing proteins from their receptors following internalization occurs with a half-time of approximately 15 min (BORDEN et al. 1990). This is consistent with the time requried for delivery of internalized molecules to late endosomes (see below). This ordered dissociation may protect many recycling molecules from degradation by lysosomal enzymes since the pH required for dissocation of enzymes from their receptors is not reached until after most recycling molecules have been removed.

Studies on virus fusion are consistent with pH-dependent events occurring within a subset of endosomes which have an appropriate pH value. Semliki forest virus coat proteins undergo a conformational change at pH 6.2 (WHITE et al. 1980) which is required for penetration of the nucleocapsid into the cytosol. Viral infections can be blocked for a few minutes after internalization by addition of weak bases or ionophores that raise the endosomal pH (MARSH et al. 1983). This suggests that it takes a few minutes for the virus to enter an endosome (for example, the early sorting endosome) that is sufficiently acidic to cause entry into the cytoplasm. Mutant viruses have been selected which fuse only at pH values near 5.5 (KIELIAN et al. 1984). The penetration of these viruses into the cytosol is slower than for wild-type virus (KIELIAN et al. 1986), as would be expected if delivery to a later, more acidic compartment (e.g., late endosomes) were reqired. Thus, as for receptor ligand dissociation, the pH dependence of the conformational change determines the type of endosome in which Semliki forest virus fusion takes place.

2. Endosome Fusion and Sorting

The preceding discussion indicates that there are functional distinctions between the various types of endosomes. This suggests that the molecular composition of the different types of endosomes should vary and that mechanisms should exist for maintaining these functional differences. At present, little is known about such mechanisms. In fact, relatively little is known about the specific proteins that make up the membrane of endosomes. It has been shown by partial purification and 2-D gel analysis that the polypeptide compositions of the different types of endosomes vary (SCHMID et al. 1988). However, at present there are no proteins that can be considered as unique markers for the endosomes, and it is not known if there necessarily are proteins that are found exclusively in the endosomes. It may be that there is such a high degree of membrane traffic between the endosomes and other compartments that all endosomal proteins are also found at significant levels in other organelles such as lysosomes, Golgi apparatus, or the plasma membrane. The search for specific endosomal membrane proteins will be an important part of the characterization of these compartments in the coming years. The existence of such proteins might provide clues about the mechanisms used to maintain endosome diversity.

Cell biological characterizations of endosomes have begun to provide some information about the basic properties of these compartments. These studies have also begun to explain how some of the sorting functions of endosomes are achieved. One of the important properties of endosomes is their ability to fuse with each other and with other organelles. In addition vesicles can bud off from endosomes (for example, the recycling endosomes which bud off from the early sorting endosomes). The discrimination between molecules that are retained as vesicles bud off and those that leave is the basis for sorting within endosomes. The basis for this sorting is not entirely known, but as described below analysis of fusion properties of endosomes leads to a basis for understanding default pathways in the sorting process.

Endosomes can fuse with each other, but there is some selectivity in the process. PASTAN and WILLINGHAM (1985) directly observed the fusion of endosomes containing internalized fluorescent tracers using image intensification fluorescence microscopy. By making exposures every 18 s, the paths of individual endosomes were tracked, and fusion events were occasionally observed.

Several types of experiments have shown that sequentially formed endosomes are able to fuse with each other but that the fusion accessibility decays with time. The data are consistent with a model in which the early sorting endosomes can fuse with newly formed endosomes, but late endosomes do not fuse efficiently with the newly formed endosomes. To demonstrate this qualitatively, cells were allowed to endocytose fluorescent LDL particles (dil-LDL) for 2 min and were then chased in the absence of ligands for various periods to allow the endocytosed dil-LDL to progress along the endocytic pathway (DUNN et al. 1989). The cells were then pulsed with fluorescein-transferrin for 2–4 min. With short intervals (2 min) between the dil-LDL pulse and the fluorescein-transferrin pulse, most of the LDL containing endosomes became labeled with fluorescein-transferrin, indicating fusion of the newly formed fluorescein-transferrin containing vesicles with the early sorting endosomes containing dil-LDL. As the interval was increased, less fusion was found. With intervals greater than 10 min, almost no fusion could be detected by this method. The loss of fusion accessibility has been quantified using a similar protocol in which fluorescein labeled proteins are chased by anti-fluorescein antibodies (SALZMAN and MAXFIELD 1988, 1989). If an endosome containing a fluorescein labeled protein fuses with an endosome containing subsequently endocytosed anti-fluorescein antibody (which enters the cell by fluid phase pinocytosis), the antibody will bind to the fluorescein and change its fluorescent properties. It was found that fluorescein-α_2m moves from a fusion-accessible compartment (early sorting endosome) to a fusion-inaccessible compartment (late endosome) with a half-time of about 8.5 min. As discussed below, the simplest explanation for this is that the α_2m is retained within an endosome that undergoes a transformation from early sorting endosome to late endosome.

Using fluorescence microscopy and digital image analysis the number of fusions during the lifetime of an early sorting endosome was determined (DUNN et al. 1989). Over a period of 10 min, approximately 40 fusions take place which result in the delivery of newly endocytosed LDL to sorting endosomes in CHO cells, and most of the LDL is retained within this compartment until it matures. The same vesicles that deliver LDL to the sorting endosome also deliver newly endocytosed transferrin, but the transferrin is rapidly exported from the sorting endosome along with its recycling receptor. The half-time for transferrin removal is less than 3 min, and the removal is accomplished by budding off recycling endosomes from the sorting endosome (SALZMAN and MAXFIED 1989). These data indicate that the sorting endosome functions by fusing with newly formed endosomes and simultaneously budding off recycling endosomes. In this way, the sorting endosome functions as an iterative fractionation apparatus, and very highly efficient sorting of recycling molecules to the surface can be achieved because the process is repeated many times. In a simple model, it was estimated that greater than 95% overall efficiency in recycling could be achieved even if each recycling endosome only captured 20%–30% of the recycling molecules present in the sorting endosome at the time it budded off (DUNN et al. 1989).

How are recycling molecules targeted to the recycling endosomes that bud off from the sorting endosome? One possibility would be that there are specific recognition signals on receptor molecules that target them for capture in the regions where recycling endosomes bud off. This would be analogous to the capture of receptors by coated pits on the cell surface. It is probable that such recognition signals are used, but no evidence for them exists. An alternative mechanism, based on the geometry of the sorting endosome, can account for much of the efficiency of sorting and would at least provide default pathways for recycling of membrane-bound molecules and delivery to lysosomes of molecules that are soluble in the endosomes.

Sorting endosomes are tubulovesicular organelles, with narrow tubules extending out from a roundish lumen that is 200–300 nm in diameter. They are similar in shape to an octopus. The recycling endosomes appear to bud off from the thin tubular extensions. Since these tubules have a high surface to volume ratio, they will remove a higher percentage of membrane than volume when they pinch off. As discussed above this pinching off is iterated many times during the lifetime of a sorting endosome, so the efficiency of sorting can become very high. Also, since the tubules contain relatively little volume, solube molecules (for example, ligands released from their receptors by the acid pH in the endosome) will tend to be retained in the rounder lumenal part of the endosome which has a low surface to volume ratio. At present there are not accurate measurements of the relative amounts of surface area and volume in the lumenal and tubular parts of the endosome, but estimates based on electron micrographs are consistent with as much as 70%–80% of the surface area of a sorting endosomes membrane being in the tubular extensions (GEUZE et al. 1983).

This model predicts that even without any sorting signals membrane-associated molecules should recycle efficiently following endocytosis. In support of this hypothesis, Pagano and co-workers have studied the endocytosis of fluorescent lipid analogues, and they found that these molecules are recycled back to the plasma membrane with 90%–95% efficiency (KOVAL and PAGANO 1989; PAGANO, personal communication). This suggests that recycling is a default pathway for internalized membrane, and the iterative fractionation provides a plausible mechanism for achieving this default pathway. The default pathway for soluble molecules is retention in the sorting endosome and delivery to lysosomes. This is seen for internalized fluid phase markers such as FITC-dextran as well as for acid-solubilized ligands. It should be noted that the efficiency for delivery to lysosomes is often considerably lower than the efficiency of recycling. Approximately 30% of internalized α_2m is returned to the surface intact and released by CHO cells (YAMASHIRO et al. 1989), and significant levels of other ligands or fluid phase markers are also released without delivery to lysosomes (BORDEN et al. 1990). The iterative fractionation which increases the efficiency of recycling will lower the efficiency of retention since small amounts of sorting endosome volume will be carried off with each recycling endosome.

3. Maturation of Endosomes

As discussed above, molecules that are soluble in the early sorting endosome (including acid-releasable ligands) tend to accumulate in the endosome for about 10 min. It is not clear at present how these retained molecules are delivered to the later endosomal compartments. One mechanism would be for the sorting endosome to undergo a maturation to a late endosome along with all of its contents. This could be accomplished, for example, by moving the endosome away from the cell surface so that fusions with incoming vesicles were halted. All molecules that had not been removed by recycling endosomes would now be in this late endosome.

An alternative mechanism for delivery to late endosomes would involve carrier vesicles that would shuttle molecules from the sorting endosome to the late endosome. In this type of a model, the sorting endosome would be a fairly stable structure from which two types of vesicles would bud. One type of vesicle (the recycling endosome) would bud off rapidly. A second type of vesicle would bud off less frequently and would preferentially carry soluble molecules for delivery to late endosomes. At present there are no data to support the existence of this second type of carrier vesicle. Further experiments will be required to distinguish between these two types of mechanisms for delivery of molecules to late endosomes. In either case, conversion of the late endosome to a hydrolytically active lysosome would occur by delivery of newly synthesized lysosomal enzymes from the trans-Golgi network.

It can be seen from this discussion that the endocytic apparatus is a complex set of organelles. The delivery of internalized molecules to specific intracellular destinations is determined by the properties of the organelles and the internalized molecules. Just as natural molecules take advantage of the unique aspects of the endosomes to achieve selective targeting, drug carriers can be designed with these properties in mind. For example, toxic drugs have been covalently attached to macromolecules via acid-sensitive linkers (SHEN and RYSER 1981). These linkers will release the drug in acidic endosomes or lysosomes much more rapidly than in the circulation.

Similarly, immunoliposomes with different pH sensitivities have been developed (COLLINS et al. 1989). These can be used to release toxins or drugs within the endocytic apparatus or via fusion with the endosome membrane into the cytosol of the target cell. Disulfide linkages are also broken within the endocytic apparatus (SHEN et al. 1985), but the site has not yet been identified.

C. Molecular Basis of Endocytosis

As discussed above, receptor-mediated endocytosis has been extensively characterized in a variety of cell culture lines using both morphological and biochemical techniques. Although a detailed picture of the intracellular pathways followed by different ligands and receptors is emerging, little is known about the molecular mechanisms of endocytosis. Elucidating the molecular mechanisms involved in the internalization, intracellular sorting, and delivery of ligands is important for understanding the physiology of the cell, both normal and pathological, and will aid in the development of strategies for the delivery of drugs, not only to specific target tissues but also to specific intracellular organelles.

Understanding endocytosis at the molecular level is presently an area of intense research. There are a number of approaches to dissecting the molecular mechanisms of this complex pathway. In this section we will review some of the recent work directed towards this goal. The intent of this section is not to serve as an exhaustive review, but to highlight the key areas of research that should eventually lead to an understanding of endocytosis at the molecular level.

I. Internalization

1. Required Receptor Sequences

A large number of genes encoding receptors that are internalized by endocytosis have been cloned and sequenced. These clones provide useful tools for performing structure/function studies of receptors. To date these studies have been most useful in providing insight into the receptor sequences required for efficient internalization through clathrin-coated pits.

The endocytic step examined in greatest molecular detail is the clustering of receptors in clathrin-coated pits. The concentration of ligand-receptor complexes in these coated pits is responsible for the rapid internalization of receptors (10%–50% of cell-surface receptors per minute), because any protein in a coated pit, as it pinches off to form an endocytic vesicle, will be internalized. Therefore, the rate at which an individual receptor is internalized is proportional to the distribution of the receptor between clathrin-coated and uncoated regions of the plasma membrane. In fibroblast cells approximately 2% of the plasma membrane is covered by clathrin-coated pits and the half-time for invagination of a coated pit is approximately 1–2 min; therefore 2%–4% of the plasma membrane can be internalized through coated pits per minute (ANDERSON et al. 1977). The significant increase in the internalization rates of receptors, over the basal rate of coated pit internalization, is the result of specific clustering of the receptors in clathrin-coated pits.

It is important to note that there are many examples of cell type specific differences in endocytic parameters; therefore caution must be exercised in generalizing specific endocytic parameters based on studies of a single cell line. For example, the percentage of the cell surface covered by clathrin-coated pits has been reported to vary from one cultured cell line to another by almost an order of magnitude (ANDERSON et al. 1977; GOLDBERG et al. 1987a). These results probably reflect differences in how specific cell types manage membrane trafficking. In this discussion we have attempted to limit ourselves to results that highlight features of endocytosis common to most cell types.

Receptor clustering in coated pits also serves as the first endocytic sorting step, since only a subclass of plasma membrane proteins are specifically concentrated in, and therefore internalized through, coated pits. Other membrane proteins are either excluded from pits (BRETSCHER et al. 1980) or are found in coated pits based on random distribution on the plasma membrane. This varying distribution of cell surface membrane proteins indicates that some proteins contain signals (or features) that are required for clustering in coated pits. The observation that different receptors can be found in a single coated pit suggested that a general "clustering signal" exists (for example, DICKSON et al. 1981, WILLINGHAM et al. 1981, CARPENTIER et al. 1982). To identify this putative "clustering signal" attention has been focused on the cytoplasmic tails of receptors, based on the assumption that these portions of the proteins would be available for interaction with the coated pit proteins. Deletion analysis of the cytoplasmic tails of a number of receptors has confirmed this prediction, with the tailless mutants being less efficiently internalized (LEHRMAN et al. 1985; LOBEL et al. 1989; McCLAIN et al. 1987; MOSTOV et al. 1986; MIETTINEN et al. 1989, PRYWES et al. 1986;

ROTHENBERGER 1987). However, the "clustering signal" is not simply a linear stretch of amino acids, but is more likely a specific protein structure, because a comparison of the sequences of the cytoplasmic domains of the endocytosed receptors has not revealed large stretches of homology, as would be anticipated if a linear amino acid sequence signal was required.

Specific amino acids on the cytoplasmic domain of receptors that are required for clustering in coated pits have been identified. The discovery that a tyrosine on the cytoplasmic domain of the human LDL receptor is required for efficient internalization proved to be the first step towards defining the sequences responsible for clustering in coated pits (DAVIS et al. 1986). Consistent with clustering in coated pits being the critical step in determining the efficiency of internalization, the LDL internalization mutants are not found clustered in coated pits to the same degree as the wild-type receptor (DAVIS et al. 1986). The requirement for a cytoplasmic tyrosine in maintaining high efficiency internalization has been extended to a number of other receptors internalized by endocytosis: LDL (DAVIS et al. 1987b); transferrin receptor (McGRAW and MAXFIELD 1990); 275 kDa Mannose-6-phosphate receptor (LOBEL et al. 1989); IgA/IgM receptor (MOSTOV et al. 1988). In each case the internalization of the mutant receptor is decreased by three- to ten-fold. We have shown that the sole tyrosine on the cytoplasmic domain of the human transferrin receptor is required for efficient internalization, but rather than being a specific requirement for a tyrosine, it is the aromatic nature of the residue that appears to be critical, as phenylalanine and tryptophan can substitute for tyrosine (McGRAW and MAXFIELD 1990). Similar results have been found for the LDL receptor (DAVIS et al. 1987b). Although these studies demonstrate that aromaticity is critical, it is of interest to note that in all receptors examined to date, the native residue critical for internalization is a tyrosine, implying that under certain conditions a tyrosine is specifically required.

A specific requirement for tyrosine has been demonstrated in one experimental system (LAZAROVITS and ROTH 1989). It was found that the substitution of a tyrosine for the native cysteine residue, six amino acids from the predicted transmembrane region in the ten amino acid cytoplasmic tail of the influenza hemagglutinin, converts this protein from a poorly to an efficiently internalized protein, whereas substitution with a phenylalanine does not promote internalization. This result can be reconciled with those of the LDL and transferrin receptors if one considers that native receptor proteins are likely to contain other signals (for example, structural features) that promote efficient internalization. In the context of these other features a phenylalanine could possibly substitute for tyrosine, whereas in the absence of these other clustering features (as in the case of the influenza hemagglutinin) there is a stringent requirement for tyrosine.

Mutagenesis studies of the LDL receptor have documented that the amino acids surrounding the tyrosine also influence the internalization rate of the receptor (CHEN et al. 1990). The sequence near the tyrosine of the LDL receptor is NPVY. Substitution of the asparagine, proline, or tyrosine with alanine results in a decrease in the internalization rate. The amino acid at the position of the valine is not critical. The sequence NPxY is found in the cytoplasmic domain of 13 cell surface membrane proteins that are either known or believed to be internalized through coated pits, indicating that this sequence might be a general internalization signal (CHEN et al. 1990). Future mutagenesis studies are needed to experimentally confirm the requirement of this sequence in the internalization of these other membrane proteins.

A number of proteins known to be internalized through coated pits, notably the transferrin and the large mannose-6-phosphate receptors, require tyrosines for efficient internalization but do not contain the NPXY sequence (MCGRAW and MAXFIELD 1990; LOBEL et al. 1989). It is likely, therefore, that tyrosine is the recognized amino acid and the NPx sequence is required, in the LDL receptor at least, for its presentation (possibly by maintaining a required local protein structure). In the transferrin and mannose-6-phosphate receptors other amino acids are likely involved in presentation of the tyrosines.

As mentioned previously, some receptors appear to be excluded from clathrin-coated pits under basal conditions and are only concentrated in coated pits (and thus internalized) under specific conditions. The best characterized example of this class of receptor is the EGF receptor, which upon binding ligand is clustered in coated pits and internalized (SCHLESSINGER 1980; DUNN and HUBBARD 1984). The binding of extracellular ligand activates, by an unknown mechanism, the intrinsic tyrosine kinase activity of the cytoplasmic domain of the receptor (CARPENTER and COHEN 1990). The kinase is capable of autophosphorylation as well as phosphorylation of other cellular substrates (CARPENTER and COHEN 1990). The roles that ligand binding, tyrosine kinase activation, and autophosphorylation play in converting this receptor from diffusely distributed to coated pit localized are presently unclear. It is known that the EGF receptor is internalized into cells through the same clathrin-coated pits as other receptors (SCHLESSINGER 1980; CARPENTIER et al. 1982). The mechanism responsible for this ligand-induced clustering is not known. It is of interest to note that, although the EGF receptor contains the NPxY "clustering signal" discussed above, deletion analysis has shown that it is not required for ligand induced internalization, suggesting that this clustering occurs by a different mechanism (GLENNEY et al. 1988).

The above discussion highlights the complexity in the first step of the specific endocytosis of a protein. A more complete understanding of the molecular and structural requirements for clustering of receptors in clathrin-coated pits and subsequent internalization of membrane proteins will come with more detailed mutagenesis studies and a determination of the 3-D structure of receptors' cytoplasmic domains.

2. Clathrin-Coated Pit Clustering Proteins

Impressive inroads have been made in identifying the features of receptors required for efficient internalization, in part because the clones of the receptors provide excellent tools for characterization. However, correspondingly little progress has been made in identifying the proteins that interact with this signal and thereby cluster receptors in coated pits. The major protein components of clathrin-coated pits have been identified, which include the clathrin heavy and light chains and a series of proteins ranging in molecular weight from 55–110 kda (ZAREMBA and KEEN 1983; PEARSE and ROBINSON 1984). These proteins have been referred to as the clathrin-associated proteins, clathrin assembly proteins, clathrin accessory proteins, and the adaptins, depending on which of their activities is being examined (VIGER et al. 1986; KEEN 1987; AHLE et al. 1988; MAHAFFEY et al. 1989). These proteins have been shown to stimulate assembly of clathrin baskets in vitro (for example, WOODWARD and ROTH 1978), have been proposed to be involved in the assembly of clathrin-coated pits in vivo (MAHAFFEY et al. 1989), and have been proposed to be required for clustering receptors in coated pits (PEARSE 1988). The latter activity is based on in vitro experiments that suggest that the adaptins bind more avidly to the cytoplasmic domains of receptors internalized by endocytosis than to those that are not efficiently internalized (PEARSE 1988; GLICKMAN et al. 1989). These in vitro results are suggestive, although the exact role of the adaptins in the in vivo clustering of receptors in coated pits needs to be experimentally documented and needs to be determined in other in vitro systems.

3. Formation of Endocytic Vesicles

The mechanism involved in the formation of an endocytic vesicle from a coated pit is not known. It is generally accepted that clathrin, possibly by its propensity to form basket structures, is requried for the pinching off of a vesicle from a coated pit. Some direct experimental evidence for the requirement of clathrin in endocytosis comes from studies in which anti-clathrin antibodies, introduced into the cytoplasm of cells, block endocytosis (DORSEY et al. 1987).

The availability of inhibitors that block internalization would provide tools useful for identifying internalization intermediates and lead to a better mechanistic understanding of this process. Unfortunately compounds that specifically block internalization have not as yet been identified. It is known that internalization is blocked at 4°C and that it requires energy (HAIGLER et al. 1980). Somewhat surprisingly, agents that disrupt microtubules (OKA and WEIGEL 1983) or actin microfilaments (WOLKOFF et al. 1984) do not prevent internalization. Other general cell treatments have also been found to affect the internalization of receptors by endocytosis. These include acidification of the cytosol to pHs < 6.5 (SANDVIG et al. 1987, 1989; DAVOUST et al. 1987; COUSSON et al. 1990), depletion of intracellular K^+ (LARKIN et al.

1983), and hypertonic shock (CARPENTIER et al. 1989; HEUSER and ANDERSON 1989). It appears as if acidification of the cytosol stabilizes coated pits on the plasma membrane, thus reducing internalization (HEUSER 1989). Potassium ion depletion and hypertonic shock appear to stabilize clathrin micro-cage structures, thereby effectively reducing the soluble pool of clathrin available for the formation of coated pits (HEUSER and ANDERSON 1989). These treatments have very general effects on cells and are probably altering a number of vesicular trafficking steps, thus limiting their usefulness in the mechanistic dissection of endocytosis. A number of in vitro/cell-free systems, attempting to reconstitute the formation of an endocytic vesicle from a coated pit, are presently being developed that should allow for a more detailed biochemical dissection of this step (for example, SMYTHE et al. 1989).

II. Intracellular Routing

The molecular signals required for the post-internalization steps (for example, delivery of receptors to lysosome vs recycling to the plasma membrane) have not been identified. As mentioned previously, there is intracellular sorting of receptors with final destinations including the trans-Golgi network, lysosomes, and the plasma membrane. The majority of proteins that are retained within the cells are eventually delivered to lysosomes. None of the mutations made in the cytoplasmic domains of the recycling receptors have been found to affect the rate or efficiency of recycling of receptors, consistent with the proposal that the bulk of receptor recycling can be viewed as a default pathway (DUNN et al. 1989).

Having the recycling pathway be the default pathway makes teleological sense since an inadvertently internalized plasma membrane protein would be returned to the cell surface rather than being degraded. As discussed in a previous section, a potential mechanism for this sorting is an iterative fractionation model in which a greater than 95% overall recycling efficiency can be achieved without requiring a specific recycling signal (DUNN et al. 1989).

The default recycling pathway does not explain all aspects of receptor sorting in endosomes. First, the recycling efficiency of receptors, including those for transferrin or LDL, are higher than 98% (GOLDSTEIN et al. 1985). This is significantly higher than for lipids and suggests that some additional aspect of the recycling molecules facilitates recycling. Second, some receptors are not recycled efficiently. The EGF receptor is one example of a molecule that is delivered to lysosomes and degraded following endocytosis (SCHLESSINGER et al. 1983).

What are the signals for retention and degradation of a membrane protein? The "signal" that diverts a membrane protein from the recycling pathway may be a physical characteristic of the protein. For example, recycling of the transferrin, LDL, or Fc receptors can be greatly reduced by binding the receptor with poly-valent antibodies (ANDERSON et al. 1982; MELLMAN and PLUTNER 1984; SCHWARTZ et al. 1986). The larger the aggregate the more serious the effect on recycling, suggesting that the oligomeric state of the protein is important in determining its final destination within the cell.

The best studied example of a native receptor sorted specifically to the lysosomal pathway is the EGF receptor. Recent studies have shown that EGF receptor sorting to the lysosomal pathway requires active EGF receptor tyrosine kinase and that receptor autophosphorylation is not required (FELDER et al. 1990). The role that the intrinsic receptor kinase plays in the intracellular sorting is not clear.

There is evidence that certain proteins can be internalized by endocytosis and sorted to the trans-Golgi network (TGN). It has been shown biochemically that internalized transferrin and transferrin receptor can be exposed to siayltransferase located in the TGN/trans-Golgi (SNIDER and ROGERS 1985). The half-time for resiaylation (hours) is very slow compared to the half-time for transferrin receptor recycling (10–20 min), thus indicating that delivery to the TGN is not the bulk endocytic pathway for transferrin. Other ligands may be more efficiently delivered to the TGN. For example, there are a number of lines of evidence demonstrating that ricin toxin is delivered to the TGN and that delivery to this site is required for cytotoxicity (see VAN DEURS et al. 1989). The intracellular compartment from which this sorting to the TGN takes place has not been identified.

A third representative of mixing between the endosomal and TGN compartments is the mannose-6-phosphate receptor (KORNFELD 1987; GRIFFITHS and SIMONS 1986). This intracellular shuttling is responsible for the delivery of newly synthesized hydrolases to the lysosomes. The efficiency of this shuttling is very high and is probably mediated by the recognition of a specific "signal" on the receptors (LOBEL et al. 1989; GLICKMAN et al. 1989). The sorting back to the TGN occurs from a late prelysosomal endosome (Fig. 2) that is distinct from the transferrin receptor containing sorting endosome, indicating the existence of at least two distinct endosomal sorting compartments (KORNFELD and MELLMAN 1989).

As is the case with the internalization step, specific inhibitors of intracellular trafficking and sorting have not been identified, although a number of less specific treatments have been shown to perturb trafficking. The delivery of ligands to lysosomes has been shown to be temperature-dependent with a block in movement of ligands from a late endosomal compartment to a lysosomal compartment observed at 16°–18°C (DUNN et al. 1980; WOLKOFF et al. 1984; MUELLER and HUBBARD 1986). This step can also be blocked by treating the cells with isotonic K^+ buffers (WARD et al. 1990). The delivery of ligands to lysosomes is dependent upon intact microtubules, as agents that disrupt microtubules have been found to reduce delivery to lysosomes, whereas intact microtubules are not required for internalization or receptor recycling. These treatments have been useful in delineating the endocytic pathway and in helping to define particular compartments, although in none of these cases is the mechanism responsible for inhibition understood.

A number of in vitro/cell-free systems have been developed to bio-chemically characterize intracellular routing (DAVEY et al. 1985; GRUENBERG and HOWELL 1986; BRAELL 1987; DIAZ et al. 1988; GRUENBERG et al. 1989). The best characterized systems are those that measure fusion of endocytic vesicles. The results of the in vitro studies correlate well with the in vivo studies of endosome fusion. The in vitro systems have shown that endosome fusion is regulated (that is, only specific subsets of endosomes can fuse), energy dependent and dependent on cytosolic factor(s). These studies have begun to elaborate the general endosomal fusion apparatus, however the molecules regulating the specific fusion among endosomal compartments have not been identified.

D. Noncoated Pit Internalization

Most of the studies of receptor specific endocytosis have focused on inter-nalization through the above discussed clathrin-coated pit pathway. There is, however, substantial evidence for an alternative non-clathrin-coated pit internalization pathway. An excellent and comprehensive review of non-clathrin-coated pit internalization has recently appeared (VAN DEURS et al. 1989). This brief discussion should only serve as a general introduction to the existence of "alternative" internalization pathways and to attest to the complexity of the overall endocytic pathway.

Internalization by non-clathrin-coated pits is often referred to as non-coated pit internalization. This is likely a misnomer, since it is not known whether there is a molecular coat required for smooth pit formation and internalization, but it is only known that a clathrin coat is not involved.

It has been known for a number of years that non-clathrin-coated pits/invaginations occur in the plasma membranes of many cells. These invagina-tions range in size from the smaller, uniformly shaped caveolae of approxi-mately 50–100 nm diameter (ORCI et al. 1978; WILLINGHAM et al. 1979; VAN DEURS et al. 1982; GOLDBERG et al. 1987a; TRAN et al. 1987; ROTHBERG et al. 1990) to the larger, more amorphously shaped smooth invaginations of approximately 150–300 nm diameter (SANDVIG et al. 1987; VAN DEURS et al. 1989). It has recently been proposed that these caveolae are involved in the concentrated uptake of small nutrients, for example uptake of folate (ROTHBERG et al. 1990). Present evidence suggests that the caveolae are more stable structures than are clathrin-coated pits, with postulated half-times for opening and closing of about 30 min. Unlike endocytic vesicles formed from coated pits, that move deeper into the cell, caveolae may not actually pinch off to form vesicles, but instead the opening of the cavoelae may transiently constrict to enclose a portion of the plasma membrane and some of the extracellular milieu (ROTHBERG et al. 1990).

Large ligands are also known to specifically be internalized by non-clathrin-coated pathways, including cholera toxin (FISHMAN 1982), tetanus toxin (MONTESANO et al. 1982), and ricin toxin (SANDVIG et al. 1987). Ricin toxin, which binds to galactose residues on the cell surface, is internalized into cells by non-clathrin-coated pits. Ricin is not found, using electron microscopy, to be clustered over clathrin-coated pits, but is concentrated over smooth invaginations of the plasma membrane. Biochemical treatments that reduce clathrin-mediated internalization do not reduce internalization of ricin toxin (SANDVIG et al. 1987), further suggesting that clathrin-coated pits are not required for its internalization. As noted above, ricin toxin is routed to the TGN. Delivery to the TGN does not seem to be specifically related to non-clathrin-coated pit internalization, but rather is a result of differences in intracellular trafficking.

The physiologically important ligand insulin has also been shown, by electron microscopy and biochemical analysis, to be internalized by a non-clathrin-coated pit pathway in adipocyte cells, demonstrating the potential physiological importance of this pathway (GOLDBERG et al. 1987a,b). It has been suggested that insulin internalized through non-clathrin-coated pits could gain access to a distinct set of intracellular compartments. Supporting this claim, in adipocyte cells, the early non-clathrin-coated internalization compartments are not mixed with the early compartments labeled by internalization through coated pits (GOLDBERG et al. 1987b). Interestingly, insulin is internalized in human lymphocyte cells by clathrin-coated pits, again illustrating the cell type specific differences in endocytosis (CARPENTIER et al. 1981).

These other internalization pathways are now receiving more attention. Future analysis will address such questions as whether the morphologically defined caveolae, observed in a number of different cells types, are similar in function or if the ligands internalized into the caveolae vary greatly among cell types, as is indicated by the studies of insulin internalization.

E. Endocytosis in Polarized Cells

Endocytosis in epithelial cells is particularly interesting because sheets of these cells provide a barrier distinguishing lumenal/exterior compartments from the serosal environment. To accomplish this the cells are polarized with tight junctions separating differentiated apical and basolateral plasma membrane domains (for review see RODRIGUEZ-BOULAN 1983). Most aspects of endocytosis in polarized cells are similar to those discussed in previous sections. The added level of complexity in polarized cells is in the intracellular sorting pathways, because receptors and ligands cannot only be recycled back to the membrane domain from which they were internalized, but can also be transported across the cell to the opposite plasma membrane domain by a process referred to as transcytosis (Fig. 3). Maintenance of po-

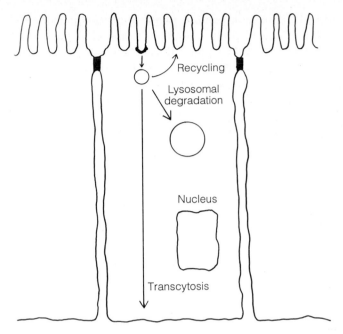

Fig. 3. Endocytic destinations in polarized cells. Ligands internalized by polarized cells can be recycled back to the surface from which they were internalized, delivered to the lysosomes (or another intracellular site), or transported across the cells and delivered to the opposite membrane domain (transcytosis). Transcytosis of proteins presents an added level of complexity in membrane trafficking by polarized cells

larity requires a cycling of proteins back to the original membrane. Transcytosis of physiological ligands and tracer molecules has been shown for a number of epithelial cell types. For example, Fc-mediated transcytosis of IgG by intestinal epithelia of neonatal rats has been documented (ABRAHAMSON and RODEWALD 1981) as has the transcytosis of fluid phase marker colloidal gold in thyroid inside-out follicles (HERZOG 1984).

The most widely used culture system for studies of membrane trafficking, both endocytosis and biogenesis, in polar cells is the Madin-Darby canine kidney (MDCK) cell line (LEIGHTON et al. 1969). These cells form tight junctions when grown on permeable supports, thereby allowing controlled access to both of the differentiated plasma membrane domains. The general endocytic pathway that has emerged from studies of MDCK cells is that the endocytic contents from both membranes (apical and basolateral) are immediately internalized into vesicles that remain near the surface from which they were internalized (BOMSEL et al. 1989). At early time points the contents of the vesicles from the opposite membrane domains do not mix. At later time points the contents mix in vivo and have been found to fuse in vitro. This mixing is dependent on the presence of an intact microtubule network, similar to the delivery of endocytosed material to lysosomes in non-polarized cells. The bulk of fluid phase material internalized from the apical membrane is either transcytosed or is recycled back to the apical membrane, whereas the bulk of fluid phase material internalized from the basolateral surface is delivered to lysosomes (BOMSEL et al. 1990).

Work has begun on characterizing the signals responsible for intracellular routing in polarized cells. Studies of the behavior of the polymeric immunoglobulin receptor expressed on MDCK cells have demonstrated that receptor phosphorylation is required for efficient transcytosis (CASANOVA et al. 1990). These studies demonstrate that molecular signaling and recognition is involved in the intracellular sorting and transport in polarized cells.

F. Summary

The objective of this chapter was to outline what is known about the basic mechanisms of endocytosis. These pathways are physiologically important because they provide the major means by which a cell interacts with and responds to its environment. A detailed understanding of endocytosis will provide insights into the normal and pathological functioning of cells. Furthermore, since endocytosis provides a specific and efficient means of internalizing molecules into cells, drugs or drug delivery systems can be developed to take advantage of this process and thereby provide for efficient and specific drug delivery.

Acknowledgements. The authors thank Lester Johnson and Kenneth Wei for their help in preparation of this manuscript.

References

Abrahamson DR, Rodewald R (1981) Evidence for the sorting of endocytic vesicle contents during the receptor-mediated transport of IgG across the new born rat intestine. J Cell Biol 91:270–280
Ahle H, Mann A, Eichelsbacher U, Ungewickel E (1988) Structural relationships between clathrin assembly proteins from the Golgi and the plasma membrane. EMBO J 7:919
Al-Awqati Q (1986) Proton-translocating ATPases. Annu Rev Cell Biol 2:179–199
Anderson RGW, Brown MS, Goldstein JL (1977) Role of coated endocytic vesicle in the uptake of receptor bound low density lipoprotein in human fibroblasts. Cell 10:351–364
Anderson RGW, Brown MS, Beisiegel U, Goldstein JL (1982) Surface distribution and recycling of the LDL receptor as visualized by anti-receptor antibodies. J Cell Biol 93:523–531
Barrett AJ (1972) Lysosomal enzymes. In: Dingle JT (ed) Lysosomes: a laboratory handbook. Elsevier North-Holland Amsterdam, pp 46–135
Blewitt MG, Chung LA, London E (1985) Effect of pH on the conformation of diphtheria toxin and its implications for membrane penetration. Biochemistry 24:5458–5464
Bomsel M, Prydz K, Parton RG, Gruenberg J, Simons K (1989) Endocytosis in filtergrown Madin-Darby canine kidney cells. J Cell Biol 109:3243

Borden LA, Einstein R, Gabel CA, Maxfield FR (1990) Acidification-dependent dissociation of endocytosed insulin precedes that of endocytosed proteins bearing the mannose-6-phosphate recognition marker. J Biol Chem 265:8497–8504

Braell WA (1987) Fusion between endocytic vesicles in a cell-free system. Proc Natl Acad Sci USA 84:1137–1141

Bretscher MS, Thompson JN, Pearse BMF (1980) Coated pits act as molecular filters. Proc Natl Acad Sci USA 77:4156–4159

Carpenter G, Cohen S (1990) Epidermal growth factor. J Biol Chem 265:7709–7712

Carpentier J-L, van Obberghen E, Gordon P, Orci L (1981) Surface redistribution of 125I-insulin in cultured human lymphocytes. J Cell Biol 91:17–25

Carpentier J-L, Gorden P, Anderson RGW, Goldstein JL, Brown MS, Cohen S, Orci L (1982) Co-localization of ^{125}I-epidermal growth factor and ferritin-low density lipoprotein in coated pits: a quantitative electron microscopy study in normal and mutant human fibroblasts. J Cell Biol 95:73–77

Carpentier J-L, Sawano F, Geiger D, Gorden P, Perrelet A, Orci L (1989) Potassium depletion and hypertonic medium reduce "non-coated" and clathrin-coated pit formation, as well as endocytosis through these gates. J Cell Physiol 138:519–526

Casanova JE, Breitfeld PP, Ross SA, Mostov KE (1990) Phosphorylation of the polymeric immunoglobulin receptor required for its efficient transcytosis. Science 248:742–745

Chen J-L, Goldstein JL, Brown MS (1990) NPXY, a sequence often found in cytoplasmic tails, is required for coated pit mediated internalization of the LDL receptor. J Biol Chem 265:3116–3123

Ciechanover A, Schwartz AL, Dautry-Varsat A, Lodish HF (1983) Kinetics of internalization and recycling of transferrin and the transferrin receptor in a human hepatoma cell line. J Biol Chem 258:9681–9689

Collins D, Maxfield FR, Huang L (1989) Immunoliposomes with different acid sensitivities as probes for the cellular endocytic pathway. Biochim Biophys Acta 987:47–55

Cousson P, de Curtis I, Pouyssegur J, Griffiths G, Davoust J (1990) Low cytoplasmic pH inhibits endocytosis and transport from the trans-Golgi network and the cell surface. J Cell Biol 108:1989

Dautry-Varsat A, Ciechanover A, Lodish HF (1983) pH and the recycling of transferrin during receptor-mediated endocytosis. Proc Natl Acad Sci USA 80:2258–2262

Davey J, Hurtley SM, Warren G (1985) Reconstitution of an endocytic fusion event in a cell-free system. Cell 43:643–652

Davis CG, Lehrman MA, Russell DW, Anderson RGW, Brown MS, Goldstein JL (1986) The J.D. mutation in familial hypercholesterolemia: amino acid substitutions in cytoplasmic domain impedes internalization of LDL receptors. Cell 45:15–24

Davis CG, Goldstein JL, Sudhof TC, Anderson RGW, Russell DW, Brown MS (1987a) Acid-dependent ligand dissociation and recycling of LDL receptor mediated by growth factor homology region. Nature 326:760–765

Davis CG, van Driel IR, Russell DW, Brown MS, Goldstein JL (1987b) The low density lipoprotein receptor. J Biol Chem 262:4075–4082

Davoust J, Gruenberg J, Howell KE (1987) Two threshhold values of low pH block endocytosis and different stages. EMBO J 6:3601–3609

Diaz R, Mayorga L, Stahl P (1988) In vitro fusion of endosomes following receptor-mediated endocytosis. J Biol Chem 263:6093–6100

Dickson RB, Willingham MC, Pastan I (1981) α_2-Macroglobulin absorbed to colloidal gold: a new probe in the study of receptor-mediated endocytosis. J Cell Biol 89:29–34

DiPaola M, Maxfield FR (1984) Conformational changes in the receptors for epidermal growth factor and asialoglycoproteins induced by the mildly acidic pH found in endocytic vesicles. J Biol Chem 259:9163–9171

Dorsey SJ, Brodskey FM, Blank GS, Helenius A (1987) Inhibition of endocytosis by anti-clathrin antobodies. Cell 50:453–463

Draper RK, Simon MI (1980) The entry of diphtheria toxin into mammalian cell cytoplasm: Evidence for lysosomal involvement. J Cell Biol 87:849–854

Draper RK, Goda Y, Brodsky FM, Pfeffer SR (1990) Antibodies to clathrin inhibit endocytosis but not recycling to the trans Golgi network in vitro. Science 248: 1539–1541

Dunn KW, McGraw TE, Maxfield FR (1989) Iterative fractionation of recycling receptors from lysosomally destined ligands in an early sorting endosome. J Cell Biol 109:3303–3314

Dunn WA, Hubbard AL (1984) Receptor-mediated endocytosis of epidermal growth factor by hepatocytes in the perfused rat liver: ligand and receptor dynamics. J Cell Biol 98:2148–2159

Dunn WA, Hubbard AL, Aronson NN Jr (1980) Low temperature selectively inhibits fusion between pinocytic vesicles and lysosomes during hetrophagy of [^{125}I]asialofetuin by the perfused rat liver. J Biol Chem 255:5971–5978

Felder S, Miller K, Moehren G, Ullrich A, Schlessinger J, Hopkins CR (1990) Kinase activity controls the sorting of the epidermal growth factor within the multivesicular body. Cell 61:623–634

Fishman PM (1982) Internalization and degradation of cholera toxin by cultured cells: relationship to toxin action. J Cell Biol 93:860–865

Geuze HJ, Slot JW, Strous G (1983) Intracellular site of asialoglycoprotein receptor-ligand uncoupling: double-label immunoelectron microscopy during receptor-mediated endocytosis. Cell 32:277–287

Glenney JR, Chen WS, Lazar CS, Walton GM, Zokas LM, Rosenfeld MG, Gill GN (1988) Ligand-induced endocytosis of the EGF receptor is blocked by mutational inactivation and by microinjection of anti-phosphotyrosine antibodies. Cell 52: 287–307

Glickman JN, Conibear E, Pearse BMF (1989) Specificity of binding of adaptors to signals on the mannsoe-6-phosphate/insulin-like growth factor II receptor. EMBO J 8:1041–1047

Goldberg RL, Smith RM, Jarrett L (1987a) Insulin and α_2-macroglobulin-methylamine undergo endocytosis by different mechanisms in rat hepatocytes. I. Comparision of cell surface events. J Cell Physiol 133:203–212

Goldberg RL, Smith RM, Jarrett L (1987b) Insulin and α_2-macroglobulin-methylamine undergo endocytosis by different mechanisms in rat hepatocytes. II. Comparision of intracellular events. J Cell Physiol 133:213–218

Goldstein JL, Brown MS, Anderson RGW, Russell DW, Schneider WJ (1985) Receptor-mediated endocytosis: concepts emerging from the LDL receptor system. Annu Rev Cell Biol 1:1–39

Griffiths G, Simons K (1986) The trans-Golgi network: sorting at the exit site of the Golgi complex. Science 234:438–443

Gruenberg JE, Howell KE (1986) Reconstitution of vesicle fusions occurring in endocytosis with a cell-free system. EMBO J 5:3091–3101

Gruenberg JH, Griffiths G, Howell KE (1989) Characterization of the early endosome and putative endocytic carrier vesicles in vivo and with an assay of vesicle fusion in vitro. J Cell Biol 108:1301–1316

Haigler HT, McKanna JA, Cohen S (1979) Rapid stimulation of pinocytosis in human carcinoma cells. A-431 by epidermal growth factor. J Cell Biol 83:82–90

Haigler HT, Maxfield FR, Willingham ML, Pastan I (1980) Dansylcadaverine inhibits internalization of ^{125}I-epidermal factor in Balb 3T3 cells. J Biol Chem 255: 1239–1241

Harding C, Heuser J, Stahl P (1983) Receptor-mediated endocytosis of transferrin and recycling of the transferrin receptor in rat reticulocytes. J Cell Biol 97: 329–339

Harford J, Bridges K, Ashwell G, Klausner RD (1983a) Intracellular dissociation of receptor-bound asialoglycoproteins in cultured hepatocytes. J Biol Chem 258: 3191–3197

Harford J, Wolkoff AW, Ashwell G, Klausner RD (1983b) Monensin inhibits intracellular dissociation of asialoglycoproteins from their receptor. J Cell Biol 96: 1824–1828

Herzog V (1984) Pathways of endocytosis in thyroid follicle cells. Int Rev of Cytol 91:107–139

Heuser J (1989) Effects of cytoplasmic pH on clathrin lattice morphology. J Cell Biol 108:410–411

Heuser J, Anderson RGW (1989) Hypertonic media inhibit receptor-mediated endocytosis by blocking clathrin-coated pit formation. J Cell Biol 108:389–400

Honegger AM, Schmidt A, Ullrich A, Schlessinger J (1990) Separate endocytic pathways of kinase-defective and -active EGF receptor mutants expressed in the same cells. J Cell Biol 110:1541–1548

Horwitz MA (1983) Formation of a novel phagosome by Legionnaire's disease bacterium (*Legionella pneumophila*) in human monocytes. J Exp Med 158: 1319–1331

Keen JH (1987) Clathrin assembly proteins: affinity purification and a model for coat assembly. J Cell Biol 105:1989

Kielian MC, Helenius A (1985) pH-induced alterations in the fusogenic spike protein of Semliki Forest virus. J Cell Biol 101:2284–2291

Kielian MC, Keränens, Kääriänen L, Helenius A (1984) Membrane fusion mutants of Semlike Forest virus. J Cell Biol 98:139–145

Kielian MC, Marsh M, Helenius A (1986) Kinetics of endosome acidification detected by mutant and wild-type Semliki Forest virus. EMBO J 5:3103–3109

Klausner RD, Ashwell G, van Renswoude J, Harford JB, Bridges KR (1983a) Binding of apotransferrin to K562 cells: explanation of the transferrin cycle. Proc Natl Acad Sci USA 80:2263–2266

Klausner RD, van Renswoude J, Ashwell G, Kempf C, Schechter AN, Dean A, Bridges KR (1983b) Receptor-mediated endocytosis of transferrin in K562 cells. J Biol Chem 258:4715–1724

Kornfeld S (1987) Trafficking of lysosomal enzymes. FASEB J 1:462–468

Kornfeld S, Mellman I (1989) The biogenesis of lysosomes. Annu Rev Cell Biol 5:483–525

Koval M, Pagano RE (1989) Lipid recycling between the plasma membrane and intracellular compartments: transport and metabolism of fluorescent sphingomyelin analogues in cultured fibroblasts. J Cell Biol 108:2169–2181

Larkin JM, Brown MS, Goldstein JL, Anderson RGW (1983) Depletion of intracellular potassium arrests coated pit formation and receptor-mediated endocytosis in fibroblasts. Cell 33:273–285

Larkin JM, Donzell WC, Anderson RGW (1985) Modulation of intracelluar potassium and ATP: effects on coated pit function in fibroblasts and hepatocytes. J Cell Biol 103:2619–2627

Lazarovits J, Roth M (1988) A single amino acid change in the cytoplasmic domain allows the influenza virus hemagglutinin to be endocytosed through coated pits. Cell 53:743–752

Lehrman MA, Goldstein JL, Brown MS, Russel DW, Schneider WJ (1985) Internalization defective LDL receptors produced by genes with nonsense and frameshift mutations that truncate the cutoplasmic domain. Cell 41:735–743

Leighton J, Brada Z, Estes LW, Justin G (1969) Secretory activity and oncogenicity of a cell line derived from canine kidney. Science 162:472–463

Lobel P, Fujimoto K, Ye RD, Griffiths G, Kornfeld S (1989) Mutations in the cytoplasmic domain of the 275 kD mannose 6-phosphate receptor differentially alter lysosomal enzyme sorting and endocytosis. Cell 57:787–796

Mahaffey DT, Moore MS, Brodsky FM, Anderson RGW (1989) Coat proteins isolated from clathrin-coated vesicles can assemble into coated pits. J Cell Biol 108:1615–1624

Marsh M (1984) The entry of enveloped viruses into cells by endocytosis. Biochem J 218:1–10 .

Marsh M, Bolzau E, Helenius A (1983) Penetration of Semliki Forest virus from acidic prelysosomal vacuoles. Cell 32:931–940

Maxfield FR (1985) Acidification of endocytic vesicles and lysosomes. In: Pastan I, Willingham MC (eds) Endocytosis. Plenum, New York, pp 235–257

Maxfield FR (1989) Measurements of vacuolar pH and cytoplasmic calcium in living cells using fluorescence microscopy. Methods Enzymol 173:745–770

McClain DA, Maegawa H, Lee J, Dull J, Ulrich, A (1987) A mutant insulin receptor with defective tyrosine kinase displays no biological activity and does not undergo endocytosis. J Biol Chem 262:14663–1467

McGraw TE, Maxfield FR (1990) Efficient internalization of the human transferrin receptor is partially dependent upon the presence of an aromatic amino acid on the cytoplasmic domain. Cell Regul 1:369–377

Mellman I, Plutner H (1984) Internalization and fate of macrophage Fc receptors bound to polyvalent immune complexes. J Cell Biol 98:1170–1177

Miettinen HM, Rose JK, Mellman I (1989) Fc receptor isoforms exhibit distinct abilities for coated pit localization as a result of cytoplasmic domain heterogeneity. Cell 58:317–327

Montesano R, Roth J, Robert A, Orci L (1982) Non-coated membrane invaginations are invovled in binding and internalization of cholera and tetanus toxins. Nature 296:651–653

Morris RE, Gerstein AS, Bonventre PF, Saelinger CB (1985) Receptor-mediated entry of diphtheria toxin into monkey kidney (Vero) cells: electron microscopic evaluation. Infect Immun 50:721–727

Mostov KE, de Bruyn Kops A, Deitcher DL (1986) Deletion of the cytoplasmic domain of the polymeric immunoglobulin receptor prevents basolateral localization and endocytosis. Cell 47:359

Mostov KE, Casanova J, Breitfeld P (1988) Transcytosis and sorting of ploymeric immunoglobulin receptor. J Cell Biol 107:439a

Mueller SC, Hubbard AL (1986) Receptor-mediated endocytosis of asialoglycoproteins by rat hepatocytes: receptor-positive and receptor-negative endosomes. J Cell Biol 102:932–942

Nelson N (1987) The vacuolar proton-ATPase of eukaryotic cells. Bioessays 7:251–254

Ohkuma S, Poole B (1978) Fluorescent probe measurement of the intralysosomal pH in living cells and the perturbation of pH by various agents. Proc Natl Acad Sci 75:3327–3331

Oka JA, Weigel PH (1983) Microtubule-depolymerizing agents inhibit asialoorosomucoid delivery to lysosomes but not its endocytosis or degradation in isolated rat hepatocytes. Biochim Biophys Acta 763: 368–376

Okada Y, Tsuchiya W, Yada T, Yano J, Yawo H (1981) Phagocytic activity and hyperpolarizing responses in L-strain mouse fibroblasts. J Physiol (Lond) 313:101–119

Orci L, Carpentier J-L, Perrlet A, Anderson RGW, Goldstein JL, Brown MS (1978) Occurrence of llow density lipoprotein within large coated pits on the surface of human fibroblasts as demonstrated by freeze-etching. Exp Cell Res 113:1–13

Pastan I, Willingham MC (1985) The pathway of endocytosis. In:Pastan I, Willingham M (eds) Endocytosis. Plenum, New York, pp 1–44

Pearse BMF (1988) Receptors compete for adaptors found in plasma membrane coated pits. EMBO J 7:3331–3336

Pearse BMF, Robinson MS (1984) Purification and preparation of 100-Kd proteins from coated vesicles and their reconstitution with clathrin. EMBO J 3:1951–1957

Prywes R, Livneh E, Ullrich A, Schlessinger, J (1986) Mutatations in the cytoplasmic domain of The EGF-R affect binding and receptor internalization. EMBO J 5:2179–2190

Rodriguez-Boulan E (1983) Membrane biogenesis, enevolped RNA viruses, and epithlial polarity. In: Satir B (ed) Modern cell biology. Liss, New York, pp 119–170

Roederer M, Bowser R, Murphy RM (1987) Kinetics and temperature dependence of exposure of endocytosed material to proteolytic enzymes and low pH: evidence for a maturation model for the formation of lysosmes. J Cell Physiol 131:200–209

Rothberg KG, Ying Y, Kolhouse JF, Kamne BA, Anderson RGW (1990) The glycophospholipid-linked folate receptor internalizes folate without entering the clathrin-coated pit endocytic pathway. J Cell Biol 110:637–649

Rothenberger S, Iacopetta BJ, Kuhn LC (1987) Endocytosis of the transferrin receptor requires the cytoplasmic domain but not its phosphorylation site. Cell 49:423–431.

Salzman NH, Maxfield FR (1989) Fusion accessibility of endocytic compartments along the recycling and lysosomal pathways in intact cells. J Cell Biol 109: 2097–2104

Salzman NH, Maxfield FR (1988) Intracellular fusion of sequentially formed endocytic compartments. J Cell Biol 106:1083–1091

Sandvig K, Olsnes S (1980) Diphtheria toxin entry into cells is facilitated by low pH. J Cell Biol 87:828–832

Sandvig K, Olsnes S, Petersen OL, van Deurs B (1987) Acidification of the cytosol inhibits the endocytosis from coated pits. J Cell Biol 105:679–689

Sandvig K, Olsnes S, Petersen OL, van Deurs B (1989) Control of coated pit function by cytoplamsic pH. Methods Cell Biol 32:365–382

Schlessinger J (1980) Mechanism of hormone-induced clustering of membrane receptors. Trends Biochem Sci 5:210–214

Schlessinger J, Schreiber AB, Levi A, Lax I, Libermann T, Yarden Y (1983) Regulation of cell proliferation by epidermal growth factor. CRC Crit Rev Biochem 14:93–111

Schmid SL, Fuchs R, Male P, Mellman I (1988) Two distinct subpopulations of endosomes involved in membrane recycling and transport to lysosomes. Cell 52:73–83

Schwartz AL, Ciechanover A, Merritt S, Turkewitz A (1986) Antibody-induced receptor loss: different fates for asialoglycoproteins and the asialoglycoprotein receptor in HepG2 cells. J Biol Chem 261:15225–15232

Shen WC, Ryser HJ (1981) Cis-aconityl spacer between daunomycin and macromolecular carriers: a model of pH-sensitive linkage releasing drug from a lysosomotropic conjugate. Biochem Biophys Res Commun 102:1048–1054

Shen WC, Ryser HJ, LaManna L (1985) Disulfide spacer between methotrexate and poly-D-lysine: a probe for exploring the reductive process in endocytosis. J Biol Chem 260:10905–10908

Silverstein SC, Steinman RM, Cohn ZA (1977) Endocytosis. Annu Rev Biochem 46:669–722

Sipe DM, Murphy RF (1987) High-resolution kinetics of transferrin acidification in BALB/c 3T3 cells: exposure to pH 6 followed by temperature-sensitive alkalinization during recycling. Proc Natl Acad Sci USA 84:7119–7123

Smythe E, Pypaert M, Lucocq J, Warren G (1989) Formation of coated vesicles from coated pits in broken A431 cells. J Cell Biol 108:843

Snider M, Rogers O (1985) Intracellular movement of cell surface receptors after endocytosis: resialyation of asialo-transferrin receptor in human erythroleukemia cells. J Cell Biol 100:826–834

Taylor SI, Leventhal S (1983) Defect in cooperatively in insulin receptors from a patient with a congenital form of extreme insulin resistance. J Clin Invest 71: 1676–1685

Tran D, Carpentier J-L, Sawano F, Gorden P, Orci L (1987) Ligands internalized through coated or noncoated invaginations follow a common intracellular pathway. Proc Natl Acad Sci USA 84:7957–7961

Tycko B, Maxfield FR (1982) Rapid acidification of endocytic vesicles containing α_2-macroglobulin. Cell 28:643–651

Tycko B, Keith CH, Maxfield RR (1983) Rapid acidification of endocytic vesicles containing asialoglycoprotein in cells of a human hepatoma line. J Cell Biol 97:1762–1776

Van Deurs B, Nilausen K, Faerdeman O, Meinertz H (1982) Coated pits and pinocytosis of cationized ferritin in human skin fibroblasts. Eur J Cell Biol 27: 270–278

Van Deurs B, Peterson OW, Olsnes S, Sandvig K (1989) The ways of endocytosis. Int Rev Cytol 117:131–177

Van Renswoude J, Bridges KR, Harford JB, Klausner RD (1982) Receptor-mediated endocytosis of transferrin and the uptake of Fe in K562 cells: identification of a non-lysosomal acidic compartment. Proc Natl Acad Sci USA 79:6186–6190

Viger A, Crowther RA, Pearse BMF (1986) Purification of the 100 kd-50 kd accessory proteins in clathrin coats. EMBO J 5:2079

Wall DA, Wilson G, Hubbard AL (1980) The galactose-specific recognition system of mammalian liver: the route of ligand internalization in hepatocytes. Cell 21:79–93

Ward DM, Hackenyos DP, Kaplan J (1990) Fusion of sequentially internalized vesicles in aveolar macrophages. J Cell Biol 110:1013–1022

Webb WW, Barak LS, Tank DW, Wu E (1982) Molecular mobility on the cell surface. Biochem Soc Symp 46:191–205

Weigel PH, Oka J (1983) The surface content of asialoglycoprotein receptors on isolated hepatocytes is reversibly modulated by changes in temperature. J Biol Chem 258:5089–5094

White JM, Wilson IA (1987) Anti-peptide antibodies detect steps in a protein conformation change: low pH activation of the influenza virus haemagglutinin. J Cell Biol 105:2887–2896

White J, Kartenbech J, Helenius A (1980) Fusion of Semliki forest virus with the plasma membrane can be induced by low pH. J Cell Biol 87:264–272

White J, Keilian M, Helenius A (1983) Membrane fusion proteins of enveloped animal viruses. Q Rev Biophys 16:151–195

Wiley HS (1985) Receptor as models for the mechanisms of membrane protein turnover and dynam,ics. Curr Top Membr Transp 24:369–412

Willingham MC, Yamada SS (1978) A mechanism for the destruction of pinosomes in cultured fibroblasts: piranhalysis. J Cell Biol 78:480–487

Willingham MC, Maxfield FR, Pastan IH (1979) α_2-Macroglobulin binding to the plasma membrane of cultured fibroblasts: diffuse binding followed by clustering in coated regions. J Cell Biol 82:614–625

Willingham MC, Pastan IH, Sahagian GG, Jourdian GW, Neufeld EF (1981) Morphologic study of the internalization of a lysosomal enzyme by the mannose-G-phosphate receptor in cultured Chinese hamster ovary cells. Proc Natl Acad Sci USA 78:6967–6971

Willingham MC, Hanover JA, Dickson RB, Pastan I (1984) Morphologic characterization of the pathway of transferrin endocytosis and recycling in human KB cells. Proc Natl Acad Sci USA 81:175–179

Wolkoff A, Klausner RD, Ashwell G, Harford J (1984) Intracellular segregation of asialoglycoproteins and their receptor. A prelysosomal event subsequent to dissociation of the ligand-receptor complex. J Cell Biol 98:375–381

Woodward MP, Roth TF (1978) Coated vesicles: characterization, selective dissociation, and reassembly. Proc Natl Acad Sci USA 75:4394–4398

Yamashiro DJ, Maxfield FR (1987a) Kinetics of endosome acidification in mutant and wild-type Chinese hamster ovary cells J Cell Biol 105:2713–2721

Yamashiro DJ, Maxfield FR (1987b) Acidification of morphologically distinct endosomes in mutant and wild-type Chinese hamster ovary cells. J Cell Biol 105: 2723–2733

Yamashiro DJ, Fluss R, Maxfield FR (1983) Acidification of endocytic vesicles by an ATP-dependent proton pump. J Cell Biol 97:929–934

Yamashiro DJ, Tycko B, Fluss SR, Maxfield FR (1984) Segregation of transferrin to a mildly acidic (pH 6.5) para-Golgi compartment in the recycling pathway. Cell 37:789–800

Yamashiro DJ, Borden LA, Maxfield FR (1989) Kinetics of α_2-macroglobulin endocytosis and degradation in mutant and wild-type Chinese hamster ovary cells. J Cell Physiol 139:377–382

Zaremb S, Keen JH (1983) Assembly polypeptides from coated vesicles mediate reassembly of unique clathrin coats. J Cell Biol 97:1339–1347

CHAPTER 3

Transport of Macromolecules
Across the Capillary Endothelium*

K.L. Audus and R.T. Borchardt

A. Introduction

The endothelial cells lining the smallest blood vessels, the capillaries or
microvessels, comprise a dynamic interface adapted for exchange of nutrients, waste products, and therapeutic substances between the blood and
the interstitial fluids (Simionescu and Simionescu 1983; Smith and Kampine
1984). This specialized vascular lining is also recognized as a heterogenous
population of cells that may perform synthetic, degradative, and receptor functions which vary depending on tissue location (Simionescu and
Simionescu 1983; Hammersen and Hammersen 1985; Fajardo 1989). Our
purpose here is to review the current understanding of several processes
that facilitate transfer of macromolecules across capillary endothelium.
We have begun by generally describing the potential pathways for macromolecule passage across capillary endothelium. Since the transport properties of endothelia vary widely from tissue to tissue, we have narrowed the
scope of subsequent discussion to one population of endothelia, the blood-
brain barrier (BBB).

B. Pathways for the Passage of Macromolecules
Across Capillary Endothelium

I. Capillary Endothelium

By definition, capillary endothelium is a single thin (0.2–0.5 μm) layer
of endothelial cells, its basement membrane, and an occasional pericyte
(Simionescu and Simionescu 1983; Smith and Kampine 1984; Hammersen
and Hammersen 1985). The basement membrane is comprised of glycoproteins and collagen which contribute to endothelial cell growth characteristics and support (Simionescu and Simionescu 1983). The pericyte's

*This work was supported by grants from the American Heart Association-National
Center, American Heart Association-Kansas Affiliate, and the Upjohn Company.

function is not completely understood although recent studies indicate a possible role in modulating endothelial cell growth (ORLIDGE and D'AMORE 1987; ANTONELLI-ORLIDGE et al. 1989). With few exceptions, the basement membrane and occasional pericytes are not considered limiting permeability barriers for the distribution of macromolecules between the blood and the interstitial tissues. Rather, it is the thin endothelial barrier which controls the distribution of macromolecules across the microvasculature (PALADE et al. 1979; RENKIN 1979; SIMIONESCU 1988; VORBRODT 1988). Factors important in macromolecule distribution across the endothelia include both the balance between osmotic and hydrostatic pressures and concentration gradients. Normally, osmotic and hydrostatic pressure forces balance to slightly favor blood to interstitial fluid transfer (SIMIONESCU and SIMIONESCU 1983).

Based upon morphology, capillary endothelium may be classified into three general types: discontinuous, fenestrated, and continuous. Discontinuous endothelium is common in the liver, spleen, and bone marrow. Typically, this endothelium has large intercellular gaps permeable to substances with effective diameters of about 1000 Å and sometimes greater. Additionally, the basement membrane is discontinuous or nonexistent. Thus, discontinuous endothelium is not an effectvie permeability barrier to macromolecules (RENKIN 1979, 1988; SIMIONESCU and SIMIONESCU 1983; SMITH and KAMPINE 1984). The movement of macromolecules across both fenestrated and continuous endothelium is dependent on specific transcellular or intercellular pathways. Accordingly, further discussion will be restricted to the potential pathways for the transfer of macromolecules across fenestrated and continuous capillary endothelium. Except for fenestra, the transcellular or intercellular pathways are similar, to some extent, in both fenestrated and continuous endothelia (RENKIN 1979, 1988). Figure 1 illustrates the possible pathways for macromolecule transfer across fenestrated and continuous capillary endothelium.

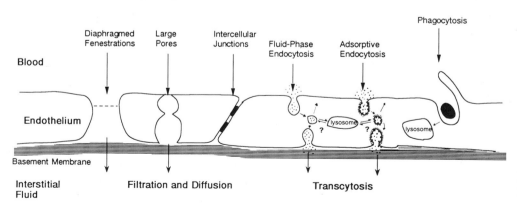

Fig. 1. Potential pathways for the transfer of blood-borne macromolecules across capillary endothelium. (From RENKIN 1979, 1988; SIMIONESCU and SIMIONESCU 1983)

II. Fenestrations

Fenestrations are circular transendothelial openings in the endothelial cell membrane that may be either open or closed over with a diaphragm. For reasons not well understood, fenestra occur in clusters at the thinnest region (i.e., luminal to abluminal thickness) of the endothelial cell (PETERS and MILICI 1983; MILICI et al. 1985). Open fenestra are typical of the renal glomerular capillaries where the openings are 600–800 Å in diameter or large enough to permit free permeation of blood-borne macromolecules. The glomerular capillary is unusual, however, in that the basement membrane is thick enough to pose a barrier to the permeation of plasma proteins and macromolecules (DEEN et al. 1983; LEVICK and SMAJE 1987). Other visceral capillary endothelia may exhibit closed or diaphragmed fenestra which, like capillary endothelia with open fenestra, are highly permeable to water, ions, and small molecules (LEVICK and SMAJE 1987). The capillary endothelium of a given tissue (e.g., intestine) may also exhibit mixtures of both closed and open fenestra (SIMIONESCU and SIMIONESCU 1983).

The diaphragm of a closed fenestration is 40–60 Å thick. Although the chemical nature of the diaphragm is not entirely clear, the luminal surface of this structure is known to be coated with heparan sulfate proteoglycans, giving the diaphragm an electronegative charge (SIMIONESCU et al. 1981, 1982, 1984). Due to the existence of a diaphragm, closed fenestrated capillary endothelia and nonfenestrated continuous capillary endothelia share similar permeability characteristics with respect to macromolecules.

Endothelial cell fenestrations with diaphragms are considered permeable to macromolecules under certain conditions. Cationic macromolecules, for instance, may be adsorbed to the surface of a fenestral diaphragm and subsequently cross the diaphragm. Polycationic substances may also neutralize the diaphragm's net negative charge, altering the overall permeability characteristics of the closed fenestra (CLEMENTI and PALADE 1969; GRANGER et al. 1986).

III. Large Pores

In nonjunctional attenuated parts of continuous and fenestrated endothelia, transient "large pores" or transendothelial channels may occur (SIMIONESCU et al. 1975). Although their frequency is low, contributions to macromolecule filtration are considered significant (RENKIN et al. 1977, RENKIN 1979; RIPPE et al. 1979). In continuous endothelia, channels are formed when chains of a few vesicles simultaneously open on both fronts of the endothelium (SIMIONESCU et al. 1975). The resulting channel has an approximate 500–700 Å opening but may be reduced to 200–300 Å, depending on the narrowness of the stricture associated with fusion of the vesicles (RENKIN 1979; PALADE et al. 1979; PALADE 1988). In fenestrated endothelia, the channel may be diaphragmed on both sides (CLEMENTI and PALADE 1969). However, the diaphragm can be distinguished from that of fenestra by the absence of a luminal anionic charge as mentioned earlier. Transendothelial channels, like fenestra, are believed to exist in clusters (PETERS and MILICI 1983; MILICI et al. 1985).

IV. Intercellular Junctions

The permeability of capillary endothelial intercellular junctions varies with tissue location (RENKIN 1988). Interjunctional diffusion or filtration of macromolecules will be limited by the effective molecular size of the particular substance. Generally, fenestrated and continuous endothelium of peripheral capillaries have intercellular junctions permeable to substances with apparent effective diameters of approximately 40–90 Å (RENKIN 1979, 1988; PALADE et al. 1979). Exceptions include the continuous endothelium forming the BBB which has "tight" intercellular junctions, excluding molecules with effective sizes greater than the lanthanum ion (Stokes radius 10 Å) (BOULDIN and KRIGMAN 1975; CSERR and BUNDGAARD 1984). For reference, serum albumin (molecular weight $\approx$ 69 000), with an effective diameter of about 72 Å, does not readily diffuse across most capillary endothelia. This is a critical feature of endothelia since albumin is a circulating protein important physiologically for maintaining the osmotic balance between the blood and the tissues (SIMIONESCU and SIMIONESCU 1983; SMITH and KAMPINE 1984; RENKIN 1988). The intercellular junction may represent the "small pore" of PAPPENHEIMER et al.'s (1951) pore model.

Interjunctional filtration or diffusion of macromolecules through endothelia may be influenced by conditions aside from simply the size limitations imposed by the width of the junctional opening. For example, lateral diffusion of plasma membrane-associated lipophilic macromolecules (e.g., chylomicrons) through intercellular junctions has been suggested (SCOW et al. 1976). Under certain pathophysiological conditions, vasoactive substances may stimulate intercellular junction alterations causing leakiness to macromolecules and water and subsequently vasogenic edema (SVENSJO and GREGA 1986). Additionally, cells of the surrounding tissues may also influence interjunctional permeability characteristics of endothelia. At the BBB, astrocytes have been shown to influence tight junction permeability of the endothelia (JANZER and RAFF 1987; TAO-CHENG et al. 1987; TRAMMEL and BORCHARDT 1989; RAUB et al. 1989).

V. Endocytosis and Phagocytosis

Endocytosis is a universal mechanism by which macromolecules may be internalized on interaction with the luminal surface of endothelia. Internalization and recycling to the cell surface, with avoidance of exposure to the lysosomal compartment, has been termed diacytosis (ROGOECZI et al.

1982). Release of internalized materials by exocytosis on the abluminal surface completes transcytosis. Based on a vesicular size range of 500–900 Å in an endothelial cell, the endocytic pathway can potentially accommodate macromolecules of substantial diameters (PALADE et al. 1979). The activity of the endocytic pathway in capillary endothelium varies, depending on tissue location, and is based on molecular size, charge, and physicochemical properties of the solute (SIMIONESCU 1988). Endocytosis may be further defined as either fluid-phase (i.e., pinocytic) or adsorptive, where the latter pathway may be either specific (e.g., receptor-mediated) or nonspecific (PASTAN and WILLINGHAM 1985).

Fluid-phase endocytosis (pinocytosis) originates through internalization of aqueous extracellular volume in either plasma membrane-derived vesicles or coated pit regions (PEARSE and CROWTHER 1987) of the plasma membrane. The rate of fluid-phase endocytosis of a molecule is directly dependent on the rate of ingestion and the extracellular concentration of the solute. This is a constitutive pathway that can be quantitatively assessed with markers (e.g., sucrose, inulin, horseradish peroxidase, fluorescein- or rhodamine-conjugated dextrans, native albumin, and native ferritin) that have limited affinity for the plasma membrane (WILLIAMS 1983; DAVIES 1984).

Adsorptive endocytosis of macromolecules by endothelia, whether specific or nonspecific, occurs in coated pit regions (PEARSE and CROWTHER 1987) of the cell surface membrane. The relationship between rate of adsorptive endocytosis of a particular solute and the extracellular concentration of solute is complex, depending on binding site capacity and affinities (WILLIAMS 1983). Also a constitutive pathway, characteristic adsorptive endocytosis by a given capillary endothelial bed varies with tissue location. Some substances that may undergo nonspecific adsorptive endocytosis include hemepeptides (GHINEA and SIMIONESCU 1985), cationized immunoglobulin G (TRIGUERO et al. 1989), and cationized albumin (KUMAGI et al. 1987; PARDRIDGE et al. 1987; SMITH and BORCHARDT 1989). These studies have demonstrated that electrostatic and carbohydrate group interactions with the endothelial cell surface are important in facilitating nonspecific adsorptive endocytosis. Receptor-mediated or specific adsorptive endocytosis is a saturable competitive process. Selected examples of macromolecules that have been shown to undergo receptor-mediated endocytosis and perhaps transcytosis in endothelia include insulin (DERNOVSEK et al. 1984; KING and Johnson 1985; PARDRIDGE et al. 1985; DUFFY and PARDRIDGE 1987; KELLER et al. 1988), albumin (SHASBY and SHASBY 1985), glycosylated albumin (SMITH and BORCHARDT 1989), ricin (RAUB and AUDUS 1987), acylated low density lipoprotein (VOYTA et al. 1984), and transferrin (FISHMAN et al. 1987; BANKS et al. 1988; NEWTON and RAUB 1988).

Endocytosis and subsequent exocytosis of substances such as proteins (SHASBY and SHASBY 1985; VORBRODT et al. 1985; BROADWELL et al. 1988) and viruses (LOMBARDI et al. 1985) may be unidirectional. Transport of some proteins and viruses apparently occurs preferentially towards the luminal surface of the endothelial cell (SHASBY and SHASBY 1985; LOMBARDI et al. 1985; VORBRODT et al. 1985; BROADWELL et al. 1988).

The endocytic activity of endothelia may be influenced by cell growth, injury, and the presence of vasoactive substances. These factors may or may not also translate to altered endothelial cell macromolecule transport (DAVIES 1984; VORBRODT et al. 1985; SVENSJO and GREGA 1986).

Endothelial cells of some vascular beds retain the capacity to phago-cytose particles on the order of micron diameters. The practical applica-tion of this route for transfer of monoclonal antibody-bearing liposomes into the endothelium has been recently considered by TRUBETSKAYA et al. (1988). Monoclonal antibodies direct liposomes to endothelia where they bind specifically and are subsequently internalized. Liposomes not bearing the monoclonal antibody are not internalized by the endothelium. In other studies, pulmonary endothelial cells have also been shown to be capable of phagocytosing polystyrene beads (RYAN 1986).

C. The Blood-Brain Barrier

Three decades ago, BENNETT et al. (1959) determined that the most restric-tive capillaries on a morphological basis are those comprising the BBB. Unlike endothelia of many peripheral tissues, the endothelia of the cerebro-vasculature have tight intercellular junctions, no fenestra, and an attenuated pinocytotic activity (REESE and KARNOVSKY 1967; BRIGHTMAN and REESE 1969). The brain capillary endothelia retain a complex glycocalyx and numer-ous enzyme systems, and have about three times more mitochondria than their peripheral counterparts, suggesting a substantial metabolic capacity (CORNFORD 1985; VORBRODT 1988). The BBB is a specialized population of endothelia with mechanisms elaborated for tightly controlling the movement of substances between the blood and the brain. As a result of these features, the BBB plays an essential role in maintaining a consistent extracellular environment for the central nervous system (CORNFORD 1985; PARDRIDGE 1987). The likely explanation for this unique elaboration appears to be at-tributable to the influence of specific cells of the central nervous system, notably astrocytes (JANZER and RAFF 1987; TAO-CHENG et al. 1987; TRAMMEL and BORCHARDT 1989; RAUB et al. 1989). A few of the basic features dis-tinguishing brain capillary from peripheral endothelium are illustrated in Fig. 2.

The apparent strategy of the BBB is to force all substances to undergo transcellular transfer between the blood and the brain. This strategy allows the BBB to regulate both the types and amounts of substances that may influence the central nervous system. While several classic transport sys-tems are available to facilitate transendothelial passage of nutrients such as hexoses, amino acids, amines, and nucleosides (OLDENDORF 1971; GOLDSTEIN and BETZ 1983; HAWKINS 1986), only a few transport mechanisms for macro-molecules have been recognized (BANKS and KASTIN 1988).

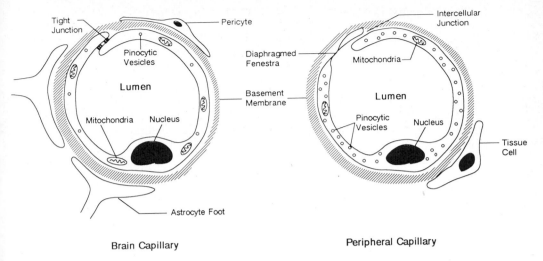

Fig. 2. Major differences between endothelium of the blood-brain barrier and the peripheral vasculature. (From SMITH and KAMPINE 1984; CORNFORD 1985; GOLDSTEIN and BETZ 1986)

The availability of an abundance of fundamental information on any of the BBB transcellular or paracellular transport processes is far from complete (CRONE 1986). However, the current interest in biotechnology products with potential applications in therapy of central nervous system maladies has created a particular need for identification of mechanisms and schemes to deliver macromolecules across the BBB. Therefore, it is not surprising that an area of microvascular research currently receiving significant attention is BBB transport and metabolism of macromolecules.

D. Experimental Model Systems

Since biochemical characterization of the permeability and matabolic properties of human capillary endothelium is not feasible for many reasons, several in vivo, in situ, and in vitro experimental model systems have been developed. In vitro or in vivo experimental model systems to study capillary permeability exist for peripheral tissues as well as those derived from special tissues such as the brain. Briefly discussed here are three representative model systems that may be used to investigate the permeability of brain capillary endothelium to macromolecules. Although the discussion here is limited to brain capillary endothelium, complementary models exist for peripheral capillary endothelium. Consequently, many of the principles and uses of the individual systems described may be analogous for peripheral capillary endothelium.

I. Brain Perfusion Model

The brain-perfusion technique or "Takasato model" (TAKASATO et al. 1984; SMITH and TAKASATO 1986) has received acceptance as one of the more versatile of several methods for characterizing brain capillary permeability in situ or in vivo (SMITH 1989). The perfusion model is established by placing a catheter in the right external carotid artery and ligating the right pterygo-palatine artery of an anesthetized animal. A syringe containing a radiolabeled impermeant vascular tracer and a radiolabeled test substance dissolved in a physiological solution (e.g., saline, plasma, blood) is connected to the cannula leading into the right external carotid artery. Immediately before initiating perfusion, the right common carotid is ligated and the perfusion solution is then infused into the carotid artery at a rate that mimics systemic blood flow into the right hemisphere. The infusion is also maintained at values that approximate normal systemic blood pressure and perfusion times can range from 5–15 s or longer. Following the perfusion, the animal is decapitated and both perfusate and brain parenchyma analyzed for radio-tracer uptake. Cerebrovascular permeability-surface area products (ml/s per g) can be readily determined for various substances (TAKASATO et al. 1984; SMITH and TAKASATO 1986).

Some advantages of this system are the reduced surgical manipulations needed, short perfusion times relative to other techniques, the absolute control over the perfusate composition, and the absence of perfusate mixing with blood which normally occurs on intravenous administration. Disadvantages of this system are the need for anesthesia, the perfusing of only one hemisphere, and the possibility of hypoxia in lengthy experiments with some perfusate solutions (TAKASATO et al. 1984; SMITH and TAKASATO 1986; SMITH 1989).

The Takasato model and related brain perfusion methods may be used to elucidate mechanisms of macromolecule transfer across brain capillary endothelium. Recently, ZLOKOVIC et al. (1987, 1989) have used a similar brain perfusion model to characterize mechanisms and kinetic parameters for leucine-enkephalin and delta sleep-inducing peptide transport across the BBB.

Descriptions and the use of other alternative in vivo or in situ type models for brain capillary endothelial transport studies have been reviewed by SMITH (1989). A number of studies on macromolecule transport across brain capillary endothelium have also been conducted with these alternative models. Some recent examples include transferrin (FISHMAN et al. 1987; BANKS et al. 1988), vasopressin (BANKS et al. 1987a), and insulin (DUFFY and PARDRIDGE 1987; BEN-SHACHAR et al. 1988).

II. Isolated Capillaries

The development of methods for the isolation of brain capillaries from animal and human brains has been a valuable resource for defining biochemical properties of the BBB. Relatively pure populations of microvessels can be conveniently obtained from the cerebral gray matter of animal or autopsy brains. Suspensions of capillary fragments are isolated by mechanical homogenization, centrifugation, and filtration through nylon meshed with approximately 200 µm openings (LIDINSKY and DREWES 1983; FRANK et al. 1986). With isolated capillaries, respiration, nutrient transport, asymmetry, enzymes, carbohydrates, lipids, and proteins associated with the BBB have been revealed (Joo 1985). In addition, isolated capillaries have been used to characterize the uptake of several macromolecules including insulin (PARDRIDGE et al. 1985; FRANK et al. 1986), chimeric peptides (KUMAGI et al. 1987; PARDRIDGE et al. 1987), and cationized immunoglobulin G (TRIGUERO et al. 1989).

Advantages of this system include availability and ease of use. Disadvantages include the inability to assess transcellular transport and the potential for metabolic deficiencies introduced by the isolation procedures (WILLIAMS et al. 1980; LASBENNES and GAYET 1984; SUSSMAN et al. 1988; McCALL et al. 1988).

III. Tissue Culture Systems

Like the isolated capillaries described above, tissue culture systems allow further characterization of the biochemical features associated with the BBB at a cellular level. Primary culture systems consisting of monolayers of brain microvessel endothelial cells can also offer the opportunity to elucidate mechanisms of the transcellular passage of substances at the BBB, an advantage over the isolated capillaries. Moreover, cultured endothelial cells do not retain metabolic deficiencies observed with freshly isolated capillaries (SUSSMAN et al. 1988; McCALL et al. 1988).

Isolation of a viable homogenous population of brain capillary endothelial cells for establishment of a tissue culture system is accomplished by a two step enzymatic digestion of cerebral gray matter and successive centrifugation over dextran and percoll gradients (BOWMAN et al. 1983; AUDUS and BORCHARDT 1986a, 1987). The development of tissue culture models can result in loss of cell features typical of the parent tissue. Thus, extensive characterization of a given tissue culture model is necessary to validate its use in transport studies. In our laboratories, primary cultures of bovine brain microvessel endothelial cell monolayers have been shown to retain morphological properties typical of the BBB in vivo such as tight intercellular junctions, attenuated pinocytosis, and no fenestra (AUDUS and BORCHARDT 1986a, 1987). Additionally, specific BBB enzyme markers, endothelial cell markers, catecholamine-degrading enzymes (AUDUS and BORCHARDT 1986a; BARANCZYK-KUZMA et al. 1986, 1989a; SCRIBA and BORCHARDT, 1989a,b), cholinesterases (TRAMMEL and BORCHARDT, unpublished observations), aminopeptidases (BARANCZYK-KUZMA and AUDUS 1987), and acid hydrolases (BARANCZYK-KUZMA et al. 1989b) are retained. All biochemical properties

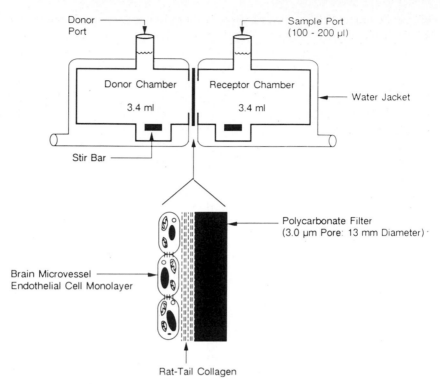

Fig. 3. The blood-brain barrier in vitro. Primary cultures of brain microvessel endothelial cells are grown to confluence on polycarbonate membranes and are then placed in a side-by-side diffusion apparatus

of the in vitro model are consistent with present understanding of the BBB in vivo.

The permeability properties of primary cultures of bovine brain microvessel endothelial cell monolayers have been characterized in a horizontal side-by-side diffusion cell apparatus diagramed in Fig. 3 (AUDUS and BORCHARDT 1987). Permeation of substances across the monolayers has been shown to be related to both lipophilicity and molecular weight in a manner consistent with the BBB in vivo (AUDUS and BORCHARDT 1986a; RIM et al. 1986; SHAH et al. 1989; AUDUS 1990). While bovine brain microvessel endothelial cell monolayers do retain tight intercellular junctions, the junctions are not identical to those observed in vivo with respect to extent or complexity. In terms of "leakiness" then, the in vitro system exceeds that of the in vivo BBB. This is a disadvantage of the tissue culture system in studying small molecule transport mechanisms. As discussed later, co-cultures with astrocytes hold promise for restoring tight junction integrity in vitro. Nonetheless, normalizing corrections for "leakiness" in the monolayers can be made with impermeant marker molecules (e.g., sucrose, fluorescein, inulin, dextrans).

Table 1. Summary listing of studies on macromolecule uptake and transport across brain capillary endothelium with tissue culture models

Peptides	References
Large	
AcLDL	VINTERS et al. (1987)
	BARANCZYK-KUZMA et al. (1989b)
Atrial natriuretic factor	SMITH et al. (1988)
Insulin, insulin-like growth factor 1,	ROSENFELD et al. (1987);
insulin-like growth factor 2	KELLER and BORCHARDT (1987)
	KELLER et al. (1988)
LDL	MERESSE et al. (1989)
Modified albumins	SMITH and BORCHARDT (1989)
Ricin	RAUB and AUDUS (1987)
Transferrin	NEWTON and RAUB (1988)
Small	
Delta sleep-inducing peptide	RAEISSI and AUDUS (1989)
Leucine-enkephalin	THOMPSON and AUDUS (1989)
Vasopressin	REARDON and AUDUS (1989);
	VAN BREE et al. (1989)

AcLDL, acetylated low density lipoprotein.

Consequently, the in vitro model can be used to study BBB carrier-mediated transport of amino acids (AUDUS and BORCHARDT 1986b), low molecular weight drugs (VAN BREE et al. 1988; CHASTAIN and BORCHARDT 1987, 1989, 1990), choline (TRAMMEL and BORCHARDT 1987), nucleosides (SHAH and BORCHARDT 1989), and macromolecules as summarized in Table 1.

E. Applications of Tissue Culture Models in the Study of Capillary Endothelial Cell Transport of Macromolecules

The transport of macromolecules across the BBB had, until recently, been considered unlikely. Accumulating evidence, however, suggests that several peptides may cross the BBB in pharmacologically significant amounts (BANKS and KASTIN 1988). Highlighted in the subsequent discussion are the applications of primary cultures of brain microvessel endothelial cells in the study of mechanisms and pathways for macromolecule transfer across the endothelia of the BBB.

I. Kinetics of Marker Molecules

The apparent absence of considerable intercellular transfer of macromolecules across brain capillary endothelium under normal conditions has stimulated interest in vesicular pathways. In efforts to further define vesicular pathways for macromolecule transfer across the BBB, marker molecules (e.g., Lucifer yellow, lectins) have been used in studies with the tissue culture model described above.

1. Lucifer Yellow

The kinetics of fluid-phase endocytosis by BBB endothelia has been assessed in the bovine brain microvessel endothelial cell monolayers (GUILLOT et al. 1990) with Lucifer yellow (LY), a fluorescent, soluble marker for fluid-phase endocytosis (SWANSON et al. 1985). The time-dependent uptake of LY by the cultured cells was observed to be biphasic with an initial rate of 233 fl/cell/h (1338 ng LY/mg protein/h, $t_{1/2}$ of 5.5 min), much slower than that observed in other representative endothelial cell types (e.g., 700 fl/cell/h for fat pad endothelium) (WILLIAMS and WAGNER 1981). The second uptake phase was slower yet, at 50 fl/cell/h (23 ng LY/mg protein/h, $t_{1/2}$ of 234 min), and tended to plateau after about 20 min. Together with other efflux and the temperature dependency data, the results suggested two endocytic compartments in these endothelia. The predominant superficial compartment (i.e., caveolae) is involved in rapid diacytosis (34 fl/cell). A second compartment within the cell has a slow turnover (6 fl/cell) and represents a compartment that slowly accumulates material from the extracellular medium. The calculated total volume turnover rate for the cultured endothelial cells was about 1.2% vol/h. For comparison, calculated total volume turnover rates for macrophages and fibroblasts are 26%–34% and 9%–15% vol/h, respectively (BESTERMAN et al. 1981). Overall results demonstrate a low level of pinocytic activity in the in vitro model (GUILLOT et al. 1990), analogous to the attenuated pinocytosis described for the BBB in vivo (REESE and KARNOVSKY 1967; BRIGHTMAN and REESE 1969).

2. Lectins

In contrast to the attenuated fluid-phase endocytic activity of primary cultures of bovine brain microvessel endothelial cells, relatively active adsorptive endocytosis of the glycoprotein ricin I is apparent (RAUB and AUDUS 1987). Internalization and recycling of radiolabeled ricin by brain microvessel endothelial cells was mediated through a binding site that was saturable with a dissociation constant of about 33 nM. Binding could be competed for with galactose and was inhibited by low temperature. Approximately 2×10^5 high affinity ricin binding sites per cell were characteristic of the cultured endothelial cells. Internalization of surface-bound ricin occurred with an initial $t_{1/2}$ of 12 min followed by a slower rate $t_{1/2}$ of 73 min. Approximately 70%–80% of internalized ricin was recycled after 2 h (RAUB and AUDUS 1987). Despite the presence of abluminal ricin binding sites (VORBRODT 1988), transcytosis of ricin does not occur, suggesting that the cultured cells were polarized with respect to membrane traffic.

Both the fluid-phase and adsorptive pathways of endocytosis at the BBB remain to be completely defined. Studies such as those described above have formed the basis for further characterization of surface lectins (RAUB and AUDUS 1987; WHITE and AUDUS 1989) and acid hydrolases (BARANCZYK-KUZMA et al. 1989b) as important features in transport of macromolecules across brain capillary endothelia. Likewise, ongoing in vitro research in our laboratories with other marker molecules and biochemical probes of endocytosis continues to pursue evidence revealing both the possible transport and metabolic fates of internalized macromolecules at the BBB.

II. Large Peptides

Among those peptides that may cross the BBB are relatively large peptides such as transferrin (FISHMAN et al. 1987; BANKS et al. 1988; NEWTON and RAUB 1988), insulin (PARDRIDGE et al. 1985; FRANK et al. 1986; KELLER et al. 1988), atrial natriuretic factor (SMITH et al. 1988), and albumin (KUMAGI et al. 1987; SMITH and BORCHARDT 1989). Each of these peptides has receptor sites on BBB endothelia, undergoes receptor-mediated internalization, and has thus been postulated to undergo subsequent transcytosis.

1. Transferrin

Primary cultures of brain microvessel endotheial cell monolayers have been shown to retain transferrin receptors and have been used to further define attributes of receptor-mediated endocytosis at the BBB (NEWTON and RAUB 1988). The number of transferrin receptors associated with brain capillary endothelial cell monolayers was observed to be 1×10^5 transferrin receptors/cell, with maximal expression at confluency. The number of transferrin receptors on the monolayers also decreased by about 40% within 2 days. Binding was saturable and the dissociation constant for transferrin binding to brain capillary endothelial cells was $5\,nM$. When compared to other kidney epithelia and adrenal endothelia, brain microvessel endothelial cells exhibited up to a twofold greater number of transferrin binding sites based on a per mg protein basis.

As might be expected for a receptor-mediated endocytic process, the internalization of radiolabeled transferrin was also saturable with an uptake constant of about $6\,nM$, could be competed for by excess unlabeled transferrin, and was inhibited by metabolic inhibitors. NEWTON and RAUB (1988) have also grown primary cultures of brain microvessel endothelial cells onto polycarbonate filters of a Transwell diffusion cell to assess the potential transcytotic passage of transferrin. In this model system, transferrin did undergo some transcytosis, however, the predominant efflux was polarized towards the apical or luminal surface (NEWTON and RAUB 1988). These findings are in good agreement with in vivo observations of FISHMAN et al. (1987) and BANKS et al. (1988) and indicate the utility of the in vitro model in characterizing transferrin receptor function at the BBB.

2. Insulin and Insulin-Like Growth Factor

Primary cultures of brain microvessel endothelial cell monolayers have also been shown to retain receptors for insulin (INS) and insulin-like growth factor 1 (IGF-1). The kinetics of receptor-mediated binding and receptor-mediated endocytosis of radiolabeled INS and IGF-1 were studied using cultured bovine brain microvessel endothelial cells (KELLER and BORCHARDT 1987; KELLER et al. 1988). Maximum specific binding at 23°C was observed to be 15% and 1.5% and, at 37°C, 5.5% and 0.9% for IGF-1 and INS, respectively. The binding of INS was not observed to vary significantly over the course of 8–11 days in culture (i.e., during the period in which the cells became a confluent monolayer). The concentraion of unlabeled peptide required to cause a 50% decrease in maximum binding (ID_{50}) was 3.8 ng/ml (0.49 nM) for IGF-1 and 6 ng/ml (1.1 nM) for INS. Unlabeled INS competed poorly for the IGF-1 receptor, requiring 2000 ng/ml (364 nM) to cause a 50% reduction in IGF-1 binding. Scatchard analysis yielded two types of binding sites for both peptides with dissociation constants (K_d) of 0.39 nM and 3.66 nM for IGF-1 and 0.82 and 19.2 nM for INS and corresponding to approximately 1.9×10^{12} and 2.4×10^{11} high affinity receptors per mg of cell protein for IGF-1 and INS, respectively. These numbers represent about 5.2×10^6 IGF-1 sites/cell and 6.6×10^5 INS sites/cell. Using an acid wash technique to assess peptide internalization, 60% of the bound INS was determined to be resistant to acid treatment within 15 min, a value which remained constant over 2 h. With IGF-1 a similar proportion of the bound material, 62%, became resistant by 30 min, but subsequently decreased to 45% by 2 h. These studies show that cultured bovine brain microvessel endothelial cells have specific receptors for INS and IGF-1 and that these receptors mediate the binding and endocytosis of these peptides. Receptors for INS or IGF-1 could mediate direct effects on the capillaries or they could mediate the transcytosis of these peptides where the peptides could produce neurologic or hormonal effects on the brain. The exact physiological function of these brain microvessel receptors for INS and IGFs have yet to be elucidated.

The specific receptors for IGF-1 and IGF-2 in cultured bovine brain microvessel endothelial cells have been partially characterized by means of affinity cross-linking techniques and specific anti-receptor antibodies. The characteristics of the receptors in the cultured bovine brain microvessel endothelial cells were compared to the receptors present in isolated rat brain microvessels and microvessel-free brain cell membranes (ROSENFELD et al. 1987). Cross-linking with radiolabeled IGF-1, followed by sodium dodecyl sulfate-polyacrylamide gel electrophoresis (SDS-PAGE), revealed an α-subunit of apparent molecular weight of 138 000 in both BBB preparations compared to 120 000 in the microvessel-free rat brain cell membrane preparation. Cross-linking was inhibited by unlabeled IGF and INS, but not by antibody directed against the IGF-2 receptor. When radiolabeled IGF-2 was cross-linked, followed by SDS-PAGE under reducing conditions, a major band of apparent molecular weight of 250 000 was identified in the microvessel-free rat brain cell membrane preparation and the two BBB preparations. Labeling of this band could be inhibited by unlabeled IGF and by antibody specific for the IGF-2 receptor. Thus, both rat and bovine brain microvessels possess classical type 1 and 2 IGF receptors. While the α subunit of the type 1 receptor of brain is smaller than that of the BBB, the type 2 receptors of brain and BBB appear to be structurally and immunologically identical.

3. Atrial Natriuretic Factor

Receptors for atrial natriuretic factor (ANF) have also been identified in isolated bovine brain microvessels (CHABRIER et al. 1987) and on cultured bovine brain microvessels (SMITH et al. 1988). ANF is produced by cardiac myocytes and is released in response to increases in atrial pressure. This 28 amino acid peptide produces natriuretic, diuretic, and hypotensive effects by acting on renal and vascular tissues (NEEDLEMAN et al. 1989).

The kinetics of binding of radiolabeled rat ANF to cultured bovine brain microvessel endothelial cells was shown to be rapid, reversible, saturable, and unaffected by the presence of hormonal peptides such as insulin, vasopressin, and angiotension II (SMITH et al. 1988). Scatchard analysis of competitive binding data indicated the presence of a single class of binding sites for ANF with a dissociation constant of $400\,pM$ and maximal binding capacity of 52 fmol/mg total cell protein. Competition of ANF fragments, atriopeptins, for specific ANF binding was determined. Binding of radiolabeled rat ANF was inhibited to varying degrees by atriopeptins I-III with atriopeptin III (5–28 amino acids of ANF) being the most potent and atriopeptin I (5–25 amino acids of ANF) being the least potent. These results suggested that the C-terminus of ANF was important for binding to the receptor. Cultured bovine brain microvessel endothelial cells were also shown to rapidly internalize rat ANF by a time- and temperature-dependent process. These results are consistent with the existence of specific receptors on the luminal surface of cultured bovine brain microvessel endothelial cells for ANF. The presence of these receptors may have several roles including direct capillary effects (e.g., regulation of water and electrolyte permeability) or neurologic or hormonal effects on the brain after receptor-mediated transcytosis of this peptide.

4. Modified Albumins

Recently, attempts have been made to use the adsorptive endocytic pathway in brain microvessel endothelial cells as a route of delivering drugs to the brain. For example, KUMAGI et al. (1987) demonstrated the enhanced binding and adsorptive-mediated endocytosis of cationized albumin and a β-endorphin-cationized albumin chimeric peptide by isolated brain capillaries. To further characterize this adsorptive endocytic pathway in brain endothelial cells, our laboratory (SMITH and BORCHARDT 1989) determined the binding, uptake and transcellular transport of bovine serum albumin (BSA), cationized BSA (cBSA), and glycosylated BSA (gBSA) in cultured bovine brain microvessel endothelial cells. The rate of radiolabeled BSA flux across the cultured endothelial cell monolayers grown onto polycarbonate membranes was linear with increasing BSA concentration and the flux could be inhibited by temperature reduction to 0°–4°C. The maximal binding of radiolabeled BSA to the cultured endothelial cells was 0.04 fmol/ mg total cell protein and it could not be inhibited by nonradiolabeled BSA.

In contrast, the binding of cBSA and gBSA was rapid and could be inhibited by nonradiolabeled cBSA or gBSA, respectively. The maximal amount bound was 1.8 fmol/mg total cell protein for cBSA and 17.4 fmol/mg total cell protein for gBSA. The dissociation constants (K_ds) were 27 ± 13 and 3.7 ± 1.1 nM for cBSA and gBSA, respectively. The flux rates of cBSA and gBSA across the endothelial cell monolayers were linear with respect to concentration and they were approximately seven times greater than those observed for BSA. Each of the proteins appeared on the antiluminal side of the endothelial cell monolayers primarily (90%) as intact protein as determined by trichloroacetic acid precipitations and SDS-PAGE. The results for BSA are similar to those observed for LY, a fluid-phase endocytic marker. In contrast to BSA, the binding and transcellular transport of cBSA and gBSA appear to proceed by an adsorptive-phase endocytic mechanism (SMITH and BORCHARDT 1989).

III. Small Peptides

Evidence suggests that several relatively small peptides may cross the BBB by saturable and competitive carrier-mediated mechanisms. These peptides include leucine-enkephalin (ZLOKOVIC et al. 1987), delta sleep-inducing peptide (DSIP) (ZLOKOVIC et al. 1989), vasopressin (BANKS et al. 1987a), small tyrosinated peptides (BANKS et al. 1987b), and D-[Ala[1]]-peptide T-amide (BARRERA et al. 1987). Some of these systems (e.g., vasopressin, small tyrosinated peptides) appear to be unidirectional, functioning to transport the peptides from brain to blood. Several aspects of the transport of these peptides across the BBB have been investigated with primary cultures of brain microvessel endothelial cell monolayers and are summarized below.

Vasopressin transfer across the BBB has been examined with primary cultures of brain microvessel endothelial cell monolayers. Evidence in vitro is analogous to the in vivo studies in that a saturable carrier system does not seem to exist for transport of vasopressin in the luminal to abluminal direction. Any transfer of vasopressin across the endothelia from the apical side appears to be passive (VAN BREE et al. 1989; REARDON and AUDUS 1989). Although confirmatory studies are required, saturable carrier-mediated abluminal to luminal transfer of vasopressin can be demonstrated to some degree in vitro (REARDON and AUDUS 1989). Both observations are consistent with the in vivo characterization of vasopressin transport (BANKS et al. 1987a).

Despite previous studies to the contrary, ZLOKOVIC et al. (1989) recently presented evidence in support of a BBB carrier for DSIP. In concurrence with the in vivo studies of KASTIN et al. (1981), our in vitro work suggests contrarily a passive transmembrane diffusion of DSIP at the BBB (RAEISSI and AUDUS 1989). By temperature dependence studies, the use of metabolic inhibitors, and analysis of possible unidirectional transport mechanisms, endocytosis and carrier system involvement in transfer of DSIP across the brain microvessel endothelial cell monolayers were ruled out. The apparent permeability coefficient for DSIP transfer across brain microvessel endothelial cell monolayers is also less than for membrane impermeant markers such as sucrose and fluorescein (RAEISSI and AUDUS 1989). On the other hand, ZLOKOVIC et al. (1989) looked at a very low concentration range to demonstrate carrier-mediated DSIP transport. Additionally, ZLOKOVIC et al. (1989) have not ruled out the possible roles of other mechanisms to differentiate their results from prior in vivo studies. Further work in our laboratories now centers on the conformational aspects of DSIP that may permit interactions with the BBB and subsequent transendothelial transfer (AUDUS and MANNING 1990). These latter studies may aid in interpretation of the nature of DSIP's transport across the BBB.

The transport of leucine-enkephalin across the BBB by a carrier-mediated mechanism has been demonstrated as mentioned above (ZLOKOVIC et al. 1987). The in vivo work of others, however, suggests that μ opioids may have the capacity to induce BBB permeability changes (BABA et al. 1988). In related studies, neurotransmitters (BANKS and KASTIN 1989) and leucine (BANKS and KASTIN 1986) too have been shown to regulate the transport of tyrosinated peptides across the BBB. Collectively, these observations suggest rather unique and complex interactions between opioids and the BBB. In the tissue culture model of the BBB , leucine-enkephalin transfer across the endothelium occurs at a relatively high rate which is consistent with a facilitating mechanism. On examination of the influence of nanomolar concentrations of the peptide on permeability to membrane impermeant markers, though, leakiness of the monolayers increases markedly (THOMPSON and AUDUS 1989). In addition, leucine-enkephalin's effects on monolayer permeability can, to some degree, be antagonized by naloxone. Therefore, our results appear in good agreement with the work of BABA et al. (1988) and have formed the basis of a more extensive inquiry into the distribution of enkephalin peptides across the BBB in the model system.

IV. Regulation of the Permeability of Capillary Endothelium

1. Astrocytes

The unique barrier characteristics of the BBB depend on the environment in which the endothelial cells grow (STEWARD and WILEY 1981). The astrocytes, the cells immediately surrounding brain microvessels, are the most likely candidate to affect the microvessel's passive permeability to solutes by modulating the formation and maintenance of the tight intercellular junctions (TJs) between the endothelial cells. Primary cultures of brain endothelium alone can form TJs (BOWMAN et al. 1983), some of which have been shown to limit the diffusion of solutes (AUDUS and BORCHARDT 1986a, 1987; DOROVINI-ZIS et al. 1984). Recently, TAO-CHENG at al. (1987) showed that when brain endothelial cells were co-cultured with astrocytes, the endothelial cell TJs were enhanced in length, width, and complexity, as seen by *en face* views of the cell membranes with freeze-fracture electron microscopy. Gap junctions, common in brain endothelium in vitro but generally absent in mature brain capillaries in vivo, were markedly diminished in area from among the enhanced TJs of co-cultures. These data suggest that, as in vivo, astrocytes in vitro play a role in the formation, extent, and configuration of the junctional complexes in brain endothelium and therefore may affect their permeability to solutes.

Recently, our laboratory (TRAMMEL and BORCHARDT 1989) reported that conditioned media from rat astrocyte cultures or C_6-glioma cell cultures decreased the permeability (>50%) of bovine brain endothelial cell monolayers to radiolabeled inulin. Co-culturing astrocytes with endothelial cells also caused a decrease in the permeability of the endothelial cell monolayer to radiolabeled inulin. However, glioma co-culture experiments increased the permeability of the endothelial cell monolayer to this solute by more than 50%. Neither the decrease nor increase in permeability of the endothelial cell monolayer was due to differences in cell count, total cellular protein, or fluid-phase endocytosis.

RAUB et al. (1989), recently reported similar results using conditioned media from C_6-glioma cells on the permeability of solutes through bovine brain endothelial cell monolayers. In addition, RAUB et al. (1989) reported that treatment of bovine brain endothelial cell monolayers with conditioned media from C_6-glioma cells increased the transendothelial electrical resistance (TEER) of this cell monolayer twofold. However, the data reported by RAUB et al. (1989) for the effects of co-culturing brain endothelial cells with C_6-glioma cells differ from those observed in our laboratory (TRAMMEL and BORCHARDT 1989). RAUB et al. (1989) reported that co-cultures of bovine brain endothelial cells with C_6-glioma cells result in a 3.75-fold increase in the TEER and a decrease in the permeability of the monolayer to solutes. In contrast, we observed a significant increase in the permeability of the endothelial cell monolayer to solutes when the cells were co-cultured with C_6-glioma cells (TRAMMEL and BORCHARDT 1989). The different experimental results with co-cultures of C_6-glioma cells may originate in the physical arrangement of the co-culture experiments. RAUB et al. (1989) did their co-culture experiments in Transwells where the C_6-glioma cells were present on the basolateral side of the endothelial cells. In contrast, our co-culture experiments were done in an arrangement where factor(s) released by the

C_6-glioma cells would only be exposed to the luminal side of the endothelial cells. Thus, changes in permeability of the endothelial cells upon co-culture with C_6-glioma cells may depend upon the cell surface exposed to the trophic factors.

From the experiments described above, it is clear that astrocytes (and glioma cells) are producing factors that can alter the formation, extent, and configuration of the junctional complexes in brain endothelium as well as their permeability. These in vitro endothelial cell culture systems will, therefore, by very useful in efforts aimed at isolation and characterization of these trophic factors.

2. Vasoactive Peptides

Under certain pathophysiological conditions, vasoactive peptides may play a significant role in mediating increases in BBB permeability. Mechanisms proposed for vasoactive peptide-induced increases in BBB permeability include modification of either transcytotic pathways, intercellular junctions, or both and/or regulation of carrier-mediated transport of nutrients (GRUBB and RAICHLE 1981; WAHL et al. 1988; BABA et al. 1988; BANKS and KASTIN 1988). Clarification of the biochemical processes controlling BBB permeability may reveal therapeutic approaches to alleviating pathological events (e.g., vasogenic edema and subsequent brain damage) and possible transcellular pathways that might be manipulated to pharmacokinetically enhance delivery of centrally acting macromolecular drugs to the brain (e.g., chemotherapy) (WAHL et al. 1988; BABA et al. 1988; BANKS and KASTIN 1988).

Vascular renin-angiotensin systems in major organs such as the brain have been directly implicated in the regulation of local blood vessel function (DZAU 1984, 1986). One of several abnormalities of the BBB in hypertension is an increased permeability. Hypertension within the cerebrovascular tree may be attributable to alterations in the local renin-angiotensin system. Although the precise mechanisms of BBB permeability changes are not known, angiotensin-induced hypertension has been shown to enhance pinocytic activity in the cerebrovasculature (JOHANSSON 1981). With this background, studies have been initiated in our laboratories with brain microvessel endothelial cell monolayers to investigate mechanisms of angiotensin peptide regulation of BBB permeability (GUILLOT and AUDUS 1989a,b,c; AUDUS 1990).

The influence of angiotensin agonists on pinocytic activity of bovine brain microvessel endothelial cell monolayers was quantitated with LY. Normally reduced uptake of LY by the monolayers, as described earlier, was found to be stimulated by 20%–30% with the agonists angiotensin II and saralasin over a nanomolar concentration range. Angiotensin II antagonists such as sarathrin had no effect on LY uptake and suggested a receptor-mediated stimulation of pinocytosis was occurring. As positive controls, bradykinin and a nonmetabolized phorbol myristate acetate also stimulated monolayer uptake of LY by about 40% and 90%, respectively. The magnitude of pinocytic uptake changes in the monolayers observed here under the different treatments were comparable to the magnitude of permeability changes produced by micromolar concentrations of norepinephrine, histamine, and serotonin in other endothelial cell model systems (BOTTARO et al. 1986).

In other experiments, brain microvessel endothelial monolayers were pretreated for 24 h with indomethacin, an inhibitor of prostaglandin synthesis. As a result of the indomethacin pretreatment, the endothelial cell monolayer uptake of LY was not stimulated above control levels by angiotensin peptides. The stimulation of LY uptake by both bradykinin and the phorbol ester, however, was unaffected by prostaglandin depletion. These latter results suggested that angiotensin peptide effects on BBB pinocytosis were probably mediated by prostaglandins. In contrast, bradykinin and phorbol ester effects on BBB pinocytosis appeared not to be mediated through prostaglandins (GUILLOT and AUDUS 1989a; AUDUS 1990). Through additional studies, including pretreatment studies with trifluoperazine and chloroquine, stimulatory effects of bradykinin and phorbol myristate acetate on LY uptake appeared to involve protein kinase C (GUILLOT and AUDUS 1989a). The role of prostanoids in mediating angiotensin-induced changes in vascular function was again consistent with current literature (BROWN and BROWN 1986; GRYGLEWSKI et al. 1988).

The effects of angiotensin peptides on the transcellular permeability of confluent bovine brain microvessel endothelial cell monolayers was studied with the side-by-side diffusion apparatus (Fig. 3). Exposure of the apical (donor or luminal) side of the monolayers to nanomolar concentrations of angiotensin agonists resulted in an 80% decrease in the flux of fluorescein-conjugated dextran (molecular weight ≈ 4000) across the monolayers in the apical to basolateral direction. On the other hand, if the basolateral (receptor or abluminal) side of the monolayers was exposed to similar concentrations of angiotensin agonists, no change in the flux of fluorescein-conjugated dextran across the monolayers in the basolateral to apical direction was observed. These results suggest that the site of responsiveness of the bovine brain microvessels' permeability to angiotensin agonists was localized on the apical or luminal side of the cells (GUILLOT and AUDUS 1989b; AUDUS 1990).

Typically, angiotensin II release in the circulation causes constriction in small vessels which is normally followed by release of vasodilatory prostaglandins (BROWN and BROWN 1986). This sequence of events has been postulated to be part of a protective mechanism in the vasculature for controlling a number of endothelial barrier functions including water and electrolyte movement and thromboresistance (GRYGLEWSKI et al. 1988). Collectively, our results have shown that angiotensin agonists stimulate fluid-phase endocytosis in a prostaglandin-dependent manner and reduce transendothelial permeability significantly. The results essentially reflect prostaglandin action in the model system. That is, following exposure to angiotens in agonists, release of prostaglandins was triggered which in turn caused a substantial decrease in monolayer permeability in the apical to basolateral direction and stimulated pinocytosis. Presumably, this response in vitro corresponds to a decrease in the blood to brain or brain to blood movement of water, ions, and macromolecules in vivo. As for the prostaglandin-dependent angiotensin-stimulated fluid-phase endocytosis, the function remains to be elucidated.

In vivo studies have also noted the increased cerebrovascular pinocytic activity in angiotensin-induced hypertension (JOHANSSON 1981). Under one hypothesis, we have ascribed the angiotensin-induced elevation in BBB pinocytic activity in vitro to prostaglandins. However, the increased pinocytic activity may be viewed differently if one considers the possibility of other physiological roles in the vasculature for angiotensin. Preliminary studies in our laboratories indicate that angiotensin undergoes receptor-mediated internalization. Along with internalization of bound material (i.e., angiotensin II), extracellular fluid containing the fluid-phase marker may also occur. Thus, vasoactive peptide stimulatory effects on fluid-phase endocytosis may alternatively depict endothelial cell sorting of the peptides to intracellular compartments for other purposes. Angiotensin, for example, has been surmised to stimulate protein synthesis and cell proliferation following internalization (RE and RARAB 1984; RE et al. 1984)

As outlined in the studies above, the in vitro model offers a potentially valuable tool to delineate cellular and biochemical pathways of vasoactive peptide regulation of capillary permeability and other fundamental functions.

F. Summary

The characteristics of macromolecular transport across capillary endothelium vary with tissue location. Possible pathways for macromolecule transport across capillary endothelium can include fenestrations, large pores, intercellular junctions, and transcytosis. For many special tissues such as the brain, however, basic transport pathways for macromolecules, in general, are not well-defined. The need for a better understanding of the macromolecular transport features of endothelia has stimulated development of appropriate in vivo and in vitro model systems. Accordingly, the emergence of tissue culture systems, as in vitro complements to the in vivo model, appears to be potentially important in the elucidation of cellular, biochemical, and molecular features of macromolecule transport across capillary endothelium.

References

Antonelli-Orlidge A, Saunders KB, Smith SR, d'Amore PA (1989) An activated form of transforming growth factor beta is produced by cocultures of endothelial cells and pericytes. Proc Natl Acad Sci USA 86:4544–4548

Audus KL (1990) Blood-brain barrier: mechanisms of peptide regulation and transport. J Control Release 11:51–59

Audus KL, Borchardt RT (1986a) Characterization of an in vitro blood-brain barrier model system for studying drug transport and metabolism. Pharm Res 3:81–87

Audus KL, Borchardt RT (1986b) Characteristics of the large neutral amino acid transport system of bovine brain microvessel endothelial cell monolayers. J Neurochem 47:484–488

Audus KL, Borchardt RT (1987) Bovine brain microvessel endothelial cell monolayers as a model for the blood-brain barrier. Ann NY Acad Sci 507:9–18

Audus KL, Manning MC (1990) In vitro studies of peptide transport through a cell culture model of the blood-brain barrier. Eur J Pharmacol 83:1636–1637

Baba M, Oishi R, Saeki K (1988) Enhancement of blood-brain barrier permeability to sodium fluorescein by stimulation of μ opioid receptors in mice. Naunyn Schmiedebergs Arch Pharmacol 337:423–428

Banks WA, Kastin AJ (1986) Modulation of the carrier-mediated transport of Tyr-MIF-1 across the blood brain barrier by essential amino acids. J Pharmacol Exp Ther 239:668–672

Banks WA, Kastin AJ (1988) Review: interactions between the blood-brain barrier and endogenous peptides: emerging clinical implications. Am J Med Sci 31: 459–465

Banks WA, Kastin AJ (1989) Effect of neurotransmitters on the system that transports Tyr-MIF-1 and the enkephalins across the blood-brain barrier: a dominant role for serotonin. Psychopharmacology (Berlin) 98:380–385

Banks WA, Kastin AJ, Horvath A, Michals EA (1987a) Carrier-mediated transport of vasopressin across the blood-brain barrier of the mouse. J Neurosci Res 18:326–332

Banks WA, Kastin AJ, Michals EA (1987b) Tyr-MIF-1 and met-enkephalin share a saturable blood-brain barrier transport system. Peptides 8:899–903

Banks WA, Kastin AJ, Fasold MB, Barrera CM, Augereau G (1988) Studies of the slow bidirectional transport of iron and transferrin across the blood-brain barrier. Brain Res Bull 21:881–885

Baranczyk-Kuzma A, Audus KL (1987) Characteristics of aminopeptidase activity from brain microvessel endothelium. J Cereb Blood Flow Metab 7:801–805

Baranczyk-Kuzma A, Audus KL, Borchardt RT (1986) Catecholamine-metabolizing enzymes of bovine brain microvessel endothelial cell monolayers. J Neurochem 46:1956–1960

Baranczyk-Kuzma A, Audus KL, Borchardt RT (1989a) Substrate specificity of phenol sulfotransferase from primary cultures of bovine brain microvessel endothelium. Neurochem Res 14:689–691

Baranczyk-Kuzma A, Raub TJ, Audus KL (1989b) Demonstration of acid hydrolase activity in primary cultures of bovine brain microvessel endothelium. J Cereb Blood Flow Metab 9:280–289

Barrera CM, Kastin AJ, Banks WA (1987) D-[Ala^1]-peptide T-amide is transported from blood to brain by a saturable system. Brain Res Bull 19:629–633

Bennett HS, Luft JH, Hampton JL (1959) Morphological classification of vertebrate blood capillaries. Am J Physiol 196:381–390

Ben-Shachar D, Yehuda S, Finberg JPM, Spanier I, Youdim MBH (1988) Selective alteration in blood-brain barrier and insulin transport in iron-deficient rats. J Neurochem 50:1434–1437

Besterman JM, Aihart JA, Woodworth RC, Low RB (1981) Exocytosis of pinocytosed fluid in cultured cells: kinetic evidence for rapid turnover and compartmentation. J Cell Biol 91:716–727

Bottaro D, Shepro D, Peterson S, Hechtman HB (1986) Serotonin, norepinephrine, and histamine mediation of endothelial cell barrier function in vitro. J Cell Physiol 128:189–194

Bouldin TW, Krigman MR (1975) Differential permeability of cerebral capillary and choroid plexus to lanthanum ions. Brain Res 99:444–448

Bowman PD, Ennis ER, Rarey KE, Betz AL, Goldstein GW (1983) Brain microvessel endothelial cells in tissue culture. A model for study of blood-brain barrier permeability. Ann Neurol 14:396–402

Brightman MW, Reese TS (1969) Junctions between intimately apposed cell membranes in the vertebrate brain. J Cell Biol 40:649–677

Broadwell RD, Balin BJ, Salcman M (1988) Transcytotic pathway for blood-borne protein through the blood-brain barrier. Proc Natl Acad Sci USA 85:7820–7824

Brown MJ, Brown J (1986) Does angiotensin-II protect against strokes? Lancet 2:427–429

Chabrier PE, Rouberi P, Braquet P (1987) Specific binding of atrial natriuretic factor in brain microvessels. Proc Natl Acad Sci USA 84:2078–2081

Chastain JE Jr, Borchardt RT (1987) Potential substrates for the large neutral amino acid transport system of bovine brain microvessel endothelial cell monolayers. J Cell Biol 105:328a

Chastain JE Jr, Borchardt RT (1989) L-α-Methyldopa transport across bovine brain microvessel endothelial cell monolayers, a model for the blood-brain barrier. Neurosci Res Commun 4:147–152

Chastain JE Jr, Borchardt RT (1990) Acivicin transport across bovine brain microvessel endothelial cell monolayers. A model of the blood-brain barrier. Neurosci Res Commun 6:51–55

Clementi F, Palade GE (1969) Intestinal capillaries. I. Permeability to peroxidase and ferritin. J Cell Biol 41:33–58

Cornford EM (1985) The blood-brain barrier, a dynamic regulatory interface. Mol Physiol 7:219–260

Crone C (1986) The blood-brain barrier as a tight epithelium: where is information lacking? Ann NY Acad Sci 481:174–185

Cserr HF, Bundgaard M (1984) Blood-brain barrier interfaces in vertebrates: a comparative approach. Am J Physiol 246:R277–R288

Davies PF (1984) Quantitative aspects of endocytosis in cultured endothelial cells. In: Jaffe EA (ed) Biology of endothelial cells. Nijhoff, Boston, p 365

Deen WM, Bridges CR, Brenner BM (1983) Biophysical basis of glomerular permeability. J Membr Biol 71:1–10

Dernovsek KD, Bar RS, Ginsberg BH, Lioubin MN (1984) Rapid transport of biologically intact insulin through cultured endothelial cells. J Clin Endocrinol Metab 58:761–763

Dorovini-Zis K, Bowman PD, Betz AL, Goldstein GW (1984) Hyperosmotic arabinose solutions open the tight junctions between brain capillary endothelial cells in tissue culture. Brain Res 302:383–386

Duffy KR, Pardridge WM (1987) Blood-brain barrier transcytosis of insulin in developing rabbits. Brain Res 420:32–38

Dzau VJ (1984) Vascular wall renin-angiotensin pathway in control of the circulation. Am J Med 77:31–36

Dzau VJ (1986) Significance of the vascular renin-angiotensin pathway. Hypertension 8:553–559

Fajardo LF (1989) The complexity of endothelial cells. Am J Clin Pathol 92:241–250

Fishman JB, Rubin JB, Handrahan JV, Connor JR, Fine RE (1987) Receptor-mediated transcytosis of transferrin across the blood-brain barrier. J Neurosci Res 18:299–304

Frank HJL, Pardridge WM, Morris WL, Rosenfeld RG, Choi TB (1986) Binding and internalization of insulin and insulin-like growth factors by isolated brain microvessels. Diabetes 35:654–661

Ghinea N, Simionescu N (1985) Anionized and cationized hemeundecapeptides as probes for cell surface charge and permeability studies: differentiated labeling of endothelial plasmalemmal vesicles. J Cell Biol 100:606–612

Goldstein GW, Betz AL (1983) Recent advances in understanding brain capillary function. Ann Neurol 14:389–395

Goldstein GW, Betz AL (1986) The blood-brain barrier. Sci Am 255:74–83

Granger DN, Kvietys PR, Perry MA, Taylor AE (1986) Charge selectivity of rat intestinal capillaries: influence of polycations. Gastroenterology 91:1443–1446

Grubb RL Jr, Raichle ME (1981) Intraventricular angiotensin II increases brain vascular permeability. Brain Res 210:426–430

Gryglewski RJ, Botting RM, Vane JR (1988) Mediators produced by the endothelial cell. Hypertension 12:530–548

Guillot FL, Audus KL (1989a) Biochemistry of angiotensin peptide-mediated effects on fluid-phase endocytosis in brain microvessel endothelial cell monolayers. J Cell Biol 107:809a

Guillot FL, Audus KL (1989b) Vasoactive peptide regulation of blood-brain barrier permeability. Pharm Res 6:S211

Guillot FL, Audus KL (1989c) Vasoactive peptide effects on brain microvessel endothelial cell membrane order. J Cell Biol 109:35a

Guillot FL, Audus KL, Raub TJ (1990) Fluid-phase endocytosis by primary cultures of bovine brain microvessel endohtelial cell monolayers. Microvasc Res 39: 1–14

Hammersen F, Hammersen E (1985) Some structural and functional aspects of endothelial cells. Basic Res Cardiol 80:491–501

Hawkins RA (1986) Transport of essential nutrients across the blood-brain barrier of individual structures. Fed Proc 45:2055–2059

Janzer RC, Raff MC (1987) Astrocytes induce blood-brain barrier properties in endothelial cells. Nature 325:253–257

Johansson BB (1981) Pharmacological modification of hypertensive blood-brain barrier opening. Acta Pharmacol Toxicol (Copenh) 48:242–247

Joo F (1985) The blood-brain barrier in vitro: ten years of research on microvessels isolated from the brain. Neurochem Int 7:1–25

Kastin AJ, Nissen C, Coy DH (1981) Permeability of the blood-brain barrier to DSIP peptides. Pharmacol Biochem Behav 15:955–959

Keller BT, Borchardt RT (1987) Cultured bovine brain capillary endothelial cells (BBCEC) – a blood-brain barrier model for studying the binding and internalization of insulin and insulin-like growth factor 1. Fed Proc 46:416

Keller BT, Smith KR, Borchardt RT (1988) Transport barriers to absorption of peptides. Pharm Weekbl [Sci] 10:38–39

King GL, Johnson SM (1985) Receptor-mediated transport of insulin across endothelial cells. Science 227:1583–1586

Kumagi AK, Eisenberg JB, Pardridge WM (1987) Adsorptive-mediated endocytosis of cationized albumin and a β-endorphin-cationized albumin chimeric peptide by isolated brain capillaries. J Biol Chem 262:15214–15219

Lasbennes F, Gayet J (1984) Capacity for energy metabolism in microvessels isolated from rat brain. Neurochem Res 9:1–10

Levick JR, Smaje LH (1987) An analysis of the permeability of a fenestra. Microvasc Res 33:233–256

Lidinsky WA, Drewes LR (1983) Characterization of the blood-brain barrier: protein composition of the capillary endothelial cell membrane. J Neurochem 41: 1341–1348

Lombardi T, Montesano R, Orci L (1985) Polarized plasma membrane domains in cultured endothelial cells. Exp Cell Res 161:242–246

McCall AL, Valente J, Cordero R, Ruderman NB, Tornhem K (1988) Metabolic characterization of isolated cerebral microvessels: ATP and ADP concentrations. Microvasc Res 35:325–333

Meresse S, Delbart C, Fruchart J-C, Cecchelli R (1989) Low-density lipoprotein receptors on endothelium of brain capillaries. J Neurochem 53:340–345

Milici AJ, L'Hernault N, Palade GE (1985) Surface densities of diaphragmed fenestrae and transendothelial channels in different murine capillary beds. Circ Res 56: 709–717

Needleman P, Blain EH, Greenwald JE, Michener ML, Saper CB, Stockman PT, Tolunay HE (1989) The biochemical pharmacology of atrial peptides. Annu Rev Pharmacol Toxicol 29:23–54

Newton CR, Raub TJ (1988) Characterization of the transferrin receptor in primary cultures of bovine brain capillary endothelial cells. J Cell Biol 107:770a

Oldendorf WH (1971) Brain uptake of radiolabeled amino acids, amines, and hexoses after arterial injection. Am J Physiol 221:1629–1639

Orlidge A, d'Amore PA (1987) Inhibition of capillary endothelial cell growth by pericytes and smooth muscle cells. J Cell Biol 105:1455–1462

Palade GE (1988) The microvascular endothelium revisited. In: Simionescu N, Simionescu M (eds) Endothelial cell biology in health and disease. Plenum, New York, p 3

Palade GE, Simionescu M, Simionescu N (1979) Structural aspects of the permeability of the microvascular endothelium. Acta Physiol Scand [Suppl] 463:11–32

Pappenheimer JR, Renkin EM, Borrero LM (1951) Filtration, diffusion and molecular sieving through peripheral capillary membranes; a contribution to the pore theory of capillary permeability. Am J Physiol 167:13–46

Pardridge WM (1987) The gate keeper: how molecules are screened for admission to the brain. The Sciences 27:50–55

Pardridge WM, Eisenberg J, Yang J (1985) Human blood-brain barrier insulin receptor. J Neurochem 44:1771–1778

Pardridge WM, Kumagi AK, Eisenberg JB (1987) Chimeric peptides as a vehicle for peptide pharmaceutical delivery through the blood-brain barrier. Biochem Biophys Res Commun 146:307–313

Pastan I, Willingham MC (1985) The pathway of endocytosis. In: Pastan I, Willingham MC (eds) Endocytosis. Plenum, New York, p 1

Pearse BMF, Crowther RA (1987) Structure and assembly of coated vesicles. Annu Rev Biophys Biophys Chem 16:49–68

Peters KR, Milici AJ (1983) High resolution SEM of the luminal surface of a fenestrated capillary endothelium. J Cell Biol 97:336a

Raeissi S, Audus KL (1989) In-vitro characterization of blood-brain barrier permeability to delta sleep-inducing peptide. J Pharm Pharmacol 41:848–852

Raub TJ, Audus KL (1987) Adsorptive endocytosis by bovine brain capillary endothelial cells in vitro. J Cell Biol 105:312a

Raub TJ, Kuentzel SL, Sawada GA (1989) Characteristics of primary bovine cerebral microvessel endothelial cell monolayers on membrane filters: permeability and glial induced changes. J Cell Biol 109:315a

Re R, Parab M (1984) Effect of angiotensin II on RNA synthesis by isolated nuclei. Life Sci 34:647–651

Re RN, Vizard DL, Brown J, Bryan SE (1984) Angiotensin II receptors in chromatin fragments generated by micrococcal nuclease. Biochem Biophys Res Commun 119:220–227

Reardon PM, Audus KL (1989) Arginine-vasopressin distribution across the in vitro blood-brain barrier. Pharm Res 6:S88

Reese TS, Karnovsky MJ (1967) Fine structural localization of a blood-brain barrier to exogenous peroxidase. J Cell Biol 34:207–217

Renkin EM (1979) Relation of capillary morphology to transport of fluid and large molecules: a review. Acta Physiol Scand [Suppl] 463:81–91

Renkin EM (1988) Transport pathways and processes. In: Simionescu N, Simionescu M (eds) Endothelial cell biology in health and disease. Plenum, New York, p 51

Renkin EM, Watson PD, Sloop CH, Joyner WL, Curry FE (1977) Transport pathways for fluid and large molecules in microvascular endothelium of the dog's
paw. Microvasc Res 14:205–214
Rim S, Audus KL, Borchardt RT (1986) Relationship of octanol/buffer and octanol/
water partition coefficients to transcellular diffusion across brain microvessel
endothelial cell monolayers. Int J Pharm 32:79–84
Rippe B, Kamiya A, Folkow B (1979) Transcapillary passage of albumin, effects of
tissue cooling and increases in filtration and plasma colloid osmotic pressure.
Acta Physiol Scand 105:171–187
Rogoeczi E, Chindemi PA, Debanne MT, Hatton MWC (1982) Dual nature of the
hepatic lectin pathway for human asialotransferrin type 3 in the rat. J Biol Chem
257:5431–5436
Rosenfeld RG, Pham H, Keller B, Borchardt RT, Pardridge WM (1987) Structural
comparison of receptors for insulin, insulin-like growth factor I and II (IGF-1
and IGF-2) in brain and blood-brain barrier. Biochem Biophys Res Commun
149:159–166
Ryan US (1986) The endothelial surface and response to injury. Fed Proc 45:
101–108
Scow RO, Blanchette-Mackie EJ, Smith LC (1976) Role of capillary endothelium in
the clearance of chylomicrons; a model for lipid transport from blood by lateral
diffusion in cell membranes. Circ Res 39:149–162
Scriba GKE, Borchardt RT (1989a) Metabolism of catecholamine esters by cultured
bovine brain microvessel endothelial cells. J Neurochem 53:610–615
Scriba GKE, Borchardt RT (1989b) Metabolism of 1-methyl-4-phenyl-1,2,3,6-
tetrahydropyridine (MPTP) by bovine brain capillary endothelial cell monolayers. Brain Res 501:175–178
Shah MV, Borchardt RT (1989) Characterization of the nucleoside transport system
in bovine brain microvessel endothelial cell (BBMEC) monolayers. Pharm
Res 6:S77
Shah MV, Audus KL, Borchardt RT (1989) The application of bovine brain microvessel endothelial cell monolayers grown onto polycarbonate membranes in
vitro to estimate the potential permeability of solutes through the blood-brain
barrier. Pharm Res 6:624–627
Shasby DM, Shasby SS (1985) Active transendothelial transport of albumin: interstitium to lumen. Circ Res 57:903–908
Simionescu M (1988) Receptor-mediated transcytosis of plasma molecules by vascular endothelium. In: Simionescu N, Simionescu M (eds) Endothelial cell
biology in health and disease. Plenum, New York, p 69
Simionescu N, Simionescu M (1983) The cardiovascular system. In: Weiss L (ed)
Histology. Elsevier, New York, p 371
Simionescu N, Simionescu M, Palade GE (1975) Permeability of muscle capillaries
to small hemepeptides: evidence for the existence of patent transendothelial
channels. J Cell Biol 64:586–607
Simionescu M, Simionescu N, Silbert JE, Palade GE (1981) Differentiated micro-
domains on the luminal surface of capillary endothelium. II. Partical charac-
terization of their anionic sites. J Cell Biol 90:614–621
Simionescu M, Simionescu N, Palade Ge (1982) Preferential distribution of anionic
sites on the basement membrane and the abluminal aspect of the endothelium
in fenestrated capillaries. J Cell Biol 95:425–434
Simionescu M, Simionescu N, Palade GE (1984) Partial chemical characterization
of the anionic sites in the basal lamina of fenestrated capillaries. Microvasc
Res 28:352–367
Smith JJ, Kampine JP (1984) Circulatory physiology. Williams and Wilkins,
Baltimore
Smith KR, Borchardt RT (1989) Permeability and mechanism of albumin, cationized
albumin and glycosylated albumin transcellular transport across monolayers of
cultured brain capillary endothelial cells. Pharm Res 6:466–473

Smith KR, Kato A, Borchardt RT (1988) Characterization of specific receptors for atrial natriuretic factor on cultured bovine brain microvessel endothelial cells. Biochem Biophys Res Commun 157:308–314

Smith QR (1989) Quantitation of blood-brain barrier permeability. In: Newelt EA (ed) Implications of the blood-brain barrier and its manipulation: basic science aspects. Plenum, New York, p 85

Smith QR, Takasato Y (1986) Kinetics of amino acid transport at the blood-brain barrier studied using an in situ brain perfusion technique. Ann NY Acad Sci 481:186–201

Stewart PA, Wiley MJ (1981) Developing nervous tissue induces formation of blood-brain barrier characteristics in invading endothelial cells: a study using quail-chick transplantation chimeras. Dev Biol 84:183–192

Sussman I, Carson MP, McCall AL, Schulz V, Ruderman NB, Tornheim K (1988) Energy state of bovine cerebral microvessels: comparison of isolation methods. Microvasc Res 35:167–178

Svensjo E, Grega GJ (1986) Evidence for endothelial cell-mediated regulation of macromolecular permeability by postcapillary venules. Fed Proc 45:89–95

Swanson JA, Yirinec BD, Silverstein SC (1985) Phorbol esters and horseradish peroxidase stimulate pinocytosis and redirect the flow of pinocytosed fluid in macrophages. J Cell Biol 100:851–859

Takasato Y, Rapoport SI, Smith QR (1984) An in situ brain perfusion technique to study cerebrovascular transport in the rat. Am J Physiol 247:H484–H493

Tao-Cheng JH, Nagy Z, Brightman MW (1987) Tight junctions of cerebral endothelium in vitro are enhanced by astroglia. J Neurosci 7:3293–3299

Thompson SE, Audus KL (1989) Aspects of leu-enkephalin transport and metabolism at the blood-brain barrier. Pharm Res 6:S175

Trammel AT, Borchardt RT (1987) Choline transport in cultured brain microvessel endothelial cells. Pharm Res 4:S41

Trammel AT, Borchardt RT (1989) The effects of astrocytes and glioma cells on the permeability of cultured brain microvessel endothelial cells. Pharm Res 6:S88

Triguero D, Buciak JB, Yang J, Pardridge WM (1989) Blood-brain barrier transport of cationized immunoglobulin G: enhanced delivery compared to native protein. Proc Natl Acad Sci USA 86:4761–4765

Trubetskaya OV, Trubetskoy VS, Domogatsky SP, Rudin AV, Popov NV, Danilov SM, Nikolayeva MN, Klibanov AL, Torchilin VP (1988) Monoclonal antibody to human endothelial cell surface internalization and liposome delivery in cell culture. FEBS Lett 228:131–134

Van Bree JMBB, Audus KL, Borchardt RT (1988) Carrier-mediated transport of baclofen across monolayers of bovine brain microvessel endothelial cells in culture. Pharm Res 5:369–371

Van Bree JMBB, de Boer AG, Verhoef JC, Danhof M, Breimer DD (1989) Transport of vasopressin fragments across the blood-brain barrier: in vitro studies using monolayer cultures of bovine brain endothelial cells. J Pharmacol Exp Ther 249:901–905

Vinters HV, Reave S, Costello P, Girvin JP, Moore SA (1987) Isolation and culture of cells derived from human cerebral microvessels. Cell Tissue Res 249:657–667

Vorbrodt AW (1988) Ultrastructural cyto-chemistry of blood-brain barrier endothelia. Prog Histochem 18:1–96

Vorbrodt AW, Lossinsky AS, Wisniewski HM, Suzuki R, Yamaguchi T, Masaoka H (1985) Ultrastructural observations on the transvascular route of protein removal in vasogenic brain edema. Acta Neuropathol (Berl) 66:265–273

Voyta JC, Via DP, Butterfield CE, Zetter BR (1984) Identification and isolation of endothelial cells based on their increased uptake of acetylated-low density lipoprotein. J Cell Biol 99:2034–2040

Wahl M, Unterberg A, Baethmann A, Schilling L (1988) Mediators of blood-brain barrier dysfunction and formation of vasogenic edema. J Cereb Blood Flow Metab 8:621–643

White EA, Audus KL (1989) Characterization of brain microvessel endothelial cell cultures: growth factors and lectin binding. J Cell Biol 109:150a
Williams SK (1983) Vesicular transport of proteins by capillary endothelium. Ann NY Acad Sci 416:457–467
Williams SK, Wagner RC (1981) Regulation of micropinocytosis in capillary endothelium by multivalent cations. Microvasc Res 21:175–182
Williams SK, Gillis JF, Matthews MA, Wagner RC, Bitensky MW (1980) Isolation and characterization of brain endothelial cells: morphology and enzyme activity. J Neurochem 35:374–381
Zlokovic BV, Lipovac MN, Begley DJ, Davson H, Rakic LJ (1987) Transport of leucine-enkephalin across the blood-brain barrier in the perfused guinea pig brain. J Neurochem 49:300–305
Zlokovic BV, Susic VT, Davson H, Begley DJ, Jankov RM, Mitrovic DM, Lipovac MN (1989) Saturable mechanism for delta sleep-inducing peptide (DSIP) at the blood-brain barrier of the vascularly perfused guinea pig brain. Peptides 10: 249–254

CHAPTER 4

Pharmacokinetics of Drug Targeting: Specific Implications for Targeting via Prodrugs

V.J. STELLA and A.S. KEARNEY

A. Introduction

Pharmacokinetics can be defined as the study of the time profiles of drugs in the body. It has largely been used to describe how a drug is handled by the body, i.e., its absorption, distribution, metabolism, and elimination. The extrapolated information is correlated to the therapeutic/toxicological effects of the drug, i.e., its pharmacodynamics. The attempt to correlate pharmacokinetic to pharmacodynamic behavior has led to the subdiscipline of applied or clinical pharmacokinetics. The vast majority of the published pharmacokinetic literature focuses on defining the clinical pharmacokinetics of drugs and toxic materials (toxicokinetics).

Early research into pharmacokinetics focused on compartmental analysis. That is, the body was viewed as being made up of a series of black boxes or compartments (WAGNER 1981). Figure 1 defines an idealized compartmental model for a drug acting at some *response* or *target site*, manifesting its toxicity at some *toxic site*, and distributing through the remainder of the body. In addition to the response and toxic sites, the drug distributes between two macroscopic compartments: (1) a series of accessible tissues that are in rapid equilibrium with the *plasma* or *central compartment* and (2) a series of less accessible tissues that are not in ready equilibrium with the plasma, the *peripheral* or *tissue compartment*. Drug input is usually viewed as occurring into the plasma or central compartment with output occurring from this same compartment. The ideal drug is one whose greatest affinity is for its response or target site and which has minimal contact with the toxic site.

For the most part, clinical applications of pharmacokinetics still focus on compartmental analyses because of their simplicity and flexibility (PECK and RODMAN 1986). The use of noncompartmental data analysis (BENET and GALEAZZI 1979; DI STEFANO 1982) has gained in popularity while physiological approaches to pharmacokinetics (HIMMELSTEIN and LUTZ 1979; JAIN and GERLOWSKI 1983 and references therein), although intuitively more representative of what might be happening in the body, are not readily applicable to clinical settings. Hybrid approaches, however, that utilize mixed classical/physiological models or so-called clearance models have proven useful for many clinical and nonclinical applications. (See the text by ROWLAND and TOZER (1989) for examples of this approach.)

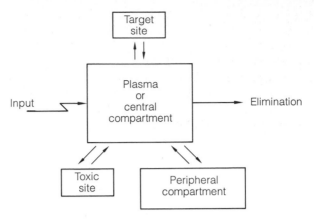

Fig. 1. Idealized compartmental pharmacokinetic model for a drug acting at a target site, manlfesting its toxicity at a toxic site and distributing throughout the remainder of the body

B. Pharmacokinetic Models and Drug Targeting

I. Defining Drug Targeting

Targeted or site-specific delivery by a chemically or physically driven drug delivery system can be defined either qualitatively or quantitatively. Targeted drug delivery by an engineered system is said to be achieved when the time profile of drug at the target site is optimized and the burden of drug to other tissues, especially tissues that may manifest toxicity, is minimized. This simple definition assumes that both activity and toxicity are related to the time profile of the intact drug at the target and toxic sites, respectively.

The assessment of targeting can be determined by comparing dose-response curves of the targeted system to the conventional or nontargeted system. Dose-response and dose-toxicity data allow one to define a term called the therapeutic index or TI. TI can be defined by Eq. 1 as the ratio of the maximum tolerated toxic dose (MTTD) to the minimum effective dose (MED):

$$TI = \frac{MTTD}{MED} \tag{1}$$

If a delivery system is now employed to target the drug, an identical term, TI′, can be defined for the targeted system:

$$TI' = \frac{MTTD'}{MED'} \tag{2}$$

The therapeutic advantage achieved from the targeted delivery system can then be defined by ratio TI′/TI. Targeting is realized when TI′/TI is significantly greater than unity. A danger here is that the targeted system may simply be changing the temporal pattern of the drug in a favorable manner relative to the non-targeted system. This point will be elaborated on later.

Targeting can also be defined quantitatively. HUNT et al., (1986) defined a term called the drug targeting index, or DTI. Assuming that the area under the site-concentration time curve (AUC) or the steady state (SS) levels at the response or target site versus the toxic site reflect the relative activity and toxicity of the drug and its delivery system, DTI can be defined by Eqs. 3 and 4:

$$DTI = \frac{AUC_{R,target}/AUC_{T,target}}{AUC_{R,nontarget}/AUC_{T,nontarget}} \qquad (3)$$

$$DTI = \frac{C_{R,SS,target}/C_{T,SS,target}}{C_{R,SS,nontarget}/C_{T,SS,nontarget}} \qquad (4)$$

where $AUC_{R,target}$, $AUC_{T,target}$, $AUC_{R,nontarget}$, and $AUC_{T,nontarget}$ represent the AUCs for the response or target site (R) and for the toxic site (T) after targeted delivery (target) and nontargeted delivery (nontarget), respectively. In Eq. 4, the terms $C_{R,SS,target}$, $C_{T,SS,target}$, $C_{R,SS,nontarget}$, and $C_{T,SS,nontarget}$ represent the steady state (SS) concentrations of drug at the response or target site (R) and at the toxic site (T) after targeted delivery (target) and nontargeted delivery (nontarget), respectively.

The use of pharmacokinetic models to help optimize drug design and delivery, especially in testing drug targeting hypotheses, has received some attention (STELLA and HIMMELSTEIN 1980, 1985a,b; NOTARI 1981; HUNT et al., 1986; SMITS and THIJSSEN 1986; and AARONS et al. 1989a,b). It is this use of pharmacokinetics that will be discussed further in this chapter. That is, can pharmacokinetic models be used to test targeting hypotheses?

II. Testing Targeting Hypotheses Using Classical or Compartmental Pharmacokinetic Models

Figure 1 described a general compartmental model that included a response or target compartment and a toxic site compartment. Models such as these can be used to test various targeting strategies. For example, consider the hypothesis: *I will achieve selective delivery of my drug by infusing the agent intra-arterially into the artery supplying blood to the target organ and, by doing so, I expect to have a significant clinical advantage over intravenous infusion administration of the same drug.* A formal compartmental model to test this hypothesis is presented in Fig. 2, a simplified form of Fig. 1. Here, the body is considered to be made up of a response or target organ and the balance of the body is made up of a single homogeneous compartment, the plasma or central compartment, and a toxic site compartment. Drug input to the response

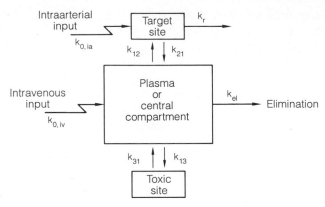

Fig. 2. Formallzed compartmental model used to test varlous targeting strategies

compartment after zero-order intravenous infusion, $k_{0,iv}$, would be by uptake via the first-order rate constant, k_{12}, which would compete with drug loss from the central compartment via elimination, k_{el}, and drug uptake by the toxic site compartment, k_{13}. Intra-arterial input can be simulated by assuming the infusion, $k_{0,ia}$, is directly into the response or target organ. It is also assumed that the drug can be eliminated from the response organ by the first-order rate constant, k_r. Competing with the response compartment is the plasma compartment, which can access drug via the first-order rate constant, k_{21}. To simplify the modeling, it will be assumed that the drug will be infused to steady state and that relative steady state levels of drug in the response and toxic organs will reflect the relative therapeutic benefit and toxicity of the two input routes, respectively.

By setting up the differential equations for each compartment, assuming conservation of mass and that the steady-state assumption holds, it can be shown that the ratio, $C_{R,SS,ia}/C_{R,SS,iv}$ can be defined by Eq. 5:

$$C_{R,SS,ia}/C_{R,SS,iv} = 1 + \left(\frac{k_{el}}{k_{12}}\right) \tag{5}$$

where the ratio, $C_{R,SS,ia}/C_{R,SS,iv}$ (or in the case of a targeted vs non targeted system, $C_{R,SS,target}/C_{R,SS,nontarget}$) has been defined as the therapeutic availability (TA):

$$TA = C_{R,SS,target}/C_{R,SS,nontarget} \tag{6}$$

TA is the dose fraction available to the response or target compartment when a targeted and a non targeted delivery system are compared. This can also be defined in terms of AUCs, (HUNT et al. 1986):

$$TA = AUC_{R,target}/AUC_{R,nontarget} \tag{7}$$

As mentioned, the equations derived for intra-arterial administration relative to intravenous administration can also pertain to a targeted drug delivery system relative to a nontargeted system. In the case of a targeted delivery system, it is hoped that the targeted system, upon systemic administration, can be preferentially delivered to the response site (as seen with intra-arterial administration) where it will release the "free" drug. Obviously, premature release of the drug from the delivery system prior to the response site will lead to a loss in the targeting ability.

Equation 5 is interesting in that it emphasizes a point that was made by numerous other researchers, that the potential for targeting is highly dependent on the properties of the drug to be targeted (STELLA and HIMMELSTEIN 1980,1985a,b; HUNT et al. 1986; SMITS and THIJSSEN 1986; AARONS et al. 1989a,b). Namely, TA will be greater than unity for direct intra-arterial infusion compared to intravenous administration of the same drug (or for a targeted compared to a nontargeted system) if the drug is rapidly eliminated from the body relative to its uptake rate by the target organ, or $k_{el} > k_{12}$. However, if $k_{12} > k_{el}$, then TA approaches unity and no therapeutic advantage would be achieved. Interestingly, rapidly eliminated drugs are not likely to be good candidates for clinical development, and drugs that are poorly taken up by the target site are also candidates likely to be discarded in the drug discovery process. In other words, drugs that are well taken up by their target site and have reasonable residence times in the body are often the candidates chosen for clinical development. It is precisely this combination of properties that makes them poor candidates for the targeting strategy tested here or for any other strategy (STELLA and HIMMELSTEIN 1980; STELLA 1989; and HUNT et al. 1986). LEVY (1987) has also qualitatively discussed this point. Another way of expressing Eq. 5 is:

$$TA = 1 + \frac{k_{el}}{R \cdot k_{21}} \tag{8}$$

where R is equal to k_{12}/k_{21}. A "good" drug would be one where $R > 1$, that is, a drug which has a higher affinity for its response compartment relative to other tissues. Such a drug is already targeted by design. If $R > 1$, then it would be more difficult for a delivery system to achieve targeting, i.e., TA will be > 1 if $k_{el} > Rk_{21}$.

The model illustrated in Fig. 2 and formulated as Eqs. 5 and 8 may not represent a meaningful comparison between intra-arterial vs intravenous drug administration in that input into the response compartment was simulated as being into the target site itself rather than the blood supplying the target site, a point to be discussed later. As simulated in this case, input is more representative of what might be called peritarget drug delivery (SMITS and THIJSSEN 1986), where drug is administered directly into the target organ or in the peritarget cavity which is the space that surrounds the target. It assumes that this peritarget administered drug is instantaneously taken up by the approximated homogeneous target site organ. Equation 8 suggests that targeting as defined by the TA will be sensitive to k_{21}, the elimination rate constant of drug from the target site. The rate of loss of drug from the target site will be determined by the membrane permeability and diffusion characteristics of the drug, the rate of drug-receptor dissociation (SADEE 1985), the direct elimination or biotransformation of the drug in the target organ, and the microperfusion or blood flow characteristics of the site (LEVY 1987).

The term TA only addresses the therapeutic availability of the drug to the target or response site. It does not address the issue of targeting as it relates to response site vs toxic site effects. That can be evaluated by the DTI. In Fig. 2, DTI can be defined by Eq. 9 (or by Eqs. 3 and 4 in the case of a targeted versus non-targeted drug delivery system):

$$\text{DTI} = \frac{C_{R,SS,ia}/C_{T,SS,ia}}{C_{R,SS,iv}/C_{T,SS,iv}} = \left(1 + \frac{k_{el}}{k_{12}}\right)\left(\frac{k_{21} + k_r}{k_{21}}\right) \tag{9}$$

If the drug is distributed to the plasma compartment from the target site faster than it is biotransformed at the target site, $k_{21} < k_r$, then DTI will be equal to TA. However, if k_r and k_{21} are comparable, then the last term on the right hand side of Eq. 9 can be described by:

$$\left(\frac{k_{21} + k_r}{k_{21}}\right) = \left(\frac{1}{F_r}\right) = \left(\frac{1}{1 - E_r}\right) \tag{10}$$

where F_r is equal to that fraction of drug released into systemic circulation that is specifically delivered to the target organ and E_r is the extraction efficiency of the target organ. If F_r was significantly less than unity (i.e., $E_r > 0$), then DTI would be greater than TA, which means that targeting would come from two sources, greater exposure of the target site to the drug and lower burden to the rest of the body which includes the toxic site (assuming the toxic site is different from the target or response site).

In discussing Eq. 8 and peritarget drug administration, it was assumed that all drug administered into a peritarget cavity was available to the target site, which presumably was not a part of the peritarget space or extravascular space. It was also assumed that drug administered into a peritarget cavity could not directly exchange with the plasma or central compartment. SMITS and THIJSSEN (1986) have discussed the possibility that the peritarget space could exchange with the plasma. Such a model is illustrated in Fig. 3. The TA for a drug administered into the peritarget cavity (zero-order input is assumed) compared to an intravenous infusion (steady state conditions also assumed) will be defined by:

$$\text{TA} = \frac{k_{21} + k_{pt}\left(1 + \dfrac{k_{el}}{k_{41}}\right)}{k_{21} + k_{pt}} \tag{11}$$

From Eq. 11, it can be seen that TA will be greater than unity only if the term, $(1 + k_{el}/k_{41})$, is very large or $k_{41} \ll k_{el}$. However, even if $(1 + k_{el}/k_{41})$

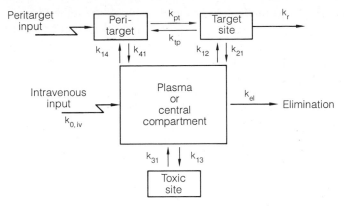

Fig. 3. Compartmental model used to test targeting strategies after peritarget administration

$\gg 1$, TA will still only approximate unity if $k_{21} \gg k_{pt}$, meaning that drug loss from the target site to the plasma or central compartment, defined by k_{21}, is fast relative to its input from the peritarget space, k_{pt}. If however, $k_{pt} \gg k_{21}$ and $(1 + k_{el}/k_{41}) \gg 1$, then TA would be greater than unity and targeting is possible. Qualitatively, targeting might be achieved after peritarget administration for drugs that are rapidly taken up by the target site relative to the plasma compartment and that have a relatively high affinity for the target site. Again, both the site and the properties of the drug determine the feasibility for targeting. Hence, drugs that readily equilibrate between the target site and plasma are not good candidates for targeting. This would probably exclude the majority of currently used therapeutic agents as candidates for targeting.

The idea that targeting could be achieved via intra-arterial versus intravenous administration is limited by the need for surgical intervention to access the artery. However, a number of physically and chemically based targeting strategies attempt to utilize this concept. For example, magnetic microsphere localization of a drug depot, drug release from biodegradable polymers injected as drug depots and trapped in the capillary bed due to size effects, and liposomes that release drug near a site such as a tumor due to pH changes or other triggering mechanisms are not unlike the intra-arterial/intravenous comparisons made here. Whereas local drug release from a depot such as a drug-containing, biodegradable matrix implanted in the intracranial space, intra-articular drug release from a drug/polymer matrix, and ophthalmic drug release from an ocular insert are not unlike the peritarget model tested above. All of these drug delivery strategies and any other strategy can be formulated as models, some more complex than those outlined above.

The problem with the steady state assumption used in evaluating the intra-arterial/intravenous comparisons is worth further discussion. Consider the hypothesis: *I will achieve targeting to a tumor by an injection of a drug entrapped in liposome whose degradation is pH dependent. Since the extracellular fluids at tumor sites are lower in pH than physiological pH, the liposome will preferentially release its drug load at the tumor site. The targeting will be affected because the drug will only be released locally.* Apart from concerns about the practical use of liposomes in general and whether liposomes are capable of escaping the vascular bed, there is nothing fundamentally wrong with this hypothesis except for what to use as a control in evaluating the hypothesis. For example, do you use a non-pH-dependent liposome, do you use an intravenous bolus or infusion dose of the drug, etc. Any one of these controls, as well as others, may not tell you if targeting was being achieved using either pharmacokinetic information or response data. Clearly, a drug delivery device like a liposome may not only change the release pattern of the drug at the site but may also change other temporal patterns of the drug (NATHANSON et al. 1983). For example, HUNT (1982) showed that the release of drugs from liposomes may mimic a slow input form of the drug; therefore, an intravenous bolus dose of the drug may not be the best control or, as stated by HUNT et al. (1986), "one cannot assign the entire observed improvement in therapeutic results to improved delivery of drug to targets by the carrier. Release of drug from the carrier before it reaches the target ('sustained release') may also contribute to the observed improvement and, in some cases, may account for all the improvement."

III. Testing Targeting Hypotheses Using Physiological Pharmacokinetic Models

A strength of the classical model approach to hypothesis testing is its simplicity. A major weakness is its inability to relate the findings or conclusions to targeting to a specific site.

1. Perfusion Models

Most pharmacokinetic based, hypothesis testing models for targeting have used physiological models or hybrid classical/physiological models rather than compartmental models. The advantage of these models is that the body can be viewed as being composed of the organs that actually make up the body and that these organs are interconnected by conduits, venous and arterial blood. The blood supply is what transports materials, nutrients, and exogenous materials to and from each organ. By considering the size or volume of each organ, blood flow to that organ in relation to cardiac output, drug binding to each organ, and the drug clearance or elimination potential at each organ, a rather sophisticated physiological view of drug absorption, distribution, metabolism, and elimination can be constructed. An incomplete physiological pharmacokinetic model of the body is shown in Fig. 4. This figure can be used to illustrate the point that drugs injected intravenously are initially

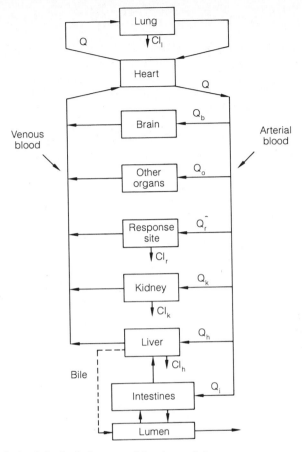

Fig. 4. Partial physiological pharmacokinetic model

carried to the heart, then to the lung, then to the heart again, and then distributed throughout the remainder of the body. So, for example, the heart and lung are unique compared to other organs in that they are "targeted" after intravenous administration rather than after intra-arterial administration.

Numerous physical and chemical means have been proposed to achieve drug targeting; however, the vast majority of these strategies have failed to live up to their proponents expectations. Why? For the most part, the hypotheses for achieving targeting fail to consider the complexity of systemic drug delivery. Already considered was the simple hypothesis for achieving drug targeting via intra-arterial drug administration into the artery supplying blood to the target site vs intravenous drug administration. This approach might be adequately termed as *passive* drug targeting. This example of a passive targeting technique is better simulated by a physiological model

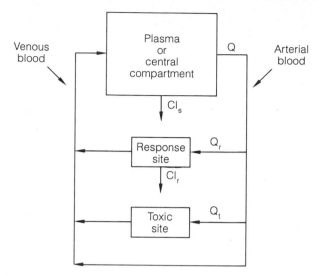

Fig. 5. Hybrid physiological pharmacokinetic model used to test targeting strategies

rather than a classical compartmental model (CHEN and GROSS 1980; OIE and HUANG 1981; SMITS and THIJSSEN 1986).

A reasonable model of this hypothesis is shown in Fig. 5. This hybrid physiological model assumes that the body is made up of a response or target compartment of volume V_r, a plasma or central compartment of volume V_p, and a toxic compartment of volume V_t. Drug is eliminated from the central compartment via a clearance Cl_s and from the target compartment via a clearance Cl_r. Clearance, having the units of flow or ml/min, represents that volume of blood carried to the organ which is cleared of drug per unit of time. Cardiac blood output is expressed as Q, blood flow to the target organ as Q_r, and to the toxic organ as Q_t. These flows also have the units of ml/min. Additionally, the assumption is made that each organ/compartment behaves as a well-mixed phase in which the drug concentration in the organ is proportional to the drug concentration in venous blood exiting the organ (this point will be expanded upon later).

If drug is now infused to steady state via intra-arterial administration into the arterial blood supplying the target site or via intravenous administration, the steady state concentration of drug entering the target organ from the two routes can be compared as per Fig. 1. As stated a priori, intra-arterial drug infusion would be expected to give superior levels of the drug in the target organ ($C_{R,ia}$) when compared to the levels obtained from intravenous drug administration, $C_{R,iv}$. The ratio $C_{R,SS,ia}/C_{R,SS,iv}$, or TA for equivalent intra-arterial and intravenous infusion rates at steady state, can be used as a measure of targeting. SMITS and THIJSSEN (1986), WEISS (1985) and CHEN and GROSS (1980) have shown that this ratio can be defined by Eq. 12. For this model, the DTI can be defined by Eq. 13:

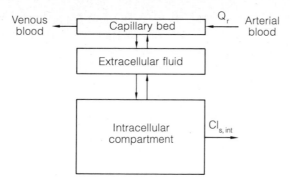

Fig. 6. Model showing that drug uptake to the intracellular space can be limited by barriers such as slow egress from the capillary bed or poor permeability across membranes separating the extracellular fluid and the intracellular compartment

$$\text{TA} = \frac{C_{\text{R,SS,ia}}}{C_{\text{R,SS,iv}}} = 1 + \frac{Cl_s}{Q_r} \tag{12}$$

$$\text{DTI} = \left(1 + \frac{Cl_s}{Q_r}\right)\left(\frac{1}{F_r}\right) = \left(1 + \frac{Cl_s}{Q_r}\right)\left(\frac{1}{1 - E_r}\right) \tag{13}$$

OIE and HUANG (1981), using a more comprehensive physiological model, developed a more general equation; however, the conclusions are essentially identical. That is, for intra-arterial administration to lead to targeting relative to intravenous drug administration, the systemic clearance of the drug must be large in relation to blood flow to the target organ. Conversely, if a drug is slowly cleared systemically and the target organ is well perfused (e.g., the liver and kidneys), there will be no significant advantage of intra-arterial drug administration over intravenous administration. As expected, these conclusion are identical to those drawn from the classical model approaches discussed earlier.

2. Trafficking and Cellular Uptake Limitations

The assumption that an organ can be considered a well-stirred tank has its limitations. Drug delivery to the target organ may not be perfusion-rate limited (ROWLAND and TOZER 1989). The mathematics of such a model can be very complex. Consider the partial model illustrated in Fig. 6. This model suggests that drug access to the intracellular space will be limited by either slow egress from the capillary bed or poor permeability across the membranes separating the extracellular fluid and the intracellular compartment.

Targeted drug delivery via particulate and macromolecular delivery systems to tumors is a good example of where passage across the endothelial cell layer (egress from the capillary bed) or basement membrane is rate limiting (WEINSTEIN et al. 1986; POZNANSKY and JULIANO 1984). BAXTER and JAIN (1989) and others have also shown that fluid transport or interstitial pressure and convection may play a very important role in determining the ability of both small and large molecules to penetrate a tumor mass. Additionally, the blood supply to a tumor mass is very heterogeneous (JAIN 1988), and a tumor, or any organ for that matter, cannot be adequately described by the simple models illustrated in Figs. 1–5.

3. Specific Examples of Models Used to Evaluate and Predict Targeting Strategies

Although drug targeting strategies have been tested experimentally in various animal models, limited efforts have been directed toward the development of mathematical models to test these strategies (STELLA and HIMMELSTEIN 1980, 1985a,b; HUNT et al. 1986; SMITS and THIJSSEN 1986; AARONS et al. 1989a,b). BAXTER and JAIN, (1989), WEINSTEIN et al. (1986), and others have developed models that attempt to explain the lack of targeting by monoclonal antibodies.

a) Model for Small Molecule Targeting via Prodrugs

STELLA and HIMMELSTEIN (1980) assessed the potential for achieving small molecule targeting via prodrugs. The initial study was followed by a number of refinements (STELLA and HIMMELSTEIN 1982, 1985a,b). The major limitations of these models were the lack of inclusion of a toxic compartment and the qualitative nature of the definition of targeting, although the 1982 paper did present their data in the form of TA, as defined by Eq. 6. Their model is presented in Fig. 7, where the body is viewed as being made up of two major compartments, the target organ and the remainder of the body. The target organ can be broken down into intra- and extracellular parts. STELLA and HIMMELSTEIN (1985a,b) assumed that access to the extracellular compartment was flow dependent but that uptake from the extracellular to the intracellular compartment need not be flow limited.

By definition, a prodrug is typically a pharmacologically inactive entity which is formed by chemical modification of the intrinsic drug molecule. The prodrug is activated (converted to the pharmacologically active parent compound) in vivo, as defined by the R terms in Fig. 7, through either enzymatically or nonenzymatically catalyzed reversion reactions. In this case drug input is from a bioreversion process rather than a physical input process.

Using this model, a number of targeting strategies were tested. The testing was limited to single bolus dose administration of drug vs prodrug using a limited number of conditions and only qualitative assessments of targeting were presented. The conclusions were drawn from relative AUCs and target site (defined as the intracellular compartment) concentration for drug input compared to prodrug input. As expected, strategies based purely on site-directed transport or site-directed bioreversion without consideration of the other parameter were shown to be shortsighted (STELLA and

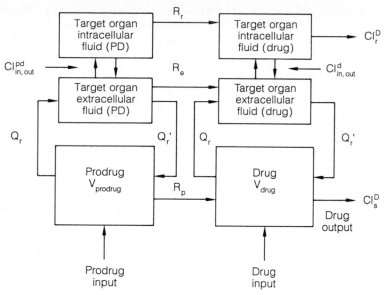

Fig. 7. Hybrid physiological pharmacokinetic model used by STELLA and HIMMELSTEIN (1985b) to test various prodrug based targeting strategies

HIMMELSTEIN 1980, 1985a,b). Novel in the findings, at that time, was the importance of the role of the properties of the parent drug to the ability to effect targeting. Like subsequent findings by HUNT et al. (1986) and LEVY (1987), site retention of the formed parent drug was critical. STELLA and HIMMELSTEIN (1985a,b) concluded that for targeting to be achieved via prodrug input, the following conditions must be met:

1. The prodrug must be readily transported to the site of action, the response compartment, and uptake at the site must be rapid, essentially perfusion-rate limited, or selective.
2. Once at the site, the prodrug must be selectively cleaved to the active drug (relative to its conversion at other sites); perhaps as important, it must be selectively cleaved at the site relative to more highly perfused tissues such as the kidneys or liver.
3. Once the active drug is generated it must be retained somewhat by the tissue.

   In short, an effective site-specific prodrug cannot be made of a parent drug which has good access to and rapid egress from the response compartment. That is, the parent drug will rapidly redistribute from the site of formation and only a minimal benefit from the prodrug input route can be expected. The findings of others, that the parent drug must also have a high systemic clearance, was not specifically recognized by STELLA and HIMMELSTEIN (1985a,b), although it was implicit in their simulations.

Interestingly, STELLA and HIMMELSTEIN (1985a,b) tested the hypothesis that targeting could be achieved via the following hypothesis: *A prodrug will be synthesized by coupling a small drug molecule to a macromolecular promoiety that will have an affinity for a cell surface determinant of a particular cell line. This prodrug, once bound to this cell surface, will be internalized via an endocytic mechanism and will be metabolized in a lysosome, thereby selectively delivering the active agent to that specific cell line.* Overall this hypothesis appears well-grounded and would seem to show promise as a targeting strategy. The idea does have some weaknesses: If the target site is in the extravascular bed, can the macromolecular-drug conjugate diffuse from the capillary vessels to its binding site? How will it fight the fluid transport or interstitial pressure as well as diffusion limitations (BAXTER and JAIN 1989) to reach all of the sites? Will the conjugate be taken up by the phagocytic cells of the reticuloendothelial system (RES) (POSTE and KIRSH 1983)? How quickly will the conjugate be metabolized systemically relative to uptake? If bound at the desired site and internalized, will lysosomal cleavage of the conjugate release the parent drug at the response site or will the drug be trapped or rapidly inactivated in the lysosome? If the drug can rapidly leave the lysosome, it may also rapidly leave the cell. Site retention of the drug then becomes a problem. Nevertheless, the simulation performed by STELLA and HIMMELSTEIN (1985a,b), which assumed that: (a) the conjugate was highly bound and accessible to the extracellular space, (b) the conjugate was internalized slowly but was selectively cleaved in the intracellular space, and (c) the formed drug had a slow egress from the intracellular space, showed that targeting was possible within the constraints placed on the system via this drug delivery technique.

b) Targeting Index Model

HUNT et al. (1986) presented a more sophisticated version of a targeting model and introduced the idea of TA and the DTI. Specifically, they introduced the important concept that not only must the optimal delivery to the response site be considered, but the possible differential delivery to toxic sites must also be recognized. A limitation of the HUNT et al. (1986) model simulations was the assumption of perfusion rate access to the target site, although this limitation was addressed qualitatively in their paper. The SMITS and THIJSSEN paper (1986) presents some useful simulations of possible applications of targeting strategies. However, their pessimism on the ability of prodrugs to effect targeting seems unwarranted. AARONS et al. (1989a,b), expanding on the work of others, examined the pharmacodynamic aspects of selective drug delivery. They concluded that the "pharmacokinetic and pharmacodynamic properties of the free drug are very important determining factors. Thus drugs with high systemic clearances which are targeted to sites of poor blood flow where the desired response is not saturated, are good candidates for targeting" and "poor selectivity cannot be easily com-

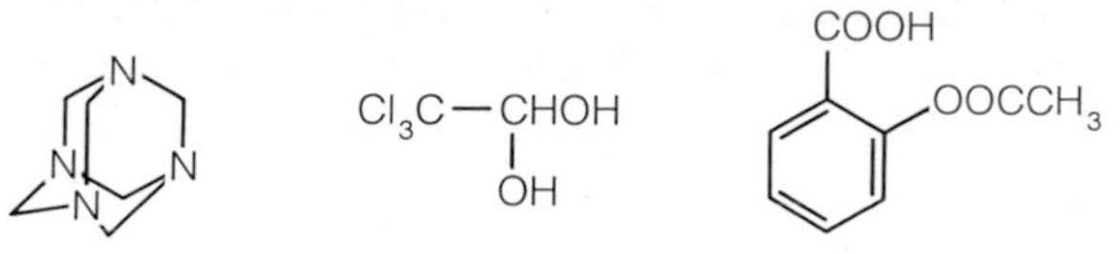

Fig. 8. Examples of early prodrugs: 1, methenamine; 2, chloral hydrate and; 3, aspirin (acetylsalicylic acid)

pensated for by adjustment of other characteristics of the drug-carrier system."

C. Prodrug-Mediated Targeted Drug Delivery

The preceding discussion of the use of pharmacokinetic modeling as a means of evaluating targeted drug delivery can, in general, be applied to any targeted drug delivery system since the equations generated above were dependent upon the concentration of the "free" drug and were independent of terms involving the specific targeting strategy. Obviously, the various delivery systems will each possess their own distinct advantages and disadvantages which will directly affect the delivery and release of the "free" drug at the target site. As a specific example of the pharmacokinetic principles mentioned previously, the ensuing discussion will deal with the merits and limitations of prodrug-mediated targeted drug delivery, which was briefly discussed in the preceding section.

I. Prodrugs in General

The prodrug or drug latentiation approach to drug delivery has been evolving over the last three decades, beginning with the work of ALBERT (1958) and HARPER (1959). Even though the concept is a relatively new one, actual examples of this drug delivery technique have been in therapeutic use for a considerably longer period of time. Methenamine, chloral hydrate, and aspirin are a few examples of prodrugs which were introduced in the nineteenth century (Fig. 8). As mentioned earlier, a prodrug is typically a pharmacologically inactive entity which is formed by chemical modification of the intrinsic drug molecule. The prodrug is activated (converted to the pharmacologically active parent compound) in vivo through either enzymatically or nonenzymatically catalyzed reversion reactions. The prodrug approach is illustrated in Fig. 9.

Through prodrug formation, improvements in the pharmaceutical and/or pharmacokinetic properties of a drug can be achieved, while the inherent pharmacologic properties of the drug remain intact. Some of the pharmaceu-

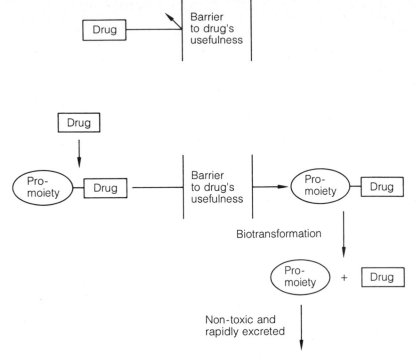

Fig. 9. Schematic representation of how prodrugs can be used to overcome various barriers to drug delivery

tical parameters which have been modified by the prodrug approach are stability, solubility, crystallinity, and taste. An especially attractive feature of the prodrug approach, when applied to physicochemical limitations, is that the associated properties can usually be altered in a predictable fashion by structurally modifying the promoiety in a predetermined way (e.g., by increasing the number of methylene units in the promoiety). This application of the prodrug approach is beyond the scope of this chapter, but it has been extensively reviewed elsewhere (SINKULA and YALKOWSKY 1975; STELLA 1975; BUNDGAARD 1985).

The prupose of this section is to discuss the potential of the use of prodrugs as a drug targeting strategy. The prodrug strategy constitutes an example of a chemically driven drug delivery system. Theoretically, as described earlier, the drug targeting concept is a simple one; however, in practice, the successful attainment of site-specific drug delivery is, at best, difficult due to the complex nature of the human body which possesses formidable barriers to drug delivery (e.g., metabolic pathways and lipoidal membranes). These barriers exist, in part, to prevent the absorption and distribution of xenobiotics.

A distinction will be made here between drug conjugates (small drug/macromolecular promoiety) and traditional prodrugs (small drug/small promoiety). In the drug conjugate case, the chemical, physical, and biological properties of the chemically modified drug entity are largely determined by the properties of the macromolecular promoiety; in the simple prodrug case, both moieties contribute to the final properties. The majority of the discussion here will focus on the ability of small drug/small promoiety prodrugs to affect targeting.

II. Site-Specific Drug Delivery via Prodrugs

Several considerations are essential to the design of prodrugs for targeting purposes: the properties of the drug, the properties of the prodrug, and the properties of the response or target compartment relative to nontarget sites. With this targeting technique, it is hoped that the prodrug will be able to preferentially deliver and release the "free" drug to the response site. Based on this reasoning, using prodrugs to alter a property such as the partition coefficient in order to enhance membrane permeability will typically lead to increased levels of drug throughout the body since it does not exploit any differences between the response and nontarget sites. There may be an increase in the therapeutic usefulness of the drug as a result of this modification; however, such an improvement does not constitute targeting.

As may be expected, the physicochemical properties of the prodrug required for optimal in vitro activity of the parent compound may not correspond to the physicochemical properties of the prodrug required for optimal in vivo delivery to the response site and for optimal formulatibility as the dosage form of interest. Consider the hypothesis: *I will achieve targeting by designing a prodrug that is a specific substrate for an enzyme that I know is present primarily at my response site. Since the prodrug will selectively regenerate the parent drug at this site, targeting will result.* Such a strategy has merit; however, it is more likely to be successful in in vitro studies than in in vivo experiments. A good example of discrepancies between the in vitro and in vivo data can be found with the peptidyl prodrugs of the anticancer compounds doxorubicin, acivicin, and phenylenediamine (CHAKRAVARTY et al. 1983a,b). It was hypothesized that the substantially elevated levels of plasminogen activators associated with many tumors (relative to normal cells) would generate higher levels of the proteolytic enzyme plasmin, which would bring about the selective activation of the peptidyl prodrugs (Fig. 10). In vitro, these prodrugs showed an improved selective activation and cytotoxicity, whereas in vivo these prodrugs failed to show any improved antitumor activity. At least two reasons can account for this failure: the peptidyl prodrugs may be too polar to reach the enzymes associated with the tumor site in therapeutically significant levels and/or a majority of the bioactivation of these prodrugs may be occurring at more highly perfused, nontarget sites possessing some protease activity, e.g., nonspecific liver esterases. This latter

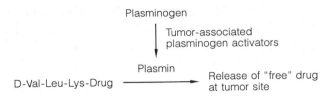

Fig. 10. Selective activation of peptide based prodrugs by plasmin triggered by tumorassociated plasminogen activators (CHAKRAVARTY et al. 1983a,b)

reason arises from the fact that an increased perfusion at nontarget sites, relative to the target site, will result in greater prodrug concentrations reaching these undersirable sites and that this may more than compensate for their potentially lower enzyme levels.

Targeted drug delivery via a delivery system can be divided into two broad classifications where the distinctions are not always clear-cut: *indirect* drug targeting and *direct* drug targeting. Useful discussions on the topic of selective drug delivery can be found in a number of earlier reviews that have been written on this subject (STELLA and HIMMELSTEIN 1980, 1982, 1985a,b; BUNDGAARD 1983).

1. Indirect Drug Targeting via Prodrugs

The majority of prodrugs which have been developed up to this point to circumvent biological constraints have attempted to achieve what might be called indirect drug targeting. This can be thought of as nonselective or improved systemic drug delivery; the drug (or prodrug) is not directed to the specific site of action but indirectly results in elevated drug delivery to the response compartment by enhancing systemic levels of the drug. This approach is consistent with traditional pharmacokinetic thinking. For example, one goal of this type of prodrug targeting is to increase the concentration of the parent drug in the systemic circulation with the belief that these elevated systemic levels will result in a proportional increase at the response site. A promoiety which modifies the limiting physicochemical properties of the drug may give rise to improvements in the pharmacokinetic and pharmacodynamic properties of the drug. Pharmacodynamically, one attempts to exploit the virtues of the Hill equation (Eq. 14) or similar models that relate concentrations of drug in the plasma and/or the response compartment to therapeutic benefits (WAGNER 1968):

$$R = \frac{R_m \, C^s}{(1/Q) + C^s} \tag{14}$$

or in a linearized form:

$$\log\left[\frac{R}{R_m - R}\right] = s \log C + \log Q \tag{15}$$

where R is the intensity of the pharmacological response due to the time dependent concentration, C, at the response site, R_m is the maximum intensity of the response, Q is a constant related to the receptor affinity for the drug, and s is a sensitivity factor. The Hill equation predicts a sigmoidal relationship between the concentration of the drug and the intensity of the pharmacological response, assuming that the drug reversibly interacts with the desired receptor. Therefore, based on this relationship, a simple increase in drug concentration in the response compartment will improve drug response. However, it may be difficult to argue that such an improvement represents targeting as defined earlier in this chapter.

Many approaches utilizing prodrugs to increase the plasma concentration of the drug have been attempted, including increasing membrane permeability and minimizing presystemic inactivation for orally administered drugs. Below are a few examples where these approaches have been used with varying degrees of success.

a) Increasing Gastrointestinal Membrane Permeability via Prodrugs

There are two major ways whereby gastrointestinal permeability can be improved via prodrugs: (1) improving passive transport of polar drugs by the synthesis of more lipophilic prodrugs and (2) designing prodrugs that utilize a specialized carrier-mediated pathway to facilitate the gastrointestinal absorption of drugs. The design of less polar prodrugs to improve passive gastrointestinal permeability has been adequately reviewed elsewhere (SINKULA and YALKOWSKY 1975; STELLA 1975; BUNDGAARD 1985) and will not be elaborated on here.

The use of carrier-mediated gastrointestinal absorption is worthy of discussion because it can be viewed as carrier-targeted delivery. An old

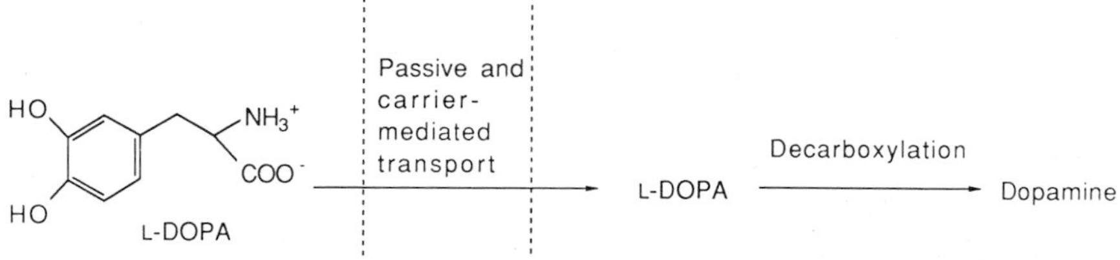

Fig. 11. Illustration of the delivery of dopamine to the brain via the prodrug, L-Dopa. L-Dopa is actively transported through the blood brain barrier via the aromatic L-amino acid transport system after which it is decarboxylated by Dopa decarboxylase

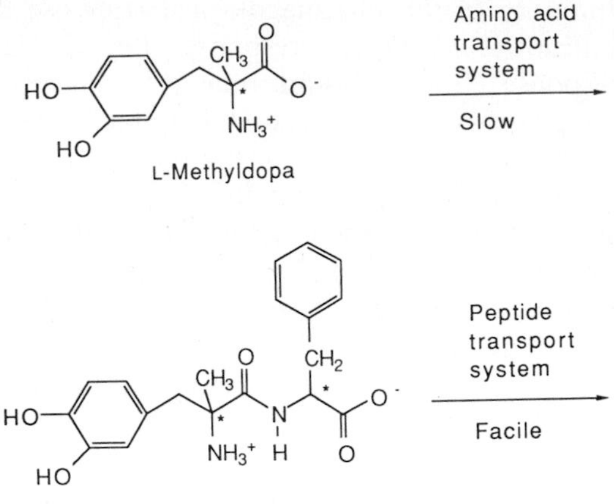

Fig. 12. L-Methyldopa and its prodrug, L-methyldopa-L-phenylalanine (Hu et al. 1989)

example of this approach is the use of L-dopa as a prodrug of dopamine. Dopamine is a very polar agent, useful in the treatment of shock and, if delivered to the brain, useful in the treatment of Parkinson's disease. L-Dopa as an L-aromatic amino acid is capable of being transported from the gastrointestinal tract by both a passive mechanism as well as by an active mechanism, the aromatic L-amino acid transport mechanism (Fig. 11). L-Dopa is transported into the brain by a similar carrier process (SHINDO et al. 1977). After reaching the systemic circulation, L-dopa can be decarboxylated to dopamine either peripherally or in the brain.

Hu et al. (1989) have used this same approach with the antihypertensive agent, L-α-methyldopa. Orally, this compound is poorly absorbed via an amino acid carrier system, i.e., it is a poorer substrate than L-dopa for the carrier process; therefore, dipeptidyl derivatives were synthesized to take advantage of the peptide carrier system (Fig. 12), which has been found to be more efficient and less structurally stringent than the amino acid carrier systems (ADIBI and KIM 1981). In situ intestinal studies revealed that these dipeptidyl prodrugs had significantly increased permeabilities relative to the parent compound. These derivatives also displayed good stability in acidified and nonacidified perfusate solutions; therefore, chemical reversion in the lumen apparently would not be a significant delivery constraint in vivo. It was suggested that the dipeptidyl derivatives may enhance the oral bioavailability of L-α-methyldopa.

Still another potential way of increasing diffusion through the gastrointestinal mucosa involves targeting enzyme systems, e.g., alkaline phosphatases and aminopeptidases associated with the brush border membrane of the intestines (AMIDON et al 1985) (Fig. 13). Oral administration of a polar

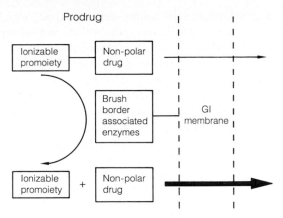

Fig. 13. A concerted metabolism/transport model proposed by AMIDON et al. (1985) for the gastrointestinal delivery of non-polar drugs via water soluble prodrugs cleaved by brush border associated enzymes

prodrug, possessing a promoiety labile to the brush border enzymes, should result in a larger percentage of the drug being released in close proximity to the lipid bilayer mucosal cell membranes. If the parent drug is relatively lipophilic it should rapidly permeate the lipoidal enterocyte membrane and enter the mucosal cell. The major advantage would be with drugs that are poorly water soluble and exhibit dissolution-rate limited bioavailability. The polar prodrug should rapidly dissolve in the milieu of the gastrointestinal tract and diffuse to the brush border area. Since the prodrug is a substrate for the brush border enzyme/s, the parent drug is released and absorbed in a concerted process. The real driving force is the increased water solubility of the prodrug relative to the parent drug; however, the specificity comes from the prodrug being a substrate for the brush border enzyme/s.

b) Minimizing Presystemic Drug Clearance via Prodrugs

The oral bioavailability of a drug can be compromised by its presystemic clearance in the gastrointestinal tract prior to absorption, in the mucosal cells during the transport from the lumen into the portal blood, or by the liver prior to reaching systemic circulation. Prodrug approaches to preventing presystemic metabolism have been dramatically unsuccessful.

One of the few reported successes has been with nalbuphine, which following oral administration undergoes extensive first-pass metabolism, including conjugation of the phenolic hydroxyl (Lo et al. 1984). Hence, the phenolic hydroxyl functionality was esterified with acetylsalicylic acid or anthranilic acid. Oral administration of these prodrugs in dogs resulted in significant increases in the bioavailability of nalbuphine (AUNGST et al. 1987). Along with these improved oral bioavailabilities, it was demonstrated that plasma levels of conjugated nalbuphine were reduced, which is consistent with a decrease in conjugative first-pass metabolism. Simlar results have been generated with oral prodrugs of other metabolically labile phenolic drugs, e.g., naltrexone and β-estradiol (HUSSAIN and SHEFTER 1988; HUSSAIN et al. 1988). The etiology of this improved delivery via the acetylsalicylate and anthranilate esters relative to the failures by other ester protecting groups has not been mechanistically addressed. It is interesting to speculate that these ester prodrugs are not substrates for esterases in the mucosal and liver cells but are substrates for deprotection at some other site within the body, since deprotection in the mucosal or liver cells should have lead to a sequential first-pass effect with ultimate conjugation of the phenolic hydroxyl.

c) Improved Endothelial Barrier Permeability

Assuming drug transport is mainly the result of non-carrier-mediated transport processes, poor permeation through biological membranes by highly polar compounds can usually be ascribed, in part, to low lipophilicity, which hinders the partitioning of the compound into the membrane of interest. For example, dopamine, administered intravenously, is unable to permeate the blood-brain barrier (BBB) in therapeutically significant quantities (Roos and STEG 1964); therefore, delivery approaches utilizing lipophilic prodrugs of dopamine have been tried. The monobenzoyl and dibenzoyl ester prodrugs of dopamine were synthesized in an attempt to improve the delivery of the parent drug, via these lipophilic prodrugs, to the brain (TEJANI-BUTT et al. 1988). A comparison of the n-octanol/phosphate buffer partition coefficients revealed that the monoester was approximately 300-fold more lipophilic and that the diester was about 20,000-fold more lipophilic than the parent compound. In addition, the monoester was found to be 28-fold more rapidly hydrolyzed than the diester at physiological pH. Following the intravenous administration of 8-^{14}C-radiolabelled esters in rats, the monobenzoyl ester was apparently unable to penetrate into the brain due to insufficient lipophilicity and/or premature bioreversion, whereas the dibenzoyl ester readily penetrated into the brain. Even though the dibenzoyl prodrug was able to reach to target site, it did not result in significant increases in the brain levels of dopamine or dihydroxyphenylacetic acid, one of its major metablites. This finding may be attributed to the prodrug having a clearance rate from the site that is more rapid than its conversion rate to the drug at the site. Similar results were obtained with the 3,4-diisobutyryl ester of the dopamine analogue N-methyldopamine, ibopamine. Following oral administration to rats, ibopamine was shown to have peripheral activity on the renal and cardiovascular systems comparable to that of intravenous dopamine (MIRAGOLI and FERRINI 1986). On the other hand, ibopamine was shown to have no significant CNS activity (MIRAGOLI et al. 1986).

These examples point out the limitations of the hypothesis: *I will achieve site directed delivery of my drug by designing a prodrug that more readily penetrates into the response compartment.* By itself, this hypothesis has some validity. It is, however, shortsighted in that, for site-directed delivery to be achieved, the prodrug must be capable of releasing the parent drug in the response compartment. L-Dopa, as an orally available form of dopamine, fits this criteria in that it more readily penetrates the (BBB) and brain dopa decarboxylase readily produces dopamine. However, in the treatment of Parkinson's disease, peripheral decarboxylation results in the production of nonbrain dopamine and side effects. This can be ameliorated by the concomitant administration of the peripheral dopa decarboxylase inhibitor, carbidopa, which is not capable of crossing the BBB. This combination product makes more dopamine available to the brain by utilizing the adequate gastrointestinal absorption and BBB transport qualities of L-dopa and by exploiting the selective brain metabolism of dopamine as a result of the peripheral inhibition of systemic decarboxylase.

d) Conclusions

Obviously, indirect drug targeting will lead to an increase in the intensity of the pharmacologic response and a potential decrease in the dose requirement. However, since the drug molecule is still freely accessible to the whole body following the systemic administration of the prodrug, the intensity of the toxic responses due to the parent molecule may also be increased. This prodrug targeting concept appears to be ideally suited for highly polar compounds that are to be administered locally at the site of interest as lipophilic prodrugs which rapidly generate the parent compound following penetration through the limiting barrier. An excellent example of this strategy is the *bis*-pivalate prodrug of epinephrine, dipivefrine, which is readily cleaved enzymatically in the eye (HUSSAIN and TRUELOVE 1976) and which was found to be much more therapeutically effective and much less cardiotoxic than epinephrine (MCCLURE 1975) (Fig. 14).

2. Direct Drug Targeting via Prodrugs

a) Pharmacokinetic Requirements

This is the area which holds the most promise from a drug delivery standpoint. Mechanistically, direct drug targeting can be achieved by combining two approaches: site-specific transport and site-specific activation. With site-specific transport, the drug can act everywhere in the body, but, as a result of the chemical modification, it is preferentially distributed to the site of action. With site-specific activation, the prodrug is widely distributed throughout the body but is preferentially activated at the site of action.

As discussed earlier, in addition to the properties of the prodrug, the pharmacokinetic behavior of the "free" drug can have a dramatic effect on its ability to be selectively delivered to the response or target site. The ideal drug

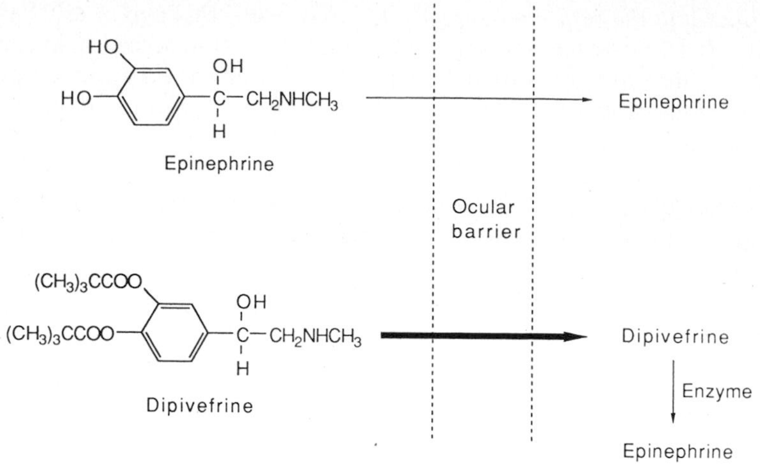

Fig. 14. Epinephrine and its prodrug, dipivefrine

cancidate for targeting is one that is poorly taken up and released by the
target site relative to non-target sites and that is rapidly eliminated from the
plasma compartment or non-target sites. That is, once released at the target
site by the targeting strategy, the "free" drug is retained, to a certain degree,
at this site since the therapeutic response is a function of the residence time of
the drug at the target site while being rapidly cleared from the rest of the
body. When a prodrug approach is used to achieve targeted drug delivery, the
pharmacokinetic behavior of the prodrug also becomes important. It has been
found previously (STELLA and HIMMELSTEIN 1980, 1982, 1985a,b; LEVY 1987)
that the prodrug must be rapidly and preferentially transported to and taken
up by the pharmacological site of action where it must be selectively activated
relative to its activation at non-target sites. It the prodrug is localized in the
target tissue and is not converted to the parent compound as readily as it
diffuses from the desired site, then the prodrug will probably result in a
pharmacologically inactive or poorly active molecule as was mentioned in the
case of the dibenzoyl ester prodrug of dompamine.

These pharmacokinetic arguments also explain why the majority of
currently marketed drugs will not achieve optimal targeting even as prodrugs.
Current pharmacological agents have been chosen because of their inherently
good transport characteristics; therefore, they are able to attain therapeutic
levels at the desired site as the unmodified compound. By chemically modifying these compounds in a bioreversible way, one can alter the properties of
various prodrug entities but not the intrinsic properties of the drug. Hence,
once the drug is regenerated at the site of action, its inherent transport
properties will result in a rapid efflux from and a short retention at the target
site.

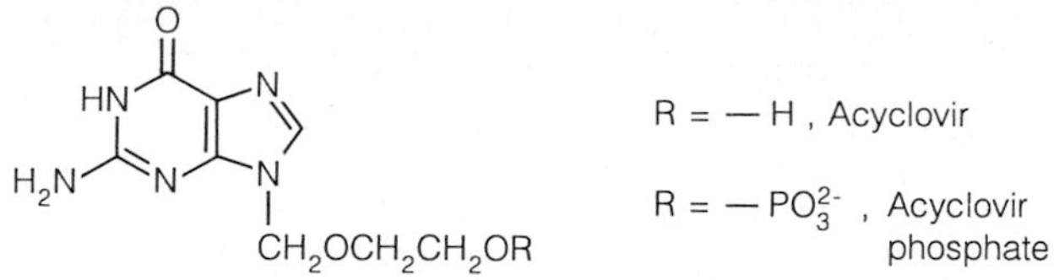

R = — H , Acyclovir

R = — PO_3^{2-} , Acyclovir phosphate

Fig. 15. Acyclovir is a prodrug of its various phosphate esters (especially the pharmacologically active triphosphate ester) that are formed in vivo in herpes infected cells

b) Targeting Viruses

One of the most successful examples of targeted drug delivery via a prodrug approach involves antiviral agents. Acyclovir, 9-(2-hydroxyethoxymethyl) guanine, displays a high therapeutic activity against herpesvirus, essentially no activity against adenovirus, minimal metabolic degradation following systemic administration, and a very low toxicity against uninfected host cells due to a site-specific activation mechanism of action (SCHAEFFER et al. 1987; ELION et al. 1977). Its remarkable selectivity is apparent when one considers the fact that a 3000-fold greater concentration of acyclovir is needed to inhibit uninfected cell multiplication when compared to the amount needed to inhibit virus multiplication. The herpesvirus encoded enzyme, pyrimidine deoxynucleoside (thymidine) kinase, is responsible for converting acyclovir to its phosphate monoester (Fig. 15). Subsequently, cellular enzymes catalyze the further conversion of the monophosphate to the di- and triphosphorylated species. This enzymatic conversion to the triphosphate occurs, to a greater extent, in the herpes infected cells. The pharmacologically active entity is the triphosphate, which functions as a chain terminator of growing viral DNA by inhibiting the herpes simplex virus DNA polymerase; cellular α-DNA polymerase is inhibited less effectively. Modifications in the acyclic side chain at position 9 of the guanine base lead to the synthesis of gancyclovir, 9-[[2-hydroxy-1 (hydroxymethyl) ethoxy] methyl] guanine which possesses the same selective mechanism of action as acyclovir (OGLIVIE et al. 1982). Recently, WINKELMANN et al. (1988) synthesized a large and diverse series of 9- and/or 6-substituted guanine derivatives. Several of their prodrugs displayed excellent in vivo activity against type I herpes simplex virus in mice. Note that the targeting comes not only from the selective activation, but also from site retention of the polar phosphorylated species.

c) Targeting the Colon

A good example of prodrugs which act selectively by a combination of targeting mechanisms, site-specific transport and site-specific activation, can be found in the work of FRIEND and CHANG (1984, 1985). As illustrated in Fig. 16, FRIEND and CHANG have developed orally administered colon-specific prodrugs by coupling a hydrophilizing promoiety, a glucose or a galactose

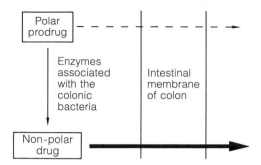

Fig. 16. Scheme proposed by FRIEND and CHANG (1984, 1985) for the selective delivery of steroids, via glycosidic prodrugs, to the colon for the treatment of lower inflammatory bowel disease

molecule, to steroids. As a result of the decreased permeability of the polar prodrugs, absorption in the small intestines is minimized, resulting in an increased concentration of the prodrug reaching the site of action, the colon. At this target site, bacterial glycosidases cleave the promoiety which releases the therapeutically active steroid. The more lipophilic parent compound can now be absorbed by the colonic mucosa and be potentially useful in the treatment of lower inflammatory bowel disease. Intragastric administration of two such steroid prodrugs, dexamethasone 21-β-D-glucoside and prednisolone 21-β-D-glucoside, in rats (FRIEND and CHANG 1985) reemphasizes the importance of the physicochemical properties of the parent compound in achieving selectivity. Even though the parent steroids are structurally similar and the promoieties are identical, about 60% of the administered does of the dexamethasone prodrug reached the cecum as compared to about 15% for the prednisolone prodrug. The properties of the parent steroid appear to determine the rate of pre-colonic hydrolysis by digestive enzymes associated with the upper intestine or the rate of precolonic hydrolysis catalyzed by acidic gastric media; both of these events will lead to premature intestinal absorption and loss of colon specificity. Also, administration of the unmodified steroids resulted in less than 1% of the dose reaching the cecum, stressing the importance of alterations in the physicochemical properties as a result of the promoiety.

An earlier example which exploits similar principles is the agent sulfsalazine (SCHRODER and CAMPBELL 1972; PEPPERCORN and GOLDMAN 1973). It is prepared by coupling diazotized 2-sulfanilamidopyridine with 5-aminosalicylic acid. Following oral administration, the unmodified sulfapyridine is readily absorbed form the small intestine, but as sulfasalazine, a large percentage of the modified drug passes into the colon intact via biliary excretion and nonabsorption in the small intestine. In the colon, sulfasalazine is cleaved to 2-sulfanilamidopyridine and 5-aminosalicylic acid by azoreductases associated with the bacterial microflora. The 5-aminosalicylic acid,

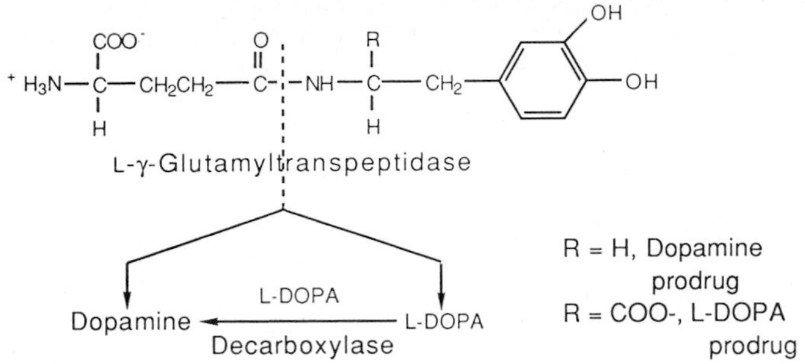

Fig. 17. Kidney selective delivery of dopamine can be achieved via the administration of L-γ-glutamyldopamine or L-γ-glutamyl-L-dopa

the active component (AZAD-KAHN et al. 1977), is now available for absorption at the site of action, while pre-colonic absorption of free sulfapyridine, which is responsible for many of the side effects, is reduced, Another potentially useful colon-specific prodrug of 5-aminosalicylic acid is azodisal (JEWEL and TRUELOVE 1981), which is formed by the diazo coupling of two 5-aminosalicylic acid molecules. This prodrug is more polar than sulfasalazine; therefore, it should be subjected to less pre-colonic absorption and possibly eliminate the side effects that may be caused by the 2-sulfanilamidopyridine. This area of targeting has recently been reviewed by RYDE (1988).

d) Targeting the Kidney

Site-specific delivery exploiting relatively high target site concentrations of an enzyme to activate the prodrug has also been achieved with delivery to the kidney. After intraperitoneal injection of γ-glutamyl L-3,4-dihydrophenylalanine (γ-glutamyl-L-dopa) to mice, dopamine (DA) selectively accumulated in the kidney via the sequential catalytic actions of two enzyme systems possessing high activity in the Kidney. First γ-glutamyl transpeptidase catalyzed the cleavage of the γ-glutamyl linkage. Then the resulting L-dopa was decarboxylated to DA by L-amino acid decarboxylase. Hence, DA was available to exert its therapeutic effect, renal vasodilation, at the target site while minimally affecting non-target sites as was demonstrated by no change in systemic blood pressure. The kidney concentration of DA was about five fold greater from the double prodrug, γ-glutamyl dopa, than from an equimolar dose of L-dopa; and administration of L-dopa resulted in a more uniform tissue distribution of DA (WILK et al. 1978). Furthermore, there is some kidney selectivity following the administration of N-acyl-γ-glutamyl prodrugs of sulfamethoxazole (WILK et al. 1980). Additionally, kidney selectivity has been achieved with L-γ-glutamyl DA, a single prodrug of DA, which requires only γ-glutamyl transpeptidase for its activation (KYNCL et al. 1979) (Fig. 17). This area of targeting has recently been reviewed by DRIEMAN (1989).

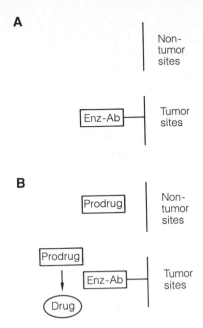

Fig. 18.A,B. Targeting unique enzymes to tumor sites in order to achieve site selective activation of prodrugs. **A** Antibody-enzyme conjugate binds to antigen-positive tumor sites. **B** The ensuing administration of the prodrug results in selective activation at the conjugate associated tumor sites relative to antigen-negative non-tumor sites. (SPRINGER et al. 1990)

e) Conclusions

As can be seen from the preceding examples, the sole use of a prodrug approach is limited unless the target site possesses a unique enzyme system, as in the case of acyclovir, or unless the target site is a highly perfused organ, as in the case of kidney-selective γ-glutamyl prodrugs of DA. Therefore, in order to optimize targeted drug delivery when the target site does not possess the above characteristics, more complex targeting approaches would appear to be the most effective way of achieving a high degree of targeting. Some of these approaches, which have been successfully exploited in the past, include the double prodrug approach (see Chap. 8); the concomitant administration of synergistic agents which compliment the prodrug approach, such as the use of L-dopa and carbidopa; the use of a prodrug in conjunction with a formulation technique, such as the coating of colon-targeted prodrugs with a pH-sensitive acrylic-based resin, Eudragit S (DEW et al. 1982); and the combination of individual targeting techniques to reap the beneficial properties of each.

In this latter category, a potentially exciting targeting approach, illustrated in Fig. 18, was recently utilized by SPRINGER et al. (1990). Since site-selective activation of prodrugs of anticancer compounds is limited because normal and diseased tissues do not exhibit sufficiently different metabolic properties, site-selective activation at the tumor site was engineered by targeting unique enzymes to the tumor sites. With this targeting system, a monoclonal antibody, which recognizes cell surface antigens preferentially expressed on the tumor, is conjugated to the unique bacterial enzyme carboxypeptidase G2. This antibody-enzyme conjugate is administered and given time to preferentially accumulate at the tumor site and to be cleared from the nontumor sites. This is followed by the administration of glutamic acid prodrugs of anticancer agents. The use of a unique enzyme should ensure that the prodrug is predominantly (or exclusively) activated at the tumor site relative to non-tumor sites. A similar technique was employed by SENTER et al. (1988). However, the major flaw associated with their system was that alkaline phosphatase was employed for the antibody-enzyme conjugate. Since alkaline phosphatase is a nonunique enzyme, activation of the phosphate monoester prodrug should occur at nontumor sites as well as at the antibody-enzyme conjugate associated tumor sites.

Finally, the findings of STELLA and HIMMELSTEIN and others, that the properties of the site, the reversion mechanism, and parent drug are critical to the targeting strategy, cannot be over emphasized. An appropriate recipe, therefore, for developing a drug targeting strategy might be:

1. Identify diseased states with well-delineated etiologies such as aberant receptors or biochemical pathways.
2. Confirm that the site of the aberration is well-defined and isolated to a single organ or cell line with clearly defined anatomical boundaries.
3. Identify any unique cell surface, membrane transporting, and metabolic properties that can be used to help effect targeting.
4. Choose a candidiate drug or agent that is known to be effective at the receptor level (receptor being broadly defined) but, because of physical/chemical properties and not other shortcomings, is poorly able to reach the receptor after in vivo administration. It is unlikely that most currently useful therapeutic agents would fit this description unless it had been established that the performance of the agent is less than ideal because it is unable to efficiently reach its site of action.
5. The drug proposed as a targeting candidate must have a "handle" in its stucture that will permit the synthesis of a derivative (prodrug) with the physical/chemical/biochemical characteristics that will allow the prodrug to reach its targeting site and, there, efficiently release the parent drug with its retentive properties.

It is at this point that we should keep in mind the comment by ALBERT (1965) that "although a detailed knowledge of permeability and enzymes can assist a designer in finding pro-agents . . . he will have in mind an organism's normal reaction to a foreign substance is to burn it up for food."

References

Aarons L, Boddy A, Petrak K (1989a) Efficiency of drug targeting: steady-state considerations using a three-compartment model. Pharm Res 6:367–372

Aarons L, Boddy A, Petrak K (1989b) Pharmacokinetic evaluation of site-specific drug delivery. In: Prescott LF, Nimmo WS (eds) Novel drug delivery. Wiley, New York

Adibi SA, Kim YS (1981) Peptide absorption and hydrolysis. In: Johnson LR (ed) Physiology of the gastrointestinal tract. Raven, New York, p 1073

Albert A (1958) Chemical aspects of selective toxicity. Nature 182:421–423

Albert A (1965) Selective toxicity, 3rd edn. Wiley, New York

Amidon GL, Fleisher D, Stewart B (1985) Design of prodrugs for improved gastro-intestinal absorption by intestinal enzyme targeting. In: Widder KJ, Green R (eds) Drug and enzyme targeting. Academic, New York, p. 360

Aungst BJ, Myers MJ, Shefter E, Shami EG (1987) Prodrugs for improved oral nalbuphine bioavailability: inter-species differences in the disposition of nal-buphine and its acetylsalicylate and anthranilate esters. Int J Pharm 38:199–209

Azad-Kahn AK, Piris J, Truelove SC (1977) An experiment to determine the active therapeutic moiety of sulphasalazine. Lancet 2:892–895

Baxter LT, Jain RK (1989) Transport of fluid and macromolecules in tumors. I. Role of interstitial pressure and convection. Microvasc Res 37:77–104

Benet L, Galeazzi R (1979) Non-compartmental determination of the steady-state volume of distribution. J Pharm Sci 68:1071–1074

Bundgaard H (1983) Drug targeting: prodrugs. In: Briemer DD, Speiser P (eds) Topics in pharmaceutical sciences. Elsevier, New York, pp 329–343

Bundgaard H (1985) Design of prodrugs. Elsevier, New York

Chakravarty PK, Carl PL, Weber MJ, Katzenellenbogen JA (1983a) Plasmin-activated prodrugs for cancer chemotherapy. II. Synthesis and biological activity of peptidyl derivatives of doxorubicin. J Med Chem 26:638–644

Chakravarty PK, Carl PL, Weber MJ, Katzenellenbogen JA (1983b) Plasmin-activated prodrugs for cancer chemotherapy. I. Synthesis and biological activity of pepti-dylacivicin and peptidylphenylenediamine. J Med Chem 26:633–638

Chen HSG, Gross JF (1980) Intra-arterial infusion of anti-cancer drugs — theoretic aspects of drug delivery and review of responses. Cancer Treat Rep 64:31–40

Dew MJ, Hughes PJ, Lee MG, Evans BK, Rhodes J (1982) An oral preparation to release drugs in the human colon. Br J Clin Pharmacol 14:405–408

DiStefano JJ (1982) Non-compartmental versus compartmental analysis: some basis for choice. Am J Physiol 243:R1–R6

Drieman JC (1989) Drug targeting to the kidney; N-acetyl-G-gutamyl derivatives as kidney-selective prodrugs. CIP-Gegevens Koninklijke Bibliotheek, Den Haag

Elion GB, Furman PA, Fyfe JA, de Miranda P, Beauchamp L, Schaeffer HJ (1977) Selectivity of action of an antiherpetic agent, 9-(2-hydroxyethoxymethyl) guanine. Proc Natl Acad Sci USA 74:5716–5720

Friend DR, Chang GW (1984) A colon-specific drug-delivery system based on drug glycosides and the glycosidases of colonic bacteria. J Med Chem 27:261–266

Friend DR, Chang GW (1985) Drug glycosides: potential prodrugs for colon-specific drug delivery. J Med Chem 28:51–57

Friend DR, Pangburn S (1987) Site-specific drug delivery. Med Res Rev 7:53–106

Harper NJ (1959) Drug latentiation. J Med Pharm Chem 1:467–500

Himmelstein KJ, Lutz RJ (1979) A review of the applications of physiologically based pharmacokinetic modeling. J Pharmacokinet Biopharm 7:127–145

Hu M, Subramanian P, Mosberg HI, Amidon GL (1989) Use of the peptide carrier system to improve the intestinal absorption of L-α-methyldopa: carrier kinetics, intestinal permeabilities, and in vitro hydrolysis of dipeptidyl derivatives of L-α-methyldopa. Pharm Res 6:66–70

Hunt CA (1982) Liposomes disposition in vivo. V. Liposome stability in plasma and implications for drug carrier function. Biochim Biophys Acta 719:450–463

Hunt CA, MacGregor RD, Siegel RA (1986) Engineering targeted in vivo drug delivery. I. The physiological and physicochemical primciples governing opportunities and limitations. Pharm Res 3:333–344

Hussain MA, Shefter E (1988) Naltrexone-3-salicylate (a prodrug of naltrexone): synthesis and pharmacokinetics in dogs. Pharm Res 5:113–115

Hussain A, Truelove JE (1976) Prodrug approaches to enhancement of physicochemical properties of drugs. IV. Novel epinephrine prodrug. J Pharm Sci 65:1510–1512

Hussain MA, Aungst BJ, Shefter E (1988) Prodrugs for improved oral β-estradiol bioavailability. Pharm Res 5:44–47

Jain RK (1988) Determinants of tumor blood flow: a review. Cancer Res 48:2641–2658

Jain RK, Gerlowski LE (1983) Physiologically based pharmacokinetic modeling: principles and applications. J Pharm Sci 72:1103–1127

Jewel DP, Truelove SC (1981) Disodium azodisalicylate in ulcerative colitis. Lancet 2:1168–1169

Kyncl JJ, Minard FN, Jones PH (1979) L-γ-glutamyl dopamine, an oral dopamine prodrug with renal selectivity. In: Imbs JL, Schwartz J (eds) Peripheral dopaminergic receptors. Permagon, New York, p 369

Levy G (1987) Targeted drug delivery – some pharmacokinetic considerations. Pharm Res 4:3–4

Lo MW, Juergens GP, Whitney CC (1984) Determination of nalbuphine in human plasma by automated high-performance liquid chromatography with electrochemical detection. Res Commun Chem Pathol Pharmacol 43:159–168

McClure DA (1975) The effect of a prodrug of epinephrine (dipivalyl epinephrine) in glaucoma – general pharmacology, toxicology, and clinical experience. In: Higuchi T, Stella V (eds) Prodrugs as novel drug delivery systems. American Chemical Society, Washington, p 224

Miragoli G, Ferrini R (1986) Effect of ibopamine on diuresis in conscious rats in normal and experimentally altered conditions. Arzneimittelforschung 36(1): 318–322

Miragoli G, Ferrini R, Sala R, Reggiani A (1986) Activity of ibopamine on central nervous system in mice and rats. Arzneimittelforschung 36(1):327–333

Nathanson MH, Hillman RS, Georgakis C (1983) Towards an optimal drug-delivery regimen for methotrexate chemotherapy. Appl Math Comput 12:99–117

Notari RE (1981) Prodrug design. Pharmacol Ther 14:25–53

Ogilvie KK, Cheriyan UO, Radatus BK, Smith KO, Galloway KS, Kennell WL (1982) Biologically active acyclonucleoside analogues. II. The synthesis of 9–[[2-hydroxy-1-(hydroxymethyl) ethoxy]methyl] guanine (BIOLF-62). Can J Chem 60:3005–3010

Oie S, Huang JD (1981) Influence of administration route on drug delivery to a target organ. J Pharm Sci 70:1344–1347

Peck CC, Rodman JH (1986) Analysis of clinical pharmacokinetic data for individualizing dru dosage regiments. In: Evans WE, Scheritag JJ, Jusko WJ (eds) Applied pharmacokinetics: principles of therapeutic drug monitoring, 2nd edn. Applied Therapeutics, Spokane

Peppercorn MA, Goldman P (1973) Distribution studies of salicylazopyridine and its metabolites. Gastroenterology 64:240–245

Poste G, Kirsh R (1983) Site specific drug delivery in cancer therapy. Biotechnology 1:869–878

Poznansky MJ, Juliano RL (1984) Biological approaches to the controlled delivery of drugs: a critical review. Pharmacol Rev 36:277–334

Roos BE, Steg G (1964) The effect of L-3,4-dihydroxyphenylalanine and DL-5-hydroxytryptophan on rigidity and tremor induced by reserpine, chlorpromazine and phenoxybenzamine. Life Sci 3:351–360

Rowland M, Tozer TN (1989) Clinical pharmacokinetics: concepts and applications, 2nd edn. Lea and Febingter, Philadelphia

Ryde EM (1988) Pharmacokinetic aspects of drugs targeted for the colon, with special reference to olsalazine. Acta Univ Up 39

Sadee W (1985) Molecular mechanism of drug action and pharmacokinetic-pharmacodynamic models. In: Borchardt RT, Repta AJ, Stella VJ (eds) Directed drug delivery: a multidisciplinary approach. Humana, Clifton, p 35

Schaeffer HJ, Beauchamp L, deMiranda P, Elion GB, Bauer DJ, Collins P (1978) 9-(2-Hydroxyethoxymethyl) guanine activity against viruses of the herpes group. Nature 272:583–585

Schroder H, Campbell DES (1972) Absorption, metabolism, and excretion of salicylazosulfapyridine in man. Clin Pharmacol Ther 13:539–551

Senter PD, Saulnier MG, Schreiber GJ, Hirschberg DL, Brown JP, Hellstrom I, Hellstrom KE (1988) Anti-tumor effects of antibody-alkaline phosphatase conjugates in combination with etoposide phosphate. Proc Natl Acad Sci USA 85:4842–4846

Shindo H, Komai T, Kawai K (1977) Mechanism of intestinal absorption and brain uptake of L-5-hydroxytryptophan in rats, as compared to those of L-3,4-dihydroxyphenylalanine. Chem Pharm Bull (Tokyo) 25:1417–1425

Sinkula AA, Yalkowsky SH (1975) Rationale for the design of biologically reversible drug derivatives: prodrugs. J Pharm Sci 64:181–210

Smits JFM, Thijssen HHW (1986) Spatial control of drug action: theoretical considerations on the pharmacokinetics of target-aimed drug delivery. In: Struyker-Boudier HAJ (ed) Rate-controlled drug administration and action. CRC, Boca Raton, p 83

Springer CJ, Antoniw P, Bagshawe KD, Searle F, Bisset GMF, Jarman M (1990) Novel prodrugs which are activated to cytotoxic alkylating agents by carboxypeptidase G2. J Med Chem 33:677–681

Stella VJ (1975) Prodrugs: an overview and definition. In: Higuchi T, Stella VJ (eds) Prodrugs as novel drug delivery systems. American Chemical Society, Washington, p 1

Stella VJ (1989) Prodrugs and site-specific drug delivery. In: Kato R, Eastabrook RW, Cayen MN (eds) Xenobiotic metabolism and disposition. Taylor and Francis, London, p 109

Stella VJ, Himmelstein KJ (1980) Prodrugs and site-specific drug delivery. J Med Chem 23:1275–1282

Stella VJ, Himmelstein KJ (1982) Critique of prodrugs and site-specific drug delivery. In: Bundgaard H, Hansen AB, Kofod H (eds) Optimization of drug delivery. Munksgaard, Copenhagen, p 134

Stella VJ, Himmelstein KJ (1985a) Site-specific drug delivery prodrugs. In: Bundgaard H (ed) Design of prodrugs. Elsevier, New York, p 177

Stella VJ, Himmelstein KJ (1985b) Prodrugs: a chemical approach to targeted drug delivery. In: Borchardt RT, Repta AJ, Stella VJ (eds) Directed drug delivery: a multidisciplinary approach. Humana, Clifton, p 247

Tejani-Butt SM, Hauptmann M, D'Mello A, Frazer A, Marcoccia JM, Brunswick DJ (1988) Evaluation of mono- and dibenzoyl esters of dopamine as potential prodrugs for dopamine in the central nervous system. Arch Pharmacol 338:497–503

Wagner JG (1968) Kinetics of pharmacologic response. J Theor Biol 20:173–201

Wagner JG (1981) History of pharmacokinetics. Pharmacol Ther 12:537–562

Weinstein JN, Black CDV, Barbet J, Eger RR, Parker RJ, Holton OD, Mulshine JL, Keenan AM, Larson SM, Sieber SM, Covell DG (1986) Selected issues in the pharmacology of monoclonal antibodies. In: Tomlinson E, Davis SS (eds) Site-specific drug delivery. Wiley, New York, chap 5

Weiss M (1985) On pharmacokinetics in target tissues. Biopharm Drug Dispos 6:57–66

Wilk S, Mizoguchi H, Orlowski M (1978) γ-Glutamyl dopa: a kidney specific dopamine precursor. J Pharmacol Exp Ther 206:227–232

Wilk S, Mizoguchi H, Orlowski M (1980) N-acly-γ-glutamyl derivatives of sulfa-methoxazole as models of kidney-selective prodrugs. J Pharmacol Exp Ther 212:167–172

Winkelmann E, Winkler I, Rolly H, Rosner M, Jahne G (1988) New prodrugs of acyclic nucleosides with antiviral activity. Arzneimittelforschung 38(2): 1545–1548

CHAPTER 5

Soluble Polymers as Targetable Drug Carriers*

N.L. Krinick and J. Kopeček[1]

A. Introduction

The efficiency of drugs would increase considerably if we were able to direct them selectively to their cellular targets. The need for targetable drug carriers was realized a long time ago. It was P. Ehrlich, in 1906, who coined the phrase "the magic bullet" describing drugs which might be selectively directed to their specific site of action. But it is only in the last 20 years that natural science has developed to such a level that several laboratories have started to try to translate this dream to reality.

It was Ringsdorf (1975) who described a new theoretical model for the development of synthetic polymers which could serve as targetable drug carriers. The consequence of attachment of low molecular weight drugs to macromolecular carriers alters their rate of excretion from the body, changes their toxicity and immunogenicity, and limits their uptake by cells via endocytosis, thus providing the opportunity to direct the drug to the particular cell type where its activity is needed.

This chapter concentrates on the rationale of using water soluble macromolecules as targetable lysosomotropic drug carriers. Rational design of lysosomotropic macromolecular drug carriers must take into account biological processes which take place when these drugs are administered into the living organism. The main objective, however, is to deliver the polymer bound drug to the particular cell type where its action is desirable. To achieve this a suitable targeting moiety-receptor (antigen) system must be known and the former has to be attached to the carrier. The polymer bound drug may interact with the cellular membrane or act intracellularly. However, there are intrinsic difficulties in targeting membrane-directed drugs. This review is therefore mainly concerned with polymeric carriers directing drugs which normally act via an intracellular site.

The bond between the drug and the carrier must be stable in the bloodstream and in the interstitial space. Upon arrival in the lysosomal compartment of the target cell the drug must be either released from the carrier by lysosomal enzymes or activated by other means, for instance by

* The support of NIH (grant DK 39544) is gratefully acknowledged.
[1] To whom correspondence should be addressed.

irradiation. The carrier itself should be totally digested in the lysosomal compartment. If a nondegradable carrier is used, its whole molecular weight distribution (MWD) must be under the renal threshold. In this case, however, not only the MWD but also the chemical structure of the carrier is of utmost importance. Its structure should be designed in such a way that, after being released from the dead cell into the bloodstream, it should be taken up by nontarget cells by fluid phase pinocytosis which is a slow process indeed. Only in this case can the capture (by receptor-mediated pinocytosis) -recapture (by adsorptive pinocytosis) cycle be broken and the carrier eliminated from the body.

All these questions will be discussed in the following sections. The interaction of water soluble macromolecules with the living organism is discussed on the cellular and subcellular levels. Factors which are important to the rational design of macromolecular carriers are described and examples of conjugates suitable to combat diseases (with the emphasis on cancer) are discussed.

B. Consequences of Drug Binding to Macromolecular Carriers: Cellular Level

Binding low MW drugs to macromolecular carriers restricts their access to the cell interior by the uptake process known as endocytosis. Endocytosis encompasses two processes: phagocytosis and pinocytosis (Table 1). In both cases, a macromolecule associates at a site on the cell surface and the membrane invaginates and pinches off inside of the cell forming an intracellular vesicle containing the macromolecule. Phagocytosis represents the process by which large particulate material enters the cell and is usually carried out by specialized phagocytic cells. Pinocytosis, on the other hand, is carried out virtually by all cells in which the cell takes in liquid or liquid containing solutes from the extracellular space.

I. Pinocytosis

There are basically three forms of pinocytosis: fluid phase, adsorptive, and receptor-mediated. The basic difference between fluid phase and adsorptive pinocytosis is found in Fig. 1. Fluid phase pinocytosis is the most general form in which soluble macromolecules and solutes enter the cell in liquid droplets. Many, if not all, nucleated cells use fluid phase pinocytosis to internalize material from the extracellular space. It is known as a "constitutive" process because it is continuous (as opposed to triggered as is phagocytosis); thus the cell is always ingesting pieces of its plasma membrane. Pinocytic vesicles are on the average of $0.1-0.3\,\mu m$, and in a typical cultured cell more than 100 are internalized per minute (TARTAKOFF 1987).

Table 1. Characteristics of pinocytosis and phagocytosis. (From LLOYD 1985)

	Pinocytosis	Phagocytosis
Substrate	Liquid (and contained solutes)	Microparticulate material
Occurrence in animal cells	In almost at cells	"Professional" phagocytes only
Stimulus required	No, constitutive phenomenon	Triggered by particle adherence
Liquid uptake	Yes	No

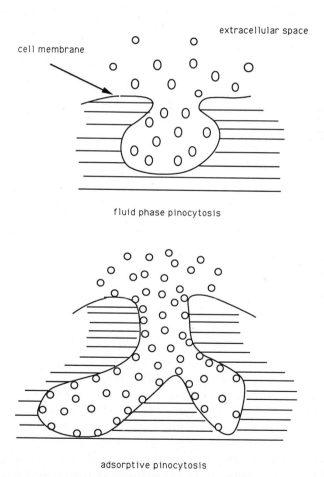

Fig. 1. Fluid phase pinocytosis vs adsorptive pinocytosis. Macromolecules are internalized by fluid phase pinocytosis as the cell "drinks" the macromolecules in the fluid surrounding the cell. On the other hand, macromolecules nonspecifically adsorb to the cell membrane in adsorptive pinocytosis

Adsorptive pinocytosis is also a relatively indiscriminate process. However, in this case a macromolecule may physically adsorb (nonspecifically) to a site on the cell membrane and then by the invagination process be taken in by the cell.

Receptor-mediated pinocytosis is by far the most specific form of pinocytosis. A macromolecule with a marker complementary to a cell surface receptor binds to that receptor and is subsequently internalized. In this way, macromolecules such as hormones, transport proteins, proteins modified for degradation, growth factors, and some antibodies are taken in by cells from the extracellular fluid. The advantage of receptor-mediated pinocytosis lies in the fact that a higher concentration of ligand may be internalized in specific cells than by the other mechanisms.

Once internalized by pinocytosis, the ultimate fate of a solute is delivery to secondary lysosomes (DE DUVE et al. 1974) where it can be degraded and distributed by the cell in various ways. Naturally, since during the process of fluid phase pinocytosis there is indiscriminate uptake of cell surface markers, the cell is equipped with the machinery to recycle essential lipids and proteins back to the cell membrane.

1. Receptor-Mediated Endocytosis

Receptor-mediated endocytosis especially receptor-mediated pinocytosis (Fig. 2), will principally be discussed, as it is the process of the cell to be exploited in drug delivery. Many macromolecules are internalized by the cell, e.g., metabolic ligands (transferrin; transcobalamin; vitellogenin; low density lipoprotein, LDL) opportunistic ligands (protein toxins, virus), growth factors (epidermal growth factor, EGF; luteinizing hormone, LH; platelet-derived growth factor, PDGF), insulin, lysosomal hydrolases, immunoglobulins, asialoglycoproteins, and α-macroglobulins (TARTAKOFF 1987). Depending upon the needs of the cell, these ligands have different fates. Although more than 50 ligands have been found to access cells by receptor-mediated endocytosis and at least 15 of the responsible receptors have been isolated, many questions regarding receptor-mediated endocytosis as well as receptor sorting and recycling remain. SHEPHERD (1989) discusses current knowledge and questions that need to be addressed which are associated with receptor-mediated endocytosis.

Some receptors are located randomly on the cell membrane while others reside in coated pits (PASTAN and WILLINGHAN 1985). The coated pit is the site at which receptor-ligand complexes first locate before entering the cell. They are so named because of their morphology; they are pits coated with the protein clathrin on the cytoplasmic side of the plasma membrane. Some receptors, such as the transferrin, LDL, asialoglycoprotein, α₂-macroglobulin, and other receptors, associate in the coated pit even when unliganded. Others such as the EGF receptor demonstrate mobility by moving into coated pits once their ligands are bound (WILLINGHAM and PASTAN 1982). This is referred

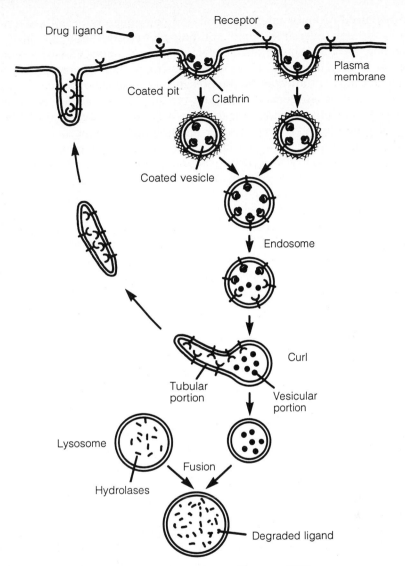

Fig. 2. Receptor-mediated pinocytosis. (From SINKULA 1987)

to as patching. It is believed that the individual steps leading to the clustering of EGF receptors in coated pits are: After a ligand binds to the EGF receptor, the protein-tyrosine kinase (inherent to the EGF receptor) is activated and the receptor is autophosphorylated. The receptors dimerize and quickly cluster by lateral movement. GLENNEY et al. (1988) studied the importance of protein-tyrosine kinase activity of EGF receptors on ligand-induced endo-cytosis. Protein-tyrosine kinase deficient EGF receptors prevented normal ligand-induced receptor internalization and consequently receptor degradation. In addition, microinjection of anti-phosphotyrosine antibodies into cells containing EGF receptors having protein kinase activity also precluded ligand-induced endocytosis. However, it was found that the receptor dimerization step was not affected by the presence or absence of protein-tyrosine kinase. Therefore, it seems that protein-tyrosine kinase activity is the main factor controlling ligand-induced endocytosis of the EGF receptor and that a phosphorylated ligand is necessary for ligand-induced endocytosis.

Many different ligands enter cells in the same coated pits, suggesting a common route of entry for receptor bound ligands (HANOVER et al. 1985). However, the specific mechanism of clustering of receptors and receptor-ligand complexes in coated pits is controversial. It is possible that ligand binding may allosterically change the conformation of the receptor in the coated pit entrapping the complex. The receptors found in coated pits may also be there as a result of recognition of their conformation by the pit (PASTAN and WILLINGHAM 1983). Another theory stems from the fact that the plasma membrane is continually under "flux" conditions in which proteins and lipids are internalized. It is thought that a "sink" mechanism ensues because the flux pattern begins at the points on the cell surface where new vesicles are delivered. The coated pit can then mediate the entry of many different kinds of receptors, complexed with a ligand or free (TARTAKOFF 1987).

Inhibition of coated pit function is a beneficial means of studying clathrin coat function. Depletion of intracellular K^+, cytoplasm acidification, and exposing cells to hypertonic media inhibits clathrin-coated pit function. It appears that both K^+ depletion and hypertonic media cause clathrin aberrant polymerization which prevents normal pit formation and hence endocytosis, however, by an unknown mechanism. Hypertonic media causes a quick dispersion of LDL receptors on fibroblasts (chick or human) which is reversible upon return to normal medium (FEUSER and ANDERSON 1989).

The cytoplasmic domain determines the selective concentration of receptors in coated pits. This was verified for the transferrin receptor by IACOPETTA et al. (1988) by comparing wild-type and cytoplasmic deletion mutant human transferrin receptors with coated pits at the surface of transfected L cell lines. They also obtained evidence that the cytoplasmic domain initiates clathrin coat assembly and offered a receptor induction model for transferrin receptor sorting.

The clathrin coat is actually an extremely complex structure. Detailed investigations of clathrin coat morphology are available in the literature (TARTAKOFF 1987; HEUSER and KIRCHHAUSEN 1985). Most investigators believe that the clathrin-coated pits pinch off and form clathrin-coated vesicles intracellularly. It is thought that intracellular protein assemblies or adaptors control the formation of clathrin-coated vesicles. These adaptors are located between the clathrin coat and the cell membrane and have many purposes: recognizing receptor tails, aiding in polymerization of clathrin, and deciding the location for this to take place. By use of adaptor specific monoclonal antibodies, CHIN et al. (1989) have shown that α 100 kDa polypeptides are directly connected with clathrin-coated vesicle assembly.

It is known that the vesicles soon shed their clathrin coating. The clathrin and associated proteins can then ultimately assemble to form new coated pits at the plasma membrane (MOORE et al. 1987). Clathrin can thereby mediate the uptake of receptor-ligand complexes by concentrating receptors (BRODSKY 1988) and efficiently transporting them to receptosomes. Receptosomes are defined as the uncoated vesicles which fuse with the endocytic vesicle derived from the clathrin-coated pit. Another theory suggests that the receptosome is formed directly from coated pits and that the coated pits are stable and always associated at the cell surface (PASTAN and WILLINGHAM 1983).

Nevertheless, after the pits pinch off, whether coated or uncoated, within about 1 min of internalization vesicles do not have a coat. The uncoating could be a result of a local change in pH or possibly an uncoating ATPase. There is also no agreement as to whether pinocytic vesicles have clathrin coats as do coated pits in receptor-mediated endocytosis.

II. Endosomes

Endosome is the more general term for receptosome. Endosomes are variable in a given cell and also vary between cell types. This renders their isolation difficult. Various methods of endosome isolation have been addressed (WILEMAN et al. 1985; COURTOY et al. 1984). Endosomal membranes were found to contain high cholesterol/phospholipid ratios and a different protein pattern than plasma or lysosomal membranes. They also contain receptors for both transferrin and mannose-6-phosphate. Endosomes have been reported as vesicles, tubular structures, trans-Golgi reticulum, and multivesicular bodies (TARTAKOFF 1987). Initially, they are small vesicles which can fuse with other endosomes creating larger endosomes (PASTAN and WILLINGHAM 1985). DIAZ et al. (1989) have determined that the N-ethylmaleimide-sensitive factor is required for early endocytic fusion. The main role of the endosome is to transport internalized material through the cell interior, ultimately to another intracellular vesicle, the lysosome.
A brief chronology of endosomal events follows:

1. During the first 2 min of cell entry, ligands leave coated vesicles and enter peripheral endosomes; the ligand remains bound to the receptor.
2. In the next 8–10 min there is intraluminal acidification and receptor-ligand dissociation.
3. The morphology changes dramatically at this time. Endosomes grow and (compartment for uncoupling of receptor and ligand) is the name given to the endosomes at this stage. It is in the CURL where the cell decides the fate of the receptor and the ligand.

4. During the next 6–15 min, the morphology changes again and the ligand ends up in multivesicular bodies. At this point, the receptors and possibly the ion pump leave the CURL. The endosome and its contents destined for degradation go to the lysosome (WILEMAN et al. 1985).

Two types of endosome were defined by HELENIUS et al. (1983): early (peripheral), which fill first and are in close proximity to the plasma membrane, and those concentrated in the Golgi-lysosomal region of the cell. The latter are spherical and larger than early endosomes and may even be a part of GERL (a structure in the area of the Golgi cisternae endoplasmic reticulum and lysosomes but its relation to the endoplasmic reticulum is not agreed upon). They house a sorting mechanism. These authors proposed two possible transport models:

1. In the *maturational model* endosomes form de novo at the cell periphery by fusion with incoming endocytic vesicles and form endosome I. This endosome moves to the perinuclear region of the cell where it becomes endosome II, containing dissociated ligands and fluid phase components. The morphology changes through condensation, reciprocal fusions, and invaginations; multivesicular bodies are formed. Ultimately, the endosome fuses with primary or secondary lysosomes. In this model, the endosome and its contents move together as the organelle undergoes maturation and ends up in the lysosome; therefore, the endosome is a transient structure.
2. In the *vesicle shuttle model* the endosomes are stable structures with well-defined and constant functions, locations, and morphology. Internalized material passes through endosomal compartments with no real change in the endosomes themselves.

The real truth probably is a combination of the two models.

Endosomes are known to have an acidic interior (pH 4-5) (TYCKO and MAXFIELD 1982; GEISOW and EVANS 1984) yet are poor in acid hydrolase content and do not degrade receptors or ligands. However, cathepsin D was found in some endosomes. Endosomes are known to have a proton pump (ATPase) which is electrogenic and controls the internal pH. Therefore acidification only takes place if an anion channel is present as well (WILEMAN et al. 1985). It is believed that the acidic environment is responsible for the dissociation of receptor-ligand complexes. Mechanisms for receptor-ligand dissociation have been studied with agents that neutralize the endosome interior. Some receptors are degraded in lysosomes while others are recycled back to the plasma membrane unharmed (HELENIUS et al. 1983). From this, it can be deduced that dissociation must take place before entry into the lysosome, therefore in endosomes (GEUZE et al. 1983, 1984; AJIOKA 1987), due to a local low pH. Consequently, endosomes represent a turning point.

There are four major pathways that internalized receptor-ligand complexes may take (SHEPHERD 1989):

1. Receptor and ligand dissociate, receptor returns to the plasma membrane, and ligands are delivered to lysosomes.
2. Both receptor and ligand recycle to the plasma membrane.
3. Both receptor and ligand are transported to the lysosome.
4. Receptor-ligand complexes are delivered to the opposite side of polarized cells where ligand is released intact.

For example, the galactose, mannose, mannose-6-phosphate, and LDL receptors target their ligands to lysosomes while transferrin and IgG are recycled to the plasma membrane. This is accomplished as vesicles bud away from the endosome and fuse with the plasma membrane, lysosomes, or elements of the Golgi apparatus. Also, transmembrane electrochemical gradients play a role in the determinants of receptor recycling. Depending on the association properties of the specific receptor-ligand complex in the acidic environment of the endosome, it may dissociate or stay bound. (WILEMAN et al. 1985). Cell type, ligand concentration, and distribution of receptors may play a significant role in determining which route a particular receptor will take (SHEPHERD 1989). It is not certain how the contents of endosomes are transferred to lysosomes. In order to learn more about the mechanism in which the cell transfers its vesicular contents between endocytic vesicles. WOODMAN and Warren (1988) studied the fusion between endocytic vesicles containing ^{125}I-transferrin and ones with anti-transferrin antibodies, as monitored by the formation of an immune complex in a cell-free medium. They found three things: fusion was irreversible, it required ATP and cytosol, and happened only between specific vesicle populations.

As can be seen, the cell maintains a complex course of taking material into the cell, transporting it intracellularly, processing it, and returning membrane components to the membrane. Differing theories of the detailed process of endocytosis can result from different methods of analysis and artifacts obtained. A few facts are known. Receptors are rapidly recycled compared to the time it takes for material to go through the lysosomal route. Also, recycling of receptors to the plasma membrane can occur at temperatures <20°C, whereas the receptor or ligand cannot enter the lysosome from the endosome at these temperatures. Specific examples of detailed recycling studies can be found in the literature (SNIDER and ROGERS 1986; WOODS et al. 1986; WILLINGHAM et al. 1984; REICHNER et al. 1988; BASU et al. 1981; WILEMAN et al. 1984).

III. Lysosomes

Pinocytosis and phagocytosis are processes by which extracellular material is brought into lysosomes, whereas autophagy, crinophagy, and possibly micro-autophagy transport organelles and macromolecules from the cytoplasm to the lysosomal compartment. The lysosome is an intracellular compartment in all eukaryotic cells containing more than 50 hydrolytic enzymes (Fig. 3) that

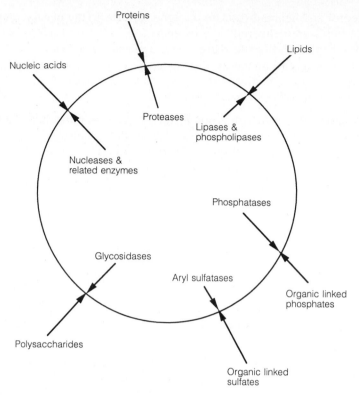

Fig. 3. Major enzymatic activities inside lysosomes

can break down molecules. It has a low pH and is impermeable to macro-molecules thereby confining acid hydrolases and preventing partially digested material from escaping (LLOYD 1986). However, small non-electrolytes have been found to diffuse across the lysosomal membrance. IVESON et al. (1989) have used an osmotic protection method to study the permeability of rat liver lysosomes; 43 organic uncharged molecules were studied (MW 62–1000). From these, three patterns were observed: little or no solute entry into the lysosome, solute entry, and very rapid solute entry. Although no correlation with MW was observed, the inverse of hydrogen binding capacity correlated with rapidity of solute entry. These results indicate that the solutes used enter lysosomes by passive diffusion. The permeability of the lysosomal membrane has been reviewed by FORSTER and LLOYD (1988). The questions which molecules can cross the lysosomal membrane, which cannot, and by which mechanism they cross were addressed.

There is evidence of carrier-mediated transport across the lysosomal membrane (LLOYD and FORSTER 1986). For instance, cystinosis is a disease that is caused by a recessively inherited genetic defect in which the efflux of cystine from the lysosome is impaired. There is reason to believe that the lysosomal membrane is missing a cystine transporter. Lysosomal accumulation of sialic acid in Salla disease may be caused by the abscence of a sialic acid transporter. Acetyltransferase is known to shuttle acetyl units into the lysosome. Cobalamin efflux is carrier-mediated. If the transporter is missing, cobalamin is trapped in the lysosome after digestion of cobalamin-transcobalamin II complex in the lysosome. This is not an exhaustive list by any means. Some substances may cross the lysosomal membrane unassisted, yet it is likely that many more carriers will be discovered in the future.

The lysosomal membrane has been studied in great detail. There is some membrane recycling, but to a very small extent. Radiolabeled galactose, covalently bound to cell surface glucoconjugates on mouse macrophage cells (P388D$_1$), was used as a marker to study the kinetics of exchange of membrane constituents between the plasma membrane and the secondary lysosomal membrane. It was found that transfer of components from plasma membrane to lysosomal membrane is very selective and accounts for only 1% of plasma membrane recycling (HAYLETT and THILO 1986). Vitamin A is a known membrane labilizer and hydrocortisone and cholesterol stabilize the lysosomal membrane (DE DUVE 1983). The membrane is also stable in isosmotic solutions of non-penetrating solvents but will burst when suspended in hypotonic solution. A permeant solute is initially stabilizing but causes osmotic imbalance and eventual bursting of the lysosome. The properties of the lysosomal membrane keep destructive enzymes from invading the rest of the cell and let catabolic products out (LLOYD 1986).

Although lysosomes mainly contain acid hydrolases, esterases, phosphatases, peptidases, and glycosidases, hydrolase stabilizing proteins, proteoglycans, and oxidoreductases are also present. A single cell may contain more than one lysosome population which could contain different densities or hydrolase activities, therefore they are polymorphic.

Lysosomal pH has been deduced by introducing dextran-fluorescein conjugates into lysosomes. The pH of 4.7 was found in mouse peritoneal macrophages. This value is in agreement with the optimal value of protein degradation by lysosomal enzymes in vitro. Most enzymes that are contained in lysosomes usually show low activity at neutral pH and optimal activity at acid pH (MAXFIELD 1985). As do endosomes, lysosomes contain an ATP controlled pump on their membranes. "Acidotropic agents," which cause a rise in endosomal lysosomal pH, such as chloroquine, natural red, and other weak bases, have been used to support the pump theory.

Lysosomes are termed residual bodies when they contain undigestible material (TARTAKOFF 1987). Vacuolation is caused by pinocytosis of some solutes in living cells in which the size of lysosomes are expanded due to the entry of undigestible solutes or solutes that can be only partially degraded and are not permeant to the membrane. On the other hand, permeant products such as nucleosides, inorganic anions, amino acids, and monosaccharides leave the lysosome by metabolic efflux. Oligopeptides such as (D-Glu)$_2$ (and possibly Glu-Glu) and tripeptides cannot traverse the lysosomal membrane.

Even small carbohydrates such as disaccharides are not permeant. Mono-nucleotides are impermeant, but they are degraded to nucleosides and inorganic phosphate which are permeant. Inorganic cations are also not able to cross the lysosomal membrane (LLOYD and FORSTER 1986).

Therefore, the lysosome is a very important organelle contained in the cell. It is responsible for killing bacteria that enter the cell by phagocytosis. It degrades hormones and transport proteins resulting in the efflux of small molecules into the cytosol making them either accessible to the cell or they may be released by the cell.

Many diseases exist in which certain enzymes are missing from lysosomes for various reasons. One reason is inefficient lysosomal trafficking (KORNFELD 1987). A naturally occurring example concerns the mannose-6-phosphate receptor. In many culture cell lines there are no or very low levels of this receptor. In these cases there is considerable loss of newly synthesized lysosomal enzymes. So, this receptor functions to somehow intracellularly target acid hydrolases to lysosomes (TARTAKOFF 1987).

The role of the 163 amino acid cytoplasmic domain of the cation-independent mannose 6-phosphate receptor was studied by LOBEL et al. (1989) in the endocytosis of extracellular lysosomal enzymes (as well as the sorting of intracellularly synthesized lysosomal enzymes). Receptor deficient mouse L cells were transfected with normal bovine cation-independent mannose 6-phosphate receptor cDNA or cDNAs mutated in the cytoplasmic domain. Depending on the degree of mutation of the receptors, different levels of inactivity of either endocytosis or intracellular sorting were apparent. It was found that the inner section of the cytoplasmic tail is necessary and sufficient for endocytosis. This is another example of the importance of the cytoplasmic domain and shows that it controls different functions through various signals.

C. Fate of Macromolecular Carriers In Vivo

The biocompatibility and consequently the clinical usefulness of a macro-molecular carrier can be impaired if it persists in the body for a long period after administration. Long-term storage in some body compartments (e.g., lysosomes) can cause adverse reactions. Three main factors influence the rate of elimination of a macromolecular carrier from the body: its chemical structure, MWD (and corresponding conformation), and biodegradability. Obviously these factors are interrelated since the chemical structure influences the biodegradability and MW influences the conformation and consequently transport across compartmental barriers.

Both biodegradable and nonbiodegadable macromolecules have been proposed as drug carriers. Both have advantages and disadvantages. It is often believed that natural macromolecules (proteins, polysaccharides) or synthetic carriers having the same structural features as natural macromolecules (synthetic polyamino acids) are the carriers of choice because they are biodegradable. However, this is not always the case and biodegradation (discussed below) is a complicated process. In addition these carriers are often immunogenic. Moreover, the biodegradability of the carrier can change dramatically when drug molecules and targeting moieties are bound. The consequence of natural carrier modification is not only a change in the rate of carrier degradation but also the degradation pattern. Degradation of a drug-modified natural carrier may not yield "monomer" units, such as amino acids and monosaccharides but fragments, oligopeptides, or oligosaccharides which may be buried in the lysosomal compartment, if they cannot penetrate the lysosomal membrane (LLOYD 1989). Moreover, they may possess biological activity. In addition, chemical modification of natural carriers (such as by binding of drugs) leads to products which are difficult to define with respect to site of substitution. Consequently, results on the relationship between the structure and degradability cannot be generalized.

Synthetic nondegradable macromolecules may sometimes be preferred, since they usually display good biocompatibility (DUNCAN and KOPEČEK 1984). They can be specifically tailored to possess properties appropriate to the biological system in which they are to be used (KOPEČEK 1982, 1984a,b). To prevent storage, the whole MWD must be under the renal threshold. Renal filtration and pinocytic capture are two processes which affect the distribution of the polymer in the body. Other processes such as penetration through capillary walls and interaction with serum proteins (OHNO et al. 1981) are important too. However, not enough data are available at the present time to evaluate them accordingly.

I. Principles of Biodegradability

Most of the enzymatically degradable carriers are either natural polymers or their structure is based on natural polymers. They usually contain peptidic, glycosidic, or phosphate bonds. In other words, to render synthetic polymers enzymatically degradable, their structure should match the active site of respective enzymes.

The active site of the enzyme is the region where the interaction with the substrate takes place. The active site plays a double role, that of binding the substrate and catalyzing the reaction. To understand the functioning of an enzyme, the structure of the enzyme-substrate complex must be known. In the investigation of the structure of the latter, there is one serious problem (FERSHT 1985): enzyme-substrate complexes react to give products in fractions of seconds whereas the acquisition of X-ray data necessary to evaluate the structure of the complex normally takes several hours. Therefore, it is normal to determine the structure of the complex of enzymes with inhibitors or substrate analogues. Supported by such data as well as kinetic measurements in solution, it is apparent that proteolytic enzymes have a considerably large active site (about 25 Å) capable of binding a number of amino acid residues. Based on the study of the cleavage of 40 diastereoisomeric peptides of alanine (Ala$_2$-Ala$_6$) by papain, SCHECHTER and BERGER (1967) suggested subdividing the active site of papain into subsites, each of which accomodates one amino acid residue of the peptide substrate (Fig. 4). The substrate aligns itself in the active center so that the -CO-NH- group being hydrolyzed always occupies the same place with respect to the remaining amino acid residues in adjacent subsites. Four subsites are located towards the NH$_2$- terminal of the substrate (denoted S$_1$, S$_2$, etc.) and three towards the COOH- terminal of the substrate (S$_1'$, S$_2'$). The amino acid residues of the substrate are denoted in a corresponding manner: P$_1$, P$_2$, . . . P$_1'$, P$_2'$, etc. The relationship between the structure of the substrate and its degradability may be conveniently described as S$_1$ − P$_1$, S$_2$ − P$_2$ interactions. This concept is generally valid for proteolytic enzymes.

Polysaccharide cleaving enzymes also have a relatively large active site. For instance, hen egg white lysozyme (MW 14 500) contains six subsites for binding the glucopyranose rings of the substrate. Upon formation of the enzyme-substrate complex the sugar ring bound to subsite S$_1$ is distorted into the sofa conformation. To avoid strain in the S$_1$ subsite, oligosaccharides frequently bind to S$_4$ − S$_2$ subsites in a nonproductive way, avoiding cleavage (FERSHT 1985).

II. Influence of Substitution on the Degradability of Natual Polymers

1. Polysaccharides

Polysaccharides are attractive candidates for use as drug carriers. If unmodified, they are in most cases, degraded to low MW units which can cross the lysosomal membrane and be eliminated from the body. It is generally

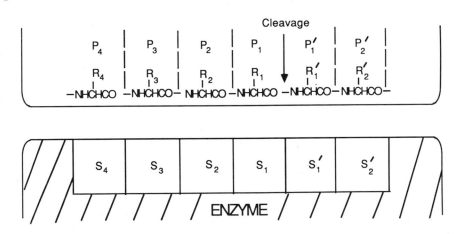

Fig. 4. The enzyme-substrate complex. (From SCHECHTER and BERGER 1967)

known that substitution of polysaccharides renders them less susceptible to enzymatic hydrolysis. Native starch is degraded in blood by amylases too rapidly to be used as a blood plasma expander. Hydroxyethylation of starch (BANKS et al. 1972) decreases the rate of its degradation. Consequently, its intravascular half-life is increased to a level acceptable for a blood plasma expander.

Dextrans are polysaccharides consisting of α-D-glucose units joined predominantly by 1–6 linkages. Partially hydrolyzed and fractionated dextran is used as a blood plasma expander (MESSMER 1988) and has been proposed as a drug carrier (SCHACHT 1987a,b; SCHACHT et al. 1988). It is cleaved by dextranases which are not present in blood, but are present in the liver (ROZENFELD et al. 1959; AMMON 1963), spleen, kidney (AMMON 1963), intestinal mucosa (FISCHER and STEIN 1960), and colon (SERRY and HEHRE 1956).

VERCAUTEREN et al. (1990) modified dextran by three methods: partial periodate oxidation and subsequent reduction of aldehyde groups; succinylation; and chloroformate activation with subsequent reaction with 2-hydroxypropylamine, ethylenediamine, and tris (2-aminoethyl)amine. The rate of degradation of derivatized dextran by dextranase decreased with increasing degree of substitution. The nature of modification had no significant effect on the rate of degradation. Similar results were obtained by others (ROSEMEYER and SELA 1984; CHAVES and ARRANZ 1985; CREPON et al. 1991). The degradation of dextran and its derivatives with isolated lysosomal enzymes (SCHACHT et al. 1988) was slower than the cleavage by dextranase. Moreover, only a minor amount of glucose was liberated. The above results clearly indicate that modification of polysaccharides has serious consequences on the rate of degradation and on the composition of degradation products. From these data it appears that the lysosomal degradation of drug-modified dextrans will produce fragments which will not permeate the lysosomal membrane. This conclusion is not suprising in light of the observation that dextran is accumulated within secondary lysosomes, particularly in the liver where it increases the liver acid phosphatase level. (MEIJER and WILLINGHAGEN 1963).

2. Polyamino Acids

There are similar drawbacks with polyamino acids, which have also been suggested as drug carriers. Data from the literature suggest that even unmodified polyamino acids yield a substantial amount of oligopeptides upon degradation. Lets discuss, as an example, the hydrolysis of polylysine by trypsin. The trypsin catalyzed hydrolysis of polylysine at pH 7.6 produced mostly di-, tri-, and tetralysine (WALEY and WATSON 1953). Using a lower concentration of trypsin (three times, i.e., 0.01 mg/ml) KATCHALSKI et al. (1961) were able to detect oligopeptides containing two to nine lysine residues in the digest during the initial stage of reaction. The longer oligopeptides and the original macromolecules disappeared from the reaction mixture when the incubation was prolonged. The final products of hydrolysis (Lys_2, Lys_3, Lys_4) were in accordance with the findings of WALEY and WATSON (1953).

It is evident that lysosomal aminopeptidases could cleave these fragments. However, due to substitution the cleavage may terminate when a modified amino acid residue is at the NH_2-terminal of the oligopeptide.

The degradability of polyamino acids depends strongly on their conformation. In synthetic polyamino acids, α, β, and random coil structures coexist in the same chain. They undergo transconformation, mimicking the self-organization of protein chains. Based on a detailed study of the degradation of polyglutamic acid and polylysine by proteolytic enzymes, MILLER (1961, 1964a,b) and MILLER and MONROE (1968) concluded that peptide bonds in the helical regions were not hydrolyzed and that in random coil regions only those peptide bonds were hydrolyzed in which the adjacent amino acid side chains were uncharged. These facts must be taken into account when designing macromolecular drug carriers.

Modification of polyamino acids further influences their susceptibility to enzymatic attack. Poly(N-hydroxyethyl)-L-glutamine is resistant to serine proteases, but the hydrophobic modification of glutamic acid side chains or the copolymerization with hydrophobic L-amino acids renders them degradable (PYTELA et al. 1989). However, the products of degradation contain fragments of a size nonpermeable through the lysosomal membrane. YAACOBI et al. (1985) studied the papain catalyzed hydrolysis of poly-L-(2-hydroxyethyl)glutamine. The final products of degradation were tetrapeptide fragments. VAN HEESWIJK et al. (1984) conjugated adriamycin to poly-α-L-glutamic acid γ-carboxyl groups via an amide bond. These conjugates were designed as macromolecular prodrugs for the selective release of free drug in tumor cells having elevated levles of γ-glutamyl transferase (GT). The authors later hypothesized (HOES and FEIJEN 1989) that after biodegradation of the polymeric carrier low MW γ-glutamyl amides of adriamycin (ADR) are formed and consequently transformed to free ADR by γ-GT. However, the conjugates were not active against B16 melanoma cells which are known to have membrane bound γ-GT (HOES et al. 1986). These results were explained by the insufficient degradability of the polymer main chain. This assumption was verified by in vitro degradation studies (HOES et al. 1985).

These examples strongly suggest that the conclusion that macromolecular carriers based on natural polymers or synthetic polyamino acids (DROBNÍK 1989; PYTELA et al. 1989; and many others) are degraded to low MW products which can cross the lysosomal membrane are premature and do not take into account the complex nature of enzymatic processes. Much more work is necessary, but the available experimental evidence suggests that, at present, it is safe to assume that any macromolecular carrier, synthetic or natural, will accumulate in the lysosomal compartment to a certain extent. Consequently, macromolecular carriers should be used only in such applications in which the aim is to kill the cell, such as cancer chemotherapy. Upon cell death, the carrier or its fragments will be released into the bloodstream and may be eliminated. From the biocompatibility point of view, it appears that the use of synthetic nondegradable carriers having suitable MWDs is preferable because products released into the bloodstream can be defined as to their chemical structure and biological properties, thereby limiting side effects. When "biodegradable" carriers are used, oligopeptide (oligosaccharide) fragments will be released (GODDARD and PETRAK 1989) which may possess unwanted biological activity. Moreover, no data are available on their detailed structure and corresponding biological activity and such data are not easy to obtain.

III. Elimination of Macromolecular Carriers from the Organism

The length of time a macromolecular drug carrier persists in the organism after fulfilling its pharmacological function is likely to influence its general toxicity, carcinogenicity, etc. (DUNCAN 1986). There are four major compartments the macromolecular drug can enter: the central compartment (blood and lymphatic system), interstitium, intestinal lumen, and lysosomes (DROBNÍK and RYPÁČEK 1984). Minor compartments are primary urine, bile, etc. There are no data available demonstrating the penetration of macromolecules into the cytoplasm, i.e., inside the cell but outside the endosomes or lysosomes (DROBNÍK 1989).

Theoretically, it is possible to use soluble macromolecules in many compartments of the organism. The drug could be released or activated outside the cells, at the cellular surface, or inside the cells in the lysosomes. Due to the endocytic activity of the majority of cells in the organism, the easiest and the experimentally most advanced target is the lysosomal compartment of the cell.

The injection route is an effective one for the introduction of soluble macromolecules into the organism (PITHA 1981) because macromolecules do not normally penetrate the skin. Another possibility is the oral route, which will be discussed in Sect.H.

After introduction into the bloodstream, macromolecules are subsequently distributed and partly excreted from the organism. Depending on the structure and MWD of the polymer, a fraction is excreted in the urine. Simultaneously, polymers are cleared from the bloodstream by endocytosis. Polymers are not able to cross the blood-brain barrier, unless the latter is osmotically opened (ARMSTRONG et al. 1989).

There are differences in the ease of penetration of macromolecules from the bloodstream into different tissues (PITHA 1980). Capillaries of the liver, spleen, and bone marrow have incomplete basal membranes and are lined with endothelial cells which are not continuously arranged. Thus, macromolecules can penetrate easily into these organs. Capillaries in endocrine glands and in muscle have a somewhat tighter arrangement, and there is an almost perfect barrier which isolates the central nervous system from circulating blood. The fate of macromolecules in the living body is schematically shown in Fig. 5.

The circulating half-life of macromolecules will depend on their hydrodynamic radius. For molecules with a radius larger than 45 Å, the rate of filtration through the kidney is nearly zero. However, these macromolecules are still capable of crossing the normal epithelium. The size of macromolecules depends on their structure and MW. Consequently, parameters such as shape, flexibility, and charge influence the transport (PETRAK and GODDARD 1989).

Changes in permeability associated with the diseased state, such as found in inflammation or tumor tissue, offer an increased opportunity for extravasation of macromolecules. The size window in such cases is believed to be in the range of 1-2 μm (PETRAK and GODDARD 1989).

1. Structural Factors Influencing the Fate of Macromolecules

a) Molecular Weight

There is clear evidence that there is a relationship between the MW (size) of macromolecules and the rate and pattern of their elimination from the organism (KOPEČEK 1981). It is better to relate the clearance of macromolecules to size, because globular proteins and synthetic macromolecules of comparable MW have different sizes. Moreover, the flexible structure of the latter permits them to pass through glomerular pores by "end-up" motion (RENNKE et al. 1979) allowing higher MW molecules to pass.

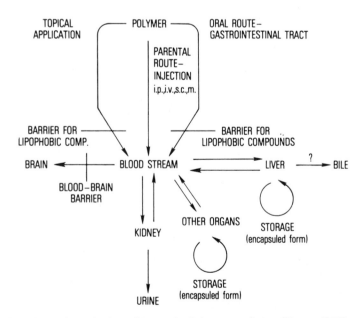

Fig. 5. The fate of synthetic polymers in living organisms. (PITHA 1981)

Unlike natural macromolecules, synthetic macromolecules are poly-disperse. Therefore, it is imperative to characterize these macromolecules not only by their average MW, but by their MWD. To be eliminated from the organism, the whole MWD must be under the threshold for glomerular filtration. The importance of the MWD was demonstrated by HESPE et al. (1977), who studied the biological fate of two preparations of [^{14}C] polyvinylpyrrolidone which were of the same average MW but had different polydispersities. The preparation with higher polydispersity (containing a fraction of macromolecules with higher MW) was found to be retained in the organs for a much longer time than the less polydisperse preparation.

SEYMOUR et al. (1987) studied the body distrbution and rate of excretion of radiolabeled poly-N-(2-hydroxypropyl)methacrylamide (HPMA) contain-ing 1 mol-% of methacryloyltyrosinamide (to permit radiolabeling) in rats. Fractions were used with narrow polydispersities ranging from 12 to 778 kDa. A MW threshold limiting glomerular filtration was identified at approximately 45 kDa. Fractions with a higher MW were lost from the bloodstream only slowly by extravasation. MW did not influence the movement of macro-molecules from the peritoneal compartment to the bloodstream after intra-peritoneal injection. Following subcutaneous administration the largest fraction (778 kDa, diameter approximately 30 nm) showed increased retention at the site of injection; approximately 20% of the dose remained there after 21 days. Smaller fractions moved readily into the bloodstream, whence they were lost in the urine, or they gradually penetrated into other tissues and organs. Long-term (21 days) body distribution of copolymers following both intraperitoneal and subcutaneous administration showed size-dependent accumulation in organs of the reticuloendothelial system.

b) Chemical Structure

Under physiological conditions cells have a negative charge on their surface. Thus introducing positive charge into the structure of macromolecular carriers leads to their nonspecific interactions with cells due to electrostatic attractive forces (ANGHILERI et al. 1976). The interactions depend on the net charge of the macromolecule and contribution or absence of hydrophobic interactions. The cell surface carbohydrates contribute to the negative charge of the cell surface but also produce a densely packed hydration sheet which effectively shields the hydrophobic cell membrane. Nonspecific interactions between macromolecules and cell surfaces arise as a consequence of long-range electrostatic forces or shorter-range hydrophobic interactions (ARTURSSON and O'MULLANE 1989), eventually by a combination of both.

McCORMICK et al. (1986) studied the interaction of a cationic HPMA copolymer with rat visceral yolk sacs in vitro and in rats in vivo. In vitro it was found that the cationic HPMA copolymer associated with the tissue. This association was primarily due to the association with the tissue surface. Following intravenous administration into rats, the clearance of the cationic copolymer from the bloodstream was rapid, the majority of the copolymer being recovered in the liver. Subcellular fractionation of the liver showed that the cationic HPMA copolymer bound initially to the membranes of liver cells. Following adsorption the copolymer was transferred slowly to the secondary lysosomes.

Another way to facilitate adsorptive pinocytosis is to incorporate hydrophobic groups into water soluble macromolecular carriers. DUNCAN et al. (1982a, 1984) have shown that incorporation of hydrophobic aromatic residues into water soluble HPMA copolymers (1984) or polyaspartamides (1982) increases the rate of pinocytosis of modified macromolecules by rat visceral yolk sacs in vitro.

Hydrophobicity of macromolecules can increase their accummulation in the kidney tubular epithelium. RYPÁČEK et al. (1982) have shown that the incorporation of a high amount (19 mol-%) of hydrophobic side chains into polyaspartamides considerably increases the affinity of the copolymer for the membrane of kidney tubular cells.

The apparent universal nature of electrostatic and hydrophobic interactions of macromolecular carriers with cell surfaces precludes the use of carriers containing large amounts of groups susceptible to these interactions for cell specific targeting of drugs. Macromolecular carriers should be designed in such a way that, if a targeting moiety is not attached, the carriers enter cells by fluid phase pinocytosis. Only in this case will there be a low probability of nonspecific recapture of the carrier after being released from a dead cell.

D. Release of Drugs

The main rationale behind the desire for designing soluble synthetic polymers for drug delivery is to increase the efficacy of drug delivery by limiting drug uptake to the pinocytic route. This insures intracellular drug delivery, reduces side effects of toxic drugs, and gives rise to the potential of drug targeting (discussed in subsequent sections). For this design to be meaningful, it is necessary to use either a drug that can be activated while attached to the polymer or a drug that is stable while bound to the polymer (such as in the bloodstream) and released intracellularly in active form. Methods for the latter will be discussed in this section. It is possible to take advantage of the intracellular environment of the diseased cell or the general environment of the target tissue to induce drug release. The pH of intracellular compartments and enzymes within the cell may be used advantageously.

I. Release of Drugs by Hydrolysis

Bonds sensitive to pH changes can be used to link drugs to polymeric carriers. These bonds are designed such that they are stable at neutral pH in the bloodstream and are hydrolyzed in an acidic intracellular environment thereby releasing the drug. Assuming that the polymer is internalized into the cell in question by pinocytosis, it will be incorporated into the endosome. The beauty of the scheme is that the drug can be released in prelysosomal compartments due to the low pH, and lysosomal fusion is not imperative However, a drawback often exists as a result of slow release of drug in the bloodstream. Examples of pH sensitive bonds follow.

A cis-aconityl spacer was used to link daunomycin (DNM), an anticancer agent, to poly-D-lysine (SHEN and RYSER 1981). Cis-aconitic anhydride was used to form this pH sensitive spacer arm. The cis-aconityl bond is acid labile due to anchimeric assistance of the cis-carboxylic acid group in the hydrolysis of the amide bond.

A similar principle was used to link a murine monoclonal antibody and the ribosome-inactivating protein gelonin via a heterobifunctional cross-linking reagent. This reagent is based on 2-methylmaleic anhydride (citraconic anhydride) which forms an acid labile link upon reaction with amino groups. The reagent was stable at pH 7 and released the fully active drug at pH 4-5 (BLÄTTLER et al. 1985).

HÖRPEL et al. (1982) have shown how the structure of the carrier can influence the rate of drug release by hydrolysis. In this study, 4-alkylthio derivatives of cyclophosphamide containing a functional group were synthesized and bound to amphiphilic copolymers prepared by amidation of polyethyleneimine with palmitic acid. The drugs were bound to these micellar block copolymers via amide bonds. The rate of drug release by hydrolysis was substantially slower when it was incorporated in the hydrophobic core of the micelle. Similar results were obtained by BADER et al. (1984) and DORN et al. (1985) on block copolymers composed of polylysine blocks substituted with palmitic acid residues and polyethyleneoxide blocks.

II. Disulfide Spacers

Another type of linkage for use in binding drugs to a polymer backbone is via a disulfide spacer (SHEN et al. 1985). Methotrexate (MTX) was bound to poly-D-lysine via a disulfide spacer. Whereas the conjugate with MTX bound directly to the polymer backbone was not cytotoxic to Chinese hamster ovary (CHO) cells, a disulfide spacer linking MTX to the polymer rendered the conjugate cytotoxic. It appears that the cleavage of the disulfide spacer occurs in prelysosomal compartments because release of drug does not require an acid pH and is not sensitive to lysosomal proteases.

III. Release of Drugs by Enzymes

In order to synthesize lysosomotropic drug-carrier conjugates, the bond between the carrier and drug should be stable in the bloodstream (during transport) and should be susceptible to enzyme catalyzed hydrolysis inside secondary lysosomes. In addition to the degradability of the bond between the drug and carrier, other important properties must be considered (SCHNEIDER 1983):

1. The drug must have chemical groups which make possible the binding to a carrier via a spacer (e.g., NH_2 or COOH groups).
2. The drug, which after penetration of the conjugate into the cell interior is liberated in secondary lysosomes, must either resist lysosomal hydrolases in the acidic pH or form pharmacologically active metabolites.
3. If the drug has to exert its pharmacological effect within lysosomes (parasitic or infectious diseases), it must be active at acid pH. If the drug has to exert its pharmacologic effect outside of lysosomes, it must be permeable to the lysosomal membrane.

It was shown that binding drugs to carriers via oligopeptide spacers fulfills the above requirements (MASQUELIER et al. 1980; KOPEČEK 1982; TROUET et al. 1982a).

1. Release of Drug Models from HPMA Copolymers by Chymotrypsin

For the first studies of the relationship between polymer-drug model conjugates and their susceptibility to enzymatic hydrolysis, α-chymotrypsin was chosen (KOPEČEK et al. 1981; KOPEČEK and REJMANOVÁ 1979) and the degradation of HPMA copolymers containing oligopeptide side chains terminating in p-nitroaniline was studied (Fig. 6). These model polymers contained three types of amide linkages: between methacrylic acid and the most proximal amino acid residue, between adjacent amino acid residues,

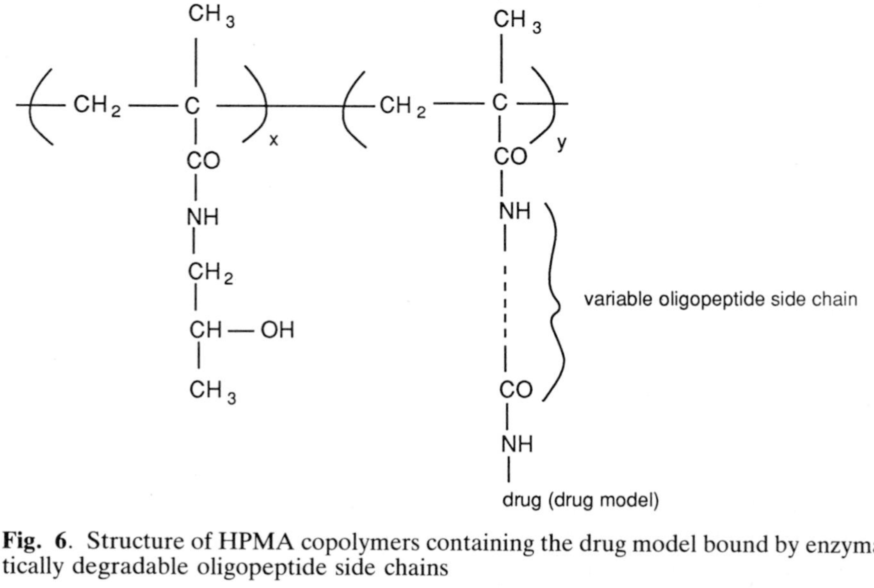

Fig. 6. Structure of HPMA copolymers containing the drug model bound by enzymatically degradable oligopeptide side chains

and between the distal amino acid residue and p-nitroaniline. Chymotrypsin is a thoroughly studied enzyme (KOPEČEK and REJMANOVÁ 1983); the detailed structure of its active site is known, along with the interactions which contribute to the binding of the substrate in the active site of the enzyme (BLOW 1974). Moreover, the chymotrypsin catalyzed hydrolysis of low MW oligopeptide p-nitroanilides was also evaluated (YAMAMOTO and IZUMIYA 1966; KASAFÍREK et al. 1976). The comparison of the cleavage of the latter with the cleavage of polymer bound forms helped to evaluate the sterical hindrance caused by the polymer chain on the formation of the enzyme-substrate complex.

The following conclusions may be drawn from the results of investigation of the kinetics of chymotrypsin catalyzed release of p-nitroaniline from the ends of oligopeptide side chains in HPMA copolymers (KOPEČEK et al. 1981; KOPEČEK 1991). In all substrates the distal amino acid residue was phenyl-alanine, a specific amino acid for chymotrypsin (Table 2).

1. Degradability of the peptide bond at the end of an oligopeptide side chain of a synthetic polymer is affected both by steric and by structural factors.
2. With increasing number of amino acid residues in the oligopeptide sequence, the rate of chymotrypsin catalyzed hydrolysis increases.
3. By choosing a suitable structure (with respect to S-P interactions), it is possible, in substrates with the same length of oligopeptide, to affect the enzymatic degradability.
4. Taking into consideration steric factors, it is possible to correlate the cleavage of side chains of polymeric substrates with the process of cleavage of low MW substrates.

Table 2. Effect of the structure of N-(2-hydroxypropyl)methacrylamide copolymer carrier on the rate of release of p-nitroaniline catalyzed by chymotrypsin. (From KOPEČEK et al. 1981)

Polymer structure	k_{cat}/K_M, $M^{-1}s^{-1}$
P-Phe-NAp	0
P-Gly-Gly-Phe-NAp	110
P-Gly-Val-Phe-NAp	245
P-Gly-Gly-Val-Phe-NAp	6 300
P-Ala-Gly-Val-Phe-NAp	14 200

Only the cleavage of the terminal bond linking the p-nitroaniline drug model was monitored.
k_{cat}/K_M represents the apparent second-order rate constant; the higher the ratio, the faster the cleavage (25°C).
P, N-(2-hydroxpropyl)methacrylamide copolymer backbone; NAp, p-nitroaniline (drug model).

0

a) Influence of Drug Loading

HPMA copolymers have a hydrophobic (C-C) backbone and hydrophilic (NH-CH$_2$-CH(OH)-CH$_3$) side chains. Oligopeptide side chains terminating in drug or drug model are usually hydrophobic. By changing the ratio of hydrophobic and hydrophilic side chains along the copolymer backbone, the solution properties of the copolymer change (ULBRICH et al. 1987). The release of *p*-nitroaniline from HPMA copolymers containing different amounts of hydrophobic Gly-Leu-Phe-NAp side chains was compared. Copolymers with more hydrophobic side chains associate in water forming micelle-like structures, the *p*-nitroaniline being inside and the polymeric chains outside. The association number (Table 3) and compactness of micelles both depend on the copolymer structure, copolymer concentration, and temperature. Micellar shells were shown to hinder the penetration of enzymes into the micellar core, thus reducing the rate of chymotrypsin catalyzed release of *p*-nitroaniline.

2. Cleavage by Lysosomal Enzymes

Within the context of the polymeric drug carrier system, the oligopeptidyl side chains of HPMA copolymers are viewed as drug attachment/release sites, and therefore their susceptibility to hydrolysis by lysosomal enzymes is important. However, there are some problems connected with controlling the release of drugs from carriers within lysosomes. Whereas for chymotrypsin (and other model enzymes) the structure of the active site and interactions taking place during the formation of the enzyme substrate complex are known in detail for every subsite, the detailed structures of active sites of lysosomal enzymes are not well-known. Thus, detailed studies on the specificity of lysosomal enzymes toward polymeric substrates are needed in order to synthesize tailor-made polymeric substrates with a controllable rate of drug (drug model) release.

Studies on the degradation of oligopeptide side chains of HPMA copolymers by a mixture of lysosomal enzymes isolated from rat liver have shown that the lysosomal cysteine proteinases are particularly important in

Table 3. Solution parameters of copolymers of *N*-(2-hydroxypropyl)methacrylamide with *N*-methacryloylglycylleucylphenylalanine *p*-nitroanilide (MA-G-L-F-NAp) determined by integral and quasielastic light scattering experiments. (From ULBRICH et al. 1987)

Content of MA-G-L-F-NAp (mol%)	$M_w \times 10^{-3}$ (g mol^{-1})	R_H (nm)	Estimated association number
6.9	130	6.1	5
3.3	54	4.6	2
1.5	42	4.2	1

the process of degradation (DUNCAN et al. 1982b, 1983). To understand the mechanism of cleavage in the lysosomes, the degradation of polymer substrates with individual cysteine proteinases had to be studied. From our studies it seems that cathepsin B (Table 4) (REJMANOVÁ et al. 1983) and cathepsin L (ŠUBR et al. 1984) are very important in releasing p-nitroaniline from oligopeptide side chains attached to HPMA copolymers.

However, the cleavage of polymer substrates with longer oligopeptide side chains is a complicated process in which a number of enzymes may be involved. It was shown that in some polymeric substrates not only the bond between the distal amino acid residue and drug model is cleaved during incubation with lysosomal enzymes (ŠUBR et al. 1988), but peptide linkages between adjacent amino acid residues can also be cleaved. The latter cleavage results in release of oligopeptide fragments. Detailed knowledge of the cleavage pattern of polymeric prodrugs is of utmost importance, because it is possible for amino acid or oligopeptide modified drug to be released from the carrier inside of secondary lysosomes. Although free drug could be released by subsequent action of enzymes having aminopeptidase (e.g., cathepsin H) or dipeptidylpeptidase (e.g., cathepsin C) activities, uncleaved drug derivatives could diffuse into the cytoplasm. In the latter case the question of different therapeutic activities of free drug and amino acid (oligopeptide) modified drug must be addressed. ŠUBR et al. (1988) studied the cleavage of

Table 4. Effect of the structure of oligopeptide side chains in N-(2-hydroxypropyl)methacrylamide copolymers on the rate of p-nitroaniline release catalyzed by cathepsin B. (From REJMANOVÁ et al. 1983)

Polymer structure	% Cleavage after 24 h of incubation
P-Acap-Leu-NAp	2
P-Gly-Val-Leu-NAp	25
P-Gly-Val-Ala-NAp	24
P-Gly-Leu-Ala-NAp	33
P-Gly-Ile-Ala-NAp	28
P-Gly-Phe-Ala-NAp	38
P-Gly-Ala-Phe-NAp	5.4
P-Gly-Phe-Leu-Gly-NAp	69
P-Gly-Phe-Tyr-Ala-NAp	52
P-Gly-Phe-Gly-Phe-NAp	6.6
P-Gly-Phe-Leu-Gly-Phe-NAp	8

Only the cleavage between the distal amino acid residue and p-nitroaniline drug model was monitored.
Conditions of cleavage: [cathepsin B] = 1.9×10^{-7} mol/l; [NAp] = 1.17×10^{-3} mol/l; $0.1 M$ phosphate buffer (KH$_2$PO$_4$/NaOH); pH = 6.0; EDTA 1 mmol/l; Cys 25 mmol/l; 40°C.
P, N-(2-hydroxypropyl)methacrylamide copolymer backbone; NAp, p-nitroaniline (drug model).

Table 5. Cleavage of *N*-(2-hydroxypropyl)methacrylamide copolymers containing various oligopeptide side chains by cathepsin D. (From ŠUBR 1986)

Polymer substrate	% cleavage after 24 h of incubation
$\downarrow$ P-Gly-Phe-Phe-NAp	4
$\downarrow$ P-Gly-Phe-Tyr-NAp	
$\downarrow$ P-Gly-Gly-Phe-Phe-NAp	
P-Gly-Phe-Gly-Phe-NAp	0
P-Gly-Gly-Val-Phe-NAp	0
P-Ala-Gly-Val-Phe-NAp	0
$\downarrow$ P-Gly-Phe-Phe-Ala-NAp	4
$\downarrow$ P-Gly-Phe-Leu-Gly-Phe-NAp	7
$\downarrow$ P-Gly-Gly-Phe-Leu-Gly-Phe-NAp	16

The bond cleaved in each case is denoted with an arrow.
Conditions of cleavage: [cathepsin D] = 2×10^{-6} mol/l; [NAp] = 1×10^{-3} mol/l; 0.2 *M* citrate buffer; pH = 4.0; 24 h; 37°C.
P, *N*-(2-hydroxypropyl)methacrylamide copolymer backbone; NAp, *p*-nitroaniline (drug model).

oligopeptide side chains attached to HPMA copolymers by artificial mixtures of lysosomal enzymes in detail.

In this process thiol-independent enzymes can also be involved. In Table 5, the cleavage of oligopeptide side chains by cathepsin D (aspartic protease) is shown (ŠUBR 1986).

A comparison of the effect of thiol proteinases B, H, and L and a mixture of lysosomal enzymes (tritosomes) on the cleavage of *p*-nitroaniline from a selected side chain (Gly-Phe-Leu-Gly-NAp) attached to an HPMA polymer is found in Fig. 7. This figure illustrates the importance of cathepsin B on the overall activity of lysosomal enzymes. Figure 8 summarizes the percent of NAp released by cathepsin B over time for a variety of oligopeptidic side chains of HPMA copolymers. It shows the influence of the detailed structure of the side chains on the rate of release of the drug model (KOPEČEK 1984b; REJMANOVÁ et al. 1983).

The rate of drug release also depends on the structure of the drug itself. The active site of proteinases usually accomodates two amino acid residues of the substrate toward the COOH terminal of the cleaved bond. Unfortunately, in polymeric prodrugs, the drug molecule occupies these positions if the oligopeptide spacer is tailor-made to be cleaved between the distal amino acid residue and the drug. Thus, the structure of the drug itself influences the interaction of the polymeric substrate with the enzyme's active site. Different

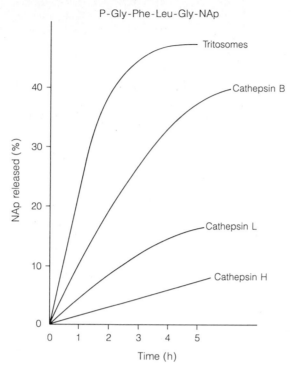

P-Gly-Phe-Leu-Gly-NAp

Fig. 7. Time dependence of *p*-nitroaniline release from P-Gly-Phe-Leu-Gly-NAp catalyzed by rat liver tritosomes, Cathepsin B, Cathepsin L, and Cathepsin H. Only the cleavage of the bond between the last amino acid residue and NAp was monitored. Tritosomes: 0.3 ml tritosomes/1 ml reaction mixture. [Cathepsin B] = 1.9 × 10⁻⁷. [Cathepsin L] = 2.4 × 10⁻⁷. [Cathepsin H] = 2.3 × 10⁻⁷.[NAp] = 1.2 × 10⁻³. 0.1 *M* phosphate buffer; pH = 6; EDTA 1 m*M*; Cys 25 m*M* (Cathepsin B) or GSH 5 m*M* (Cathepsins L, H); 40°C. (From KOPEČEK 1984b; results of REJMANOVÁ et al. 1983)

drugs bound to the very same polymeric carrier will have different rates of release. The influence of the structure of the leaving group on its rate of release is shown in Fig. 9 (KOPEČEK et al. 1985). The fast release of puromycin may be due to the fact that its structure in the vicinity of the NH₂ groups (attachment site) is similar to that of aromatic amino acids. Thus, from the three leaving groups compared above, puromycin may fit into the active site of thiol proteinases most easily.

IV. Relationship Between Susceptibility to Enzymatically Catalyzed Hydrolysis and Biological Activity

The results obtained in vitro using cell cultures and in vivo are consistent with the concept of intralysosomal delivery. TROUET et al. (1982a,b) studied the activity of DNM, coupled covalently to succinylated bovine serum albumin

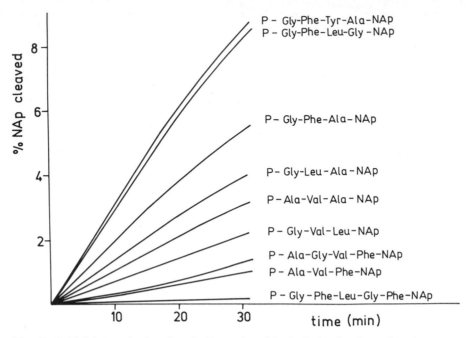

Fig. 8. Initial interval of cathepsin B catalyzed hydrolysis of polymeric substrates. Conditions of cleavage see Fig. 7. (From Kopeček 1984b)

via oligopeptide spacers composed of one to four amino acid residues, against L1210 leukemia in mice. The activity of the conjugate without the spacer or with one amino acid residue was negligible, whereas the conjugates with longer spacers were more active. The increase in biological activity corresponded to the increase in the rate of DNM release by lysosomal enzymes.

Říhová and Kopeček (1985) and Říhová et al. (1988) studied the immunosuppressive activity of DNM-HPMA copolymer-anti Thy 1.2 antibody conjugates in mice. The cytotoxicity of these conjugates was dependent on the degradability of the oligopeptide spacer. When the drug was bound via a nondegradable (Gly-Gly) spacer the conjugates were inactive, whereas incorporation of a degradable spacer (Gly-Phe-Leu-Gly) rendered them biologically active (Table 6). Similar results were obtained with HPMA copolymer-DNM (or ADR) conjugates containing fucosylamine or galactosamine as targeting moieties. These conjugates were active against mouse leukemia L1210 in vivo only when the oligopeptide linking the drug to the polymeric backbone was susceptible to lysosomal degradation (Kopeček and Duncan 1987; Duncan et al. 1988, 1989).

HPMA copolymers modified with galactosamine interact with the asialoglycoprotein receptor on hepatocytes. Subcellular fractionation of liver cells after administration of these copolymers to rats confirmed that they were

Polymer Structure	% drug released after 5 h incubation with tritosomes	Drug Structure
P-G-F-L-G-PRM	62	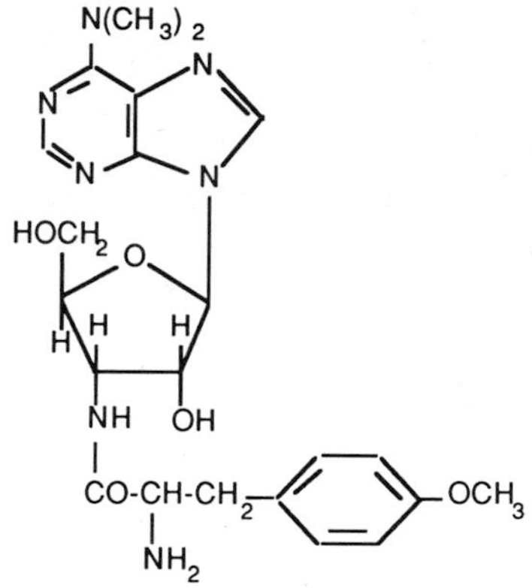
P-G-F-L-G-NAp	45	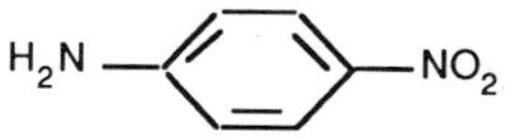
P-G-F-L-G-DNM	12	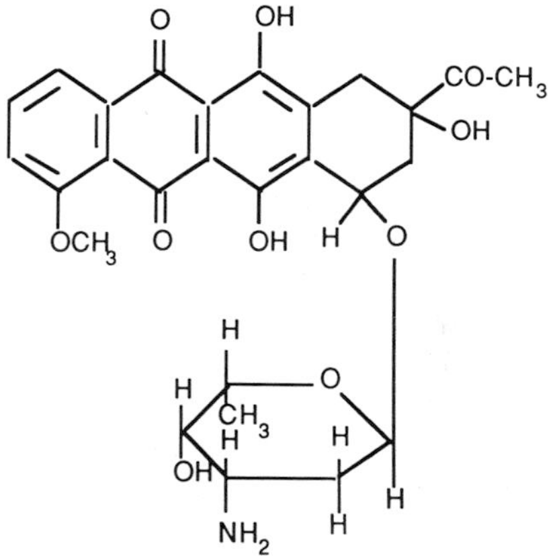

Fig. 9. Relation between the structure of drug and the rate of its release from the carrier by a mixture of tritosomes isolated from rat liver. PRM, puromycin; NAp, *p*-nitroaniline; DNM, daunomycin. Conditions of cleavage: phosphate/citrate buffer pH 5.5; 1 m*M* EDTA; 0.2% triton X-100; 4 mg substrate/ml; 300 µl tritosomes/ml/37°C. (From KOPEČEK et al. 1985)

Table 6. In vivo suppression of sheep red blood cell antibody response. (From ŘíHOVÁ et al. 1988)

Polymer structure	Total dose per mouse		Suppression (% of control)
	Immunoglobulin (mg)	DNM (mg)	
P⟨Gly-Phe-Leu-Gly-DNM / Gly-Phe-Leu-Gly-ATS	3.0	0.4	98
P⟨Gly-Gly-DNM / Gly-Gly-ATS	3.0	0.6	0

Suppression is determined by the number of plaque-forming cells.
P, N-(2-hydroxypropyl)methacrylamide copolymer backbone; DNM, daunomycin; ATS, anti-Thy 1.2 antibodies.

internalized by hepatocytes and that radiolabeled model drug was liberated intralysosomally and passed out of the lysosome across its membrane (DUNCAN et al. 1986).

E. Targeting

I. Principles of Targeting

Current methods of chemotherapy are not optimal due to nonspecific uptake of drug in tissue other than that which the drug is intended to cure. In addition, large doses are often required to produce a therapeutic effect. Hence many undesirable side effects often result. For example, ADR, an anthracycline antibiotic, has shown a wide variety of activity in the treatment of nonlymphocytic leukemia, lymphomas, and human solid tumors including those of the breast, lung, ovary, head, bladder, prostate, and soft tissue sarcomas. However, toxic effects of ADR include myelosuppression, cardiomyopathy, nausea, vomitting, and hair loss (YOUNG et al. 1981). Myelosuppression is the acute dose-limiting toxicity, while cardiomyopathy is the cumulative dose-limiting toxicity. The incidence of congestive heart failure is proportional to the total dose (LEFRAK et al. 1973). Attempts have been made to sequester higher levels of drug in the diseased tissue than in the normal tissue to increase pharmacologic activity and to decrease side effects. Binding a low MW drug to a polymeric carrier changes its characteristics such that it can enter cells by fluid phase pinocytosis, a slow process. Some types of cancer cells maintain a higher endocytic rate than other cells. This difference in rate in these particular systems may be taken advantage of to accumulate more polymer bound drug in cancer cells than normal cells. LAGUEUX et al. (1984) used a DNM-albumin conjugate to target mouse P388D1 leukemia in CDF1 mice. These cells have a high endocytic rate and the conjugate was effective against them both in vivo and in vitro. Although the conjugate proved more efficacious than the free drug, nonspecific uptake remained a problem. Targeting drugs with targeting moieties to cell surface receptors or antigens on specific cells is a more promising approach, which should decrease undesirable side effects from the interaction of drugs with healthy cells. Consequently, the pharmacologic activity should be increased by having a greater amount of drug in the target tissue than in normal tissue.

Targeting moieties such as carbohydrates and hormones specific for cell surface receptors and antibodies specific for cell surface antigens have been suggested to direct polymeric drug carriers to specific cell subsets. (For informative reviews on polymeric antitumor drugs see Dorn et al. 1985, Ferrutti and Tanzi 1986, Sezaki et al, 1989 and Hoes and Feijen 1989.) The main criteria to be followed in designing these targetable polymer conjugates are (Schneider et al. 1984):

1. The carrier must be able to penetrate anatomical barriers in order to reach the target tissue where it must be recognized by the target tissue and internalized into cells by pinocytosis.
2. The conjugate must be inactive during transport and only activated upon drug release (e.g., lysosomal) or activation at the target tissue.
3. The carrier must be nontoxic, nonimmunogenic, and ideally biodegradable.

Targeting polymeric drug carriers to intracellular organelles, for instance lysosomes, is advantageous. Fortuitously, the lysosome is the natural target of endocytosed macromolecules within the cell. Polymers can be designed with spacer arms that require lysosomal enzymes for drug release and ultimately drug activation. Also, it is often the case that the drug to be targeted is actually a lysosomal enzyme for the therapy of lysosomal storage diseases.

II. Obstacles to Targeted Drug Delivery

There are a number of barriers to selective drug delivery in vivo (Poznansky and Juliano 1984; Tomlinson 1987). There is an endothelial barrier between the lumen of the vasculature and the extravascular compartment. It is not well-understood how solutes are transported from the plasma to tissue fluid. However, there is a relatively high permeability to water soluble macromolecules. The vascular endothelium contains plasmalemmal vesicles that are derived from the plasma membrane luminal side of the capillary. They originate by a process identical to pinocytosis. The vesicles are then transcytosed and avoid the lysosome. A hypothesis exists that there are receptors on the luminal face of the endothelial cell that are responsible for transporting proteins; however, details of the specificity of this system are unknown. The capillary endothelium is supported by a basement membrane, the basal lamina. The ability of this material to ultrafilter macromolecules is a concern. Size, charge, and binding characteristics of the macromolecule are factors.

The reticuloendothelial system is also an obstacle to drug delivery using macromolecular drugs. The liver Kupffer cells, macrophages of the spleen, blood phagocytes and monocytes, and tissue and alveolar macrophages are phagocytic and sequester macromolecules. The macrophages have Fc receptors as well as receptors for at least two complement components (C3b and C5b). Different IgG isotypes in drug conjugates can bind to macrophages through protease sensitive F_c receptors.

Protein carriers themselves may be immunogenic in which case anti-carrier antibodies are formed causing complex formation and subsequent elimination by the reticuloendothelial system. It is possible as well for polymeric drug carriers, especially if complex carbohydrates are involved, to activate the complement system. If complement components are activated, especially C3b could remain attached to the carrier and the complex could be taken up via C3b receptors of the macrophage. All these sequestering mechanisms by the reticuloendothelial system would cause drug to be eliminated before reaching its destination

Extravasation into target tissue is a major concern when using polymer bound drugs (especially targeted by antibodies). Normally, the high hydrostatic pressure at the arterial end of the capillary forces proteinaceous fluid through the capillary wall. At the venular end, the hydrostatic pressure is lower and the colloid osmotic pressure of plasma proteins causes the readsorption of water and electrolytes. However, protein cannot be readsorbed and, along with some water and electrolytes, is drained by the lymph system. Macromolecular drugs may not circulate and distribute in the same way as plasma protein, even if they are the same size. Specific shape, electrostatic charge, and carbohydrate content all contribute. Small changes can make a plasma protein seem totally foreign.

Targeting, especially targeting anticancer drugs to cancer cells, is a problem for many reasons (BAGSHAWE 1989; PIMM 1988). Different molecules can be exploited for targeting such as antibodies, saccharides, growth factors, protein or peptide hormones. In vitro the targeting systems are effective, but once attempted in vivo they are not as promising. Cancer cells in particular have unique problems in terms of determining targeting moieties particular to target cells. Loss of specific receptors, down-regulation of tumor associated antigens, and antibody shedding into body fluids are processes inherent to cancer cells. The fact that tumor cells contain a heterogeneous distribution of receptors and also continually change or mutate might make it more feasible to use a cocktail of monoclonal antibodies instead of a single monoclonal against one single antigen. In the future it would be worthwhile to devise targeting strategies against transformational states of the cancer cell that may not be subjected to barriers known so far. For example, oncogenes themselves, regulatory genetic elements associated with oncogenes, or initial transcription or translation products may be targeted (POZNANSKY and JULIANO 1984).

There are also issues of molecular size, clearance, penetration, lipo-philicity, and dwell time. HAGAN et al. (1986) studied the effect of tumor size on the incorporation of monoclonal antibodies in human tumors grown in nude mice. The results sustain that radiopharmaceuticals taken up by tumors are inversely proportional to tumor size. These results were independent of antibody class, type of tumor, target antigen, or antigen mobility. This suggests that the antibodies may be reaching the tumor surface but penetra-tion is a problem.

1. Multidrug Resistance

An obstacle to drug delivery in chemotherapy found with low MW drugs is multidrug resistance. It has been the subject of intense study in recent years. Multidrug resistance (MDR) is a complex phenotype involving resistance to a variety of unrelated low MW drugs. A wide variety of biochemical changes have been detected in MDR cell lines (LING 1987). The most constant alteration found is the overexpression of the P-glycoprotein and gene amplifi-cation (RIORDAN and LING 1985).

P-glycoprotein is a plasma membrane glycoprotein of about 170 kD. It functions as an energy-dependent export pump to reduce intracellular levels of anticancer drugs. The cytoplasmic domain probably couples energy from ATP to export drugs through a channel formed by the transmembrane segments of P-glycoprotein (LING et al. 1988). Studies with monoclonal antibodies against P-glycoprotein indicate that it is conserved in size and immunogenicity. The degree of drug resistance that a cell offers correlates with the amount of P-glycoprotein on the cell surface. Gene amplification seems to be the foundation of P-glycoprotein overexpression.

In changing the transport properties of the drug by binding it to a polymer carrier, it may be possible to overcome MDR in some cases. Also, it may be possible to use the P-glycoprotein on the surface of MDR cells as a target. However, at this point, not enough is known to decide if an intra-cellularly acting or a surface active drug should be used in designing these conjugates.

III. Targeting Lysosomes with Carbohydrate Moieties

Carbohydrates were suggested as targeting moieties for polymer bound drugs following the discovery of a number of natural recognition systems. Desialated serum glycoproteins were found to be cleared from the circulation rapidly because their exposed carbohydrate residues could be recognized by recep-tors which mediate their clearance. In addition, in nature, lysosomal enzymes are sequestered into the lysosomes of cells upon their synthesis, also by receptors which recognize carbohydrate residues. Synthetic polymers and glycoconjugates have been designed with pendant carbohydrate groups to exploit the natural recognition systems to allow incorporation of the drug into cells with specificity for those carbohydrate groups.

1. Asialoglycoproteins

Glycoconjugates (glycoproteins and glycolipids) are known to be essential components of plasma membranes of all mammalian cells. Membrane glyco-conjugates are natural receptors of viruses, bacteria, parasites, bacterial and plant toxins, lectins, and antibodies (MONSIGNY et al. 1983). ASHWELL and MORELL (1974) discovered that desialated serum glycoproteins have reduced survival times in the circulation compared to the native form of the same proteins. Desialating serum glycoproteins exposes galactosyl residues which causes rapid removal and sequestration of the proteins by the liver. A specific receptor (asialoglycoprotein receptor) (ASHWELL and HARFORD 1982) was found on the cell surface of hepatocytes that actually controls the clearance of the desialated serum glycoproteins. The receptor recognizes both galactose and N-acetyl-galactosamine. Upon binding, the protein enters the cell by receptor-mediated endocytosis and ends up in the lysosome. Five recognition systems have been evaluated (NEUFELD and ASHWELL 1980):

1. Galactose/mammalian hepatocytes
2. L-fucose/mammalian macrophages
3. N-acetylglucosamine/avian hepatocytes
4. N-acetylglucosamine or mannose/mammalian reticuloendothelial cells
5. Mannose-6-phosphate/human fibroblasts.

For the hepatocytes in both systems, Ca^{+2} is required in order to bind nonreducing carbohydrate moieties of circulating proteins (NEUFELD and ASHWELL 1980). These carbohydrate recognition systems are very specific. In fact, in the alveolar macrophage system, mannose α-1,6 binds to the receptor, while α-1,3 or α-1,2 do not. It may be the case that a more complex structure is recognized, composed of more than one sugar (STAHL et al. 1978).

2. Lysosomal Hydrolases

In the normal cell, lysosomal enzymes are glycoproteins that are synthesized in the rough endoplasmic reticulum; they are modified by glycosylation during or just after their cotranslational translocation into the lumen of the endoplasmic reticulum. Carbohydrate modification happens during transit through both the endoplasmic reticulum and the Golgi apparatus. The enzymes are then transported somehow from the *trans* side of the Golgi to the lysosome. In fibroblasts, a recognition system has been discovered in which the sequestration of lysosomal enzymes is dependent on a membrane receptor that recognizes mannose 6-phosphate residues on lysosomal enzymes. The receptor and enzyme are separated in a prelysosomal compartment. The receptor is recycled and the enzyme enters the lysosome.

3. Glycoconjugates

Neoglycoproteins are synthetic glycoconjugates in which synthetic or natural carbohydrates are coupled to proteins. These are advantageous in studying the role of carbohydrates in the binding and cellular uptake of glycoproteins because naturally occurring glycoproteins are difficult to acquire in pure form. It is also desirable to study the differences in uptake characteristics of the same protein containing different sugar residues. If natural glycoproteins are used, terminal carbohydrate residues must be sequentially removed to reveal different carbohydrate structures. Again, pure products are difficult to obtain. Lee and Lee (1982) reviewed the various chemistries used in the synthesis of neoglycoproteins with regard to mild reaction conditions, control of reaction, availability and stability of reagents, versatility, and linkage characteristics. The use of these probes in in vitro and in vivo uptake studies was also discussed.

L-Fucose terminated glycoconjugates are recognized and internalized by macrophages via the same receptor that mediates the plasma clearance and uptake of lysosomal glycosidases. The macrophage receptor is capable of binding a number of glycoconjugates, especially those bearing mannose or fucose residues. ^{125}I-L-fucose-albumin and rat β-glucuronidase were cleared at a high rate from the plasma circulation after i.v. administration. However, β-glucuronidase is not cleared if L-fucose-albumin or D-mannose-albumin are administered. The results indicate that L-fucose or L-fucose-oligosaccharides are good ligands and inhibitors of macrophage receptors when coupled to albumin. It was found that the receptor that binds the L-fucose conjugate is identical to the one that binds D-mannose glycoconjugates (Shepherd et al. 1981).

Galactose terminated residues are endocytosed into hepatocytes via receptor-mediated pinocytosis. Limet et al. (1985) followed the internalization process of galactosylated serum albumin and polymeric IgA in the hepatocytes of rat liver. The two compounds were internalized by two different receptor systems, but they were internalized together. Both ligands were found to localize in similar coated pits, coated vesicles, and electron lucent vesicles. It was concluded that, because the galactosylated serum albumin ended up in the lysosome and the polymeric IgA ended up in bile, a sorting process must be taking place. Studies of this type are important in order to learn the intracellular fate of drug carriers targeted with carbohydrate moieties.

An MTX conjugate of a neoglycoprotein, mannosyl bovine serum albumin (BSA), was targeted efficiently to the surface mannosyl receptors of murine peritoneal macrophages (Chakraborty et al. 1990). The conjugate (containing 30 moles of MTX per mole of neoglycoprotein) strongly inhibited the growth of *Leishmania donovani* inside macrophages. The targetable conjugate was 100 times more active than free MTX, whereas MTX bound to

BSA or nonspecific neoglycoproteins, e.g., galactosyl BSA and glucosyl BSA, had leishmanicidal effects comparable to free MTX.

Adenine-9-β-D-arabinofuranoside (ara-A) is a drug currently used for the treatment of chronic hepatitis B. Its mechanism of action reduces serum levels of virus DNA polymerase causing the disappearance of infectivity and disease reduction. Side effects of this drug include gastrointestinal and neurological disorders. In addition, bone marrow depression is apparent with high doses. FIUME et al. (1982) selectively delivered this agent using asialofetuin or galactosaminated serum albumin to mouse hepatocytes in vivo to eliminate side effects due to nonspecific uptake. In another study (FIUME et al. 1983), ara-A was coupled to asialofetuin (AF) and lactosaminated serum albumin. The activity of the conjugates was evaluated in mice infected by the ectromelia virus. The quantity of ara-A required to inhibit DNA synthesis in liver was about ten times smaller when the compound was conjugated to lactosaminated serum albumin than when it was administered as free drug. The targeted delivery of antiviral drugs was recently reviewed (FIUME et al. 1988).

MONSIGNY et al. (1983) reviewed the use of lectins and related substances as toxins and drug carriers. Plant toxins such as ricin, abrin, and modeccin bind to cell surface glycoproteins having an exposed galactose residue. These plant toxins consist of an A and a B chain. The A chain is an enzyme that catalyzes the transfer of ADP ribose from NAD to cytosolic protein elongation factor II and is responsible for the toxicity of the toxin. The B chain is involved in the specific binding of the toxin to cell surface glycoconjugates and enables cell entry. Only the A unit is needed to block protein synthesis and, due to its toxicity, only one molecule is required for specific targeting (MONSIGNY et al. 1983).

Many glycoproteins have been used to target the A chain to specific cell types. A disulfide bond was used to link the fragment A of diphtheria toxin (DTA) to AF (CAWLEY et al. 1981). It was found that this conjugate was 600- and 1800-fold more effective in inhibiting protein synthesis in rat hepatocytes than either whole diphtheria toxin or DTA, respectively. Concentration dependence studies showed that the conjugate, at a concentration as low as 10 pM, still showed an effect. AF was also used as a carrier to target primaquine to hepatocytes to treat the exoerythrocytic stage of malaria. Another example was delivering DNM to hepatocytes in vivo and to hepatoma (Hep G2) cells in vitro with a human serum albumin-DNM-galactose conjugate. Pharmacokinetic studies after i.v. administration of the conjugate in mice and rats showed a plasma half-life of 12 minutes and nearly complete uptake of the conjugate in the liver (TROUET and JOLLES 1984).

4. Synthetic and Natural Polymers

It was shown that HPMA copolymers modified with galactosamine interact with the asialoglycoprotein receptor on hepatocytes (DUNCAN et al. 1986; CARTLIDGE et al. 1987) very efficiently. The influence of the structure of

HPMA copolymers and the manner of administration on their activity in vivo was established. Subcellular fractionation of the liver (and isolation of hepatocytes) after administration of galactosamine modified HPMA copolymers to rats (DUNCAN et al. 1986) confirmed that they were internalized by hepatocytes and localized in the lysosomal compartment.

HPMA copolymers containing a tetrapeptide side chain (Gly-Phe-Leu-Gly) terminated in ADR and, optionally, galactosamine, as a targeting moiety (KOPEČEK et al. 1985), were recently approved in the United Kingdom for phase I/phase II clinical trials to treat primary hepatoma. Similarly, HPMA copolymers containing the anthracycline antibiotics, DNM (DUNCAN et al. 1987, 1988) and ADR (DUNCAN et al. 1989) were modified with fucosylamine, and it was shown that they interact with the receptor on L1210 cells in vitro and in vivo. Subsequent experiments were performed to test the pharmacologic activity of these conjugates in vivo against L1210 leukemia in DBA$_2$ mice. Two localizations of tumor were chosen: intraperitoneal and subcutaneous. In both cases, experimental animals were treated intraperitoneally with free drug or drug-HPMA copolymer conjugates. HPMA copolymers containing anthracycline antibiotics showed therapeutic effects only when the oligopeptide sequence between the drug and the polymeric carrier was biodegradable (Gly-Phe-Leu-Gly) in the lysosomal compartment of the cell. HPMA copolymer conjugates which contained a nondegradable oligopeptide sequence (Gly-Gly) were not active. HPMA copolymer prodrugs produced increased life spans and an increased number of long-term survivors (KOPEČEK and DUNCAN 1987; DUNCAN et al. 1987, 1988, 1989) depending on the structure of the conjugate, timing of administration, and number of doses (Table 7).

In addition, an HPMA copolymer has been synthesized with the incorporation of chlorin e$_6$ (a photosensitizer) and galactosamine (targeting moiety) into its side chains. This conjugate was tested for biological activity in vitro on a human hepatoma cell line PLC/PRF/5 (Alexander cells) containing asialoglycoprotein receptors; the conjugate was more active than a similar conjugate without targeting moiety (galactosamine). Both polymeric conjugates were less dark toxic than free chlorin e$_6$ (KRINICK et al. 1988). HPMA copolymers can therefore be very versatile carriers. By incorporation of different drugs and carbohydrate moieties they can direct drugs to specific cell subsets for specific purposes (KOPEČEK 1984b, 1988, 1990).

SCHACHT et al. (1988) also took advantage of the asialoglycoprotein receptor system in hepatocytes. Galactose (mono, di, or tri) was linked to chloroformate activated dextrans of varying MWs. Although the data is preliminary, they found that all dextran conjugates of MW 40000 were taken up by Kupffer cells in rat liver. Lower (6000) MW conjugates were preferentially sequestered by hepatocytes only if substituted with monogalactose ligands. Surprisingly, none of the conjugates of intermediate MW were taken up by the liver at all. Therefore, the combination of polymer and targeting moiety affects preferential uptake by selected cell types.

Table 7. Effect of intravenous N-(2-hydroxypropyl)methacrylamide copolymer-adriamycin administration on DBA$_2$ mice bearing L1210 leukemia. (From DUNCAN et al. 1989)

Experiment	Treatment	Dose (mg/kg)	Day of administration	Day of death	Mean survival time ± SE	Long-term survivors
L1210 (i.p.)	None	–	–	14, 14, 15, 16, 16, 17, 17, 18, 40	18 ± 2.4	0/10
	P-Gly-Phe-Leu-Gly-ADR	–	–	17, 18, 19, 25	19.8 ± 1.8*	1/5
	P<Gly-Phe-Leu-Gly-Gal	5	1	14, 15, 16, 20, 24	17.8 ± 1.8^{NS}	0/5
	P<Gly-Phe-Leu-Gly-ADR / Gly-Phe-Leu-Gly-fuc	5	1	16, 18, 47	27 ± 10.0^{NS}	2/5
L1210 (i.p.)	None	–	–	10, 14, 14, 15, 15, 15, 15, 15	14.1 ± 0.6	0/8
	P-Gly-Phe-Leu-Gly-ADR	10	1	15, 17, 19, 35	21.5 ± 4.6*	0/4
	P-Gly-Phe-Leu-Gly-ADR	20	1	21, 21, 24, 38	26.0 ± 4.1**	1/5
	P-Gly-Phe-Leu-Gly-ADR	40	1	26, 35, 40, 47	37.0 ± 4.4***	1/5
	P<Gly-Phe-Leu-Gly-ADR / Gly-Phe-Leu-Gly-Gal	10	1	16, 16, 42	24.7 ± 8.7*	0/3
	P<Gly-Phe-Leu-Gly-ADR / Gly-Phe-Leu-Gly-Gal	20	1	20, 23	21.5	3/5
	P<Gly-Phe-Leu-Gly-ADR / Gly-Phe-Leu-Gly-Gal	40	1	20, 26, 48	33.5 ± 6.4*	1/5

* $p < 0.05$; ** $p < 0.01$; *** $p < 0.001$.

IV. Antibodies

A great amount of work has been done with antibodies to target drugs to specific cells, especially for cancer therapy. Theoretically, targeting with antibodies is ideal because antibody-antigen interactions are very specific. There are basically three types of antigens that can be used as targeting moieties for antibodies: organotypic, tumor associated antigens (TAA), and tumor specific antigens. Organotypic antigens would restrict the uptake of the drug-antibody conjugate to one cell type; however, it would not restrict uptake to the tumor cell. TAAs are present on the surface of embryonic cells and reappear in the course of malignant transformations or exist in small amounts on normal cells and in large amounts on tumor cells. Tumor specific antigens may be expressed during malignant transformations and are expressed at the surface of tumor cells (SCHNEIDER et al. 1984).

Monoclonal antibodies have been produced which react with a wide range of human cancers, including carcinomas of the colon, rectum, breast, ovary, lung, pancreas, and bladder, malignant melanomas, bone and soft tissue sarcomas, and leukemias. The absolute tumor specificity of many antitumor monoclonal antibodies is hard to define, and only with antibodies to idiotypes on B cell tumors is it virtually certain that tumor specificity has been obtained (PIMM 1988).

Saccharides of the cell surface are important tumor associated and differentiation antigens (FEIZI 1984). They belong to a family of carbohydrates which also includes the major blood group antigens: A,B, H, Le^a, and Le^b. The expression of these carbohydrates varies during different stages of embryogenesis, differentiation, and oncogenesis. The availability of donor substrates, activity of glycosyl transferases, or genes that code for the biosynthesis of these enzymes, can be factors in the changes found in the carbohydrate structures. Monoclonals are useful in the detection of glycosylation changes and to study the biochemistry of these changes; however, their performance in tumor localization did not meet expectations.

1. Antibody-Drug Conjugates

Antibody linked drugs enter cells by receptor-mediated endocytosis and eventually end up in the cell lysosome. Although there is limited success in binding drugs directly to an antibody, there are several disadvantages. Antibody solubility may be altered by binding hydrophobic drugs. This restricts the number of drug molecules that can be delivered by an antibody molecule. Also, antibody activity may be effected by binding drugs; the degree of loss of activity differs depending on the binding method.

TROUET and JOLLÉS (1984) have tried various drug carriers including antibodies against tumor specific antigens, antibodies against TAA, and antibodies to tissue specific antigens as tumor vectors. One example is in the human breast cell system. Primary tumor and metastases have organotypic antigens. An antibody against human milk fat globule membrane (HMFGM) that is recognized by both normal and tumor breast cells as a drug carrier was used. This antibody (7F11C7) was tested against normal and tumoral tissues and reacted with 19 out of 19 tested breast carcinomas as well as with lymph and lymph node metastatic cells. There was, however, some cross-reaction with normal epithelial cells of nonbreast origin. The binding, uptake, and subcellular distribution was studied on a human breast carcinoma cell line (MCF-7). The antibody was internalized by receptor-mediated pinocytosis and gained access to lysosomes. A DNM-antibody conjugate was synthesized. However, only three drug molecules could be bound to the antibody without altering its activity. It was concluded that there is a need for developing a high ratio of drug molecule to IgG molecule in order to introduce a cell killing effect before antigenic modulation may occur (TROUET and JOLLÉS 1984). This again stresses the importance of an intermediate polymeric carrier.

DNM was linked covalently to monoclonal antibodies against carcino-embryonic antigen (CEA). The conjugate was tested in vitro for thymidine incorporation in human colon adenocarcinoma cells which express CEA. The conjugate was more active than either drug or antibody alone. Combinations were also less effective than the conjugate. Preliminary data on the in vivo pharmacologic activity of DNM-anti-CEA conjugates, using CEA producing LoVo cells grafted in nude mice, confirmed the in vitro experiments (PAGE and EMOND 1983).

DURRANT et al. (1987) studied colorectal cancer in which many cell lines are resistant to most cytotoxic drugs. Monoclonal 791T/36 antibodies against osteogenic sarcoma cells were used. Dividing cells have been isolated from primary colorectal tumors and their response to free drug or 791/T36 antibody-drug conjugates studied. Eight different cell lines were investigated; they were sensitive in varying degrees to different drugs (MTX, 5-fluorouracil, and DNM) bound to the antibody. The results have shown that cell lines which were resistant to MTX were more sensitive to antibody-MTX conjugates. This very important study shows that newly established cell lines that are resistant to classical chemotherapeutic agents are rendered sensitive when the drug enters the cell as a drug-antibody conjugate.

a) Antibody Binding Methods

The method of antibody binding is important in terms of preserving antibody and drug activity. Examples of five different types of antibody activation methods are shown in Fig. 10. HURWITZ et al. (1975) bound DNM and ADR to immunoglobulins via three different methods using the aminosugar moiety of the drug as the binding site: (1) the bond between C-3 and C-4 of the aminosugar was oxidized by periodate. The formed carbonyl group reacted with amino groups of the IgG forming azomethine bonds which were reduced with sodium borohydride; (2) drugs and IgG were conjugated via glu-taraldehyde; (3) drugs and IgG were conjugated using a water soluble carbodiimide   (1-ethyl-3-(3-dimethylaminopropyl)carbodiimide·HCl).   The

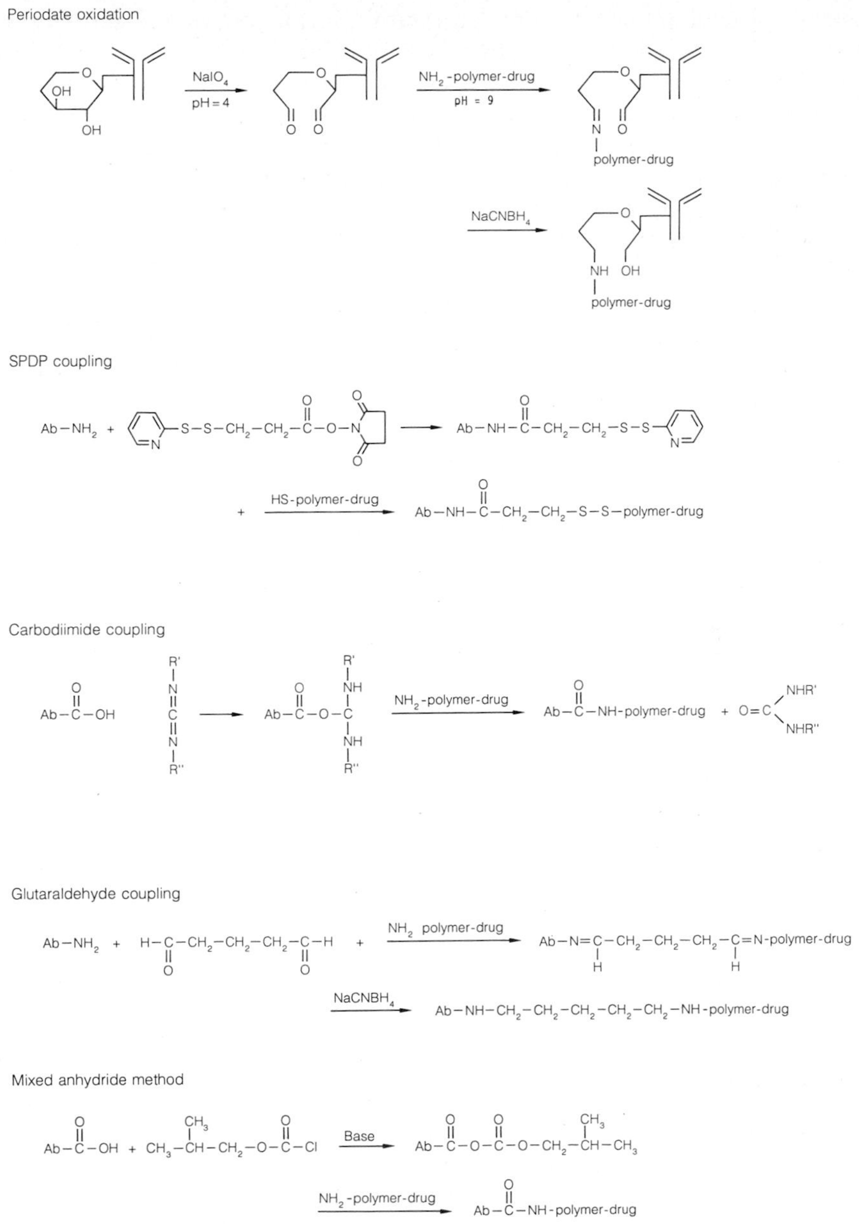

Periodate oxidation

SPDP coupling

Carbodiimide coupling

Glutaraldehyde coupling

Mixed anhydride method

Fig. 10. Antibody activation methods of binding of polymeric drug carriers

inhibition of [^{3}H] uridine incorporation into target cells (B cell leukemia) was used to quantitate the activity of conjugates. Other target cells were tested including other tumor lines, such as YAC, Moloney virus induced lymphoma in A/J mice, and PC5, a Balb/c plasmocytoma. The drug activity was best preserved with method (2) and least with (3). The activity of antibody was best preserved using the periodate oxidation (method 1).

RODWELL et al. (1986) compared the method of antibody oxidation of carbohydrate moieties with other methods. The oxidation method yielded active antibody (mouse monoclonal anti-phosphocholine IgM). However, in using lysine, aspartic acid, or glutamic acid side chains for binding, binding was found to be heterogeneous and antibody affinity was decreased. An antibody with an ^{125}I-labeled peptide or a diethylenetriaminopentaacetic acid chelate of ^{111}In bound in the carbohydrate position localized better in a tumor in vivo (nude mice/subcutaneous xenograft) than if the tyrosines or lysines of the antibody were labeled. Similarly, in preliminary experiments it was found that when HPMA copolymers containing chlorin e_6 and an anti-Thy 1.2 antibody bound via carbohydrate moieties were more photodynamically active against (A/J mice) T lymphocytes in vitro than when binding was via free N^ε-amino lysine residues of the antibody molecule (KRINCK et al. 1990). Therefore the method of antibody binding is critical in the overall efficacy of the conjugate. It appears that the oligosaccharide modification of antibodies is a preferred mehtod for the preparation of conjugates.

ALVAREZ et al. (1986) used ^{111}In-labeled antibodies for tumor imaging and found minimal nonspecific uptake when the antibody was modified at carbohydrate residues. With other methods, problems were encountered such as hepatic uptake, aggregated or denatured antibodies, instability of the radiolabel, binding of antibodies to F_c receptors mainly in the liver, and clearance by the reticuloendothelial system. Monoclonal antibodies against rat surface alloantigens were used to image a subcutaneous Brown Norway (BN) rat lymphoma implanted in nude mice. Excellent imaging was produced.

Another method of binding drugs to an antibody molecule is with carbodiimide coupling. SHEN et al. (1986) synthesized an MTX anti-SSEA-1 (stage specific embryonic antigen) antibody conjugate with this method. They found no change in antibody activity. The conjugate released MTX intracellularly in vitro and inhibited the growth of F-9 teratocarcinoma cells containing the SSEA-1 antigen. Since the antibody was a monoclonal IgM, it was possible to bind 45 drug molecules per antibody molecule. It has ten binding sites, so the chance of reducing activity is much less than for an IgG with only two binding sites per molecule. However, size is a drawback using IgMs.

The method of antibody binding may also have an effect on the clearance of the antibody from the circulation. WORRELL et al. (1986) studied three different ricin A chain-antibody conjugates. They differed in their linking structures: (a) a disulfide linkage using N-succinimidyl-3-(2-pyridyldithio)-propionate cross-linker; (b) a protected disulfide spacer (a methyl group was substituted on the C atom of the bridging structure next to the disulfide linkages), and (c) a sulfide linkage using N-succinimidyl 4-(iodoacetylamino) benzoate. The first compound was more reducible than the second, and the third was not reducible. When administered to animals, all three displayed biphasic kinetics. However, the degree of reducibility had no effect on the early disappearance of the conjugate from the circulation. At later times, the degree of reduction correlated with the rapidity of disappearance. In this study, all three conjugates were cleared from the circulation faster than the unconjugated antibody.

Ricin A chain was linked to a monoclonal IgM against human breast carcinoma via disulfide bonds without altering toxin toxicity or antibody activity (KROLICK et al. 1981). Similarly, BYERS et al. (1988) conjugated the ricin A chain with anti-CEA (228RTA). They found that, by introducing other antibodies against different CEA epitopes, the effects can be potentiated. This in fact led to an increase in retention at the tumor cell surface (198 and B14B8 potentiating antibodies). It was shown that enhanced antibody affinity leads to increased endocytosis of the immunoconjugate and potentiation of cytotoxicity.

KRALOVEC et al. (1989) used a regiospecific coupling method to bind MTX to a mouse anti-human renal cancer monoclonal IgG (Dal K-20). Two conjugates were synthesized. In both cases MTX was bound via γ-carboxyl groups. In one case it was attached to amino groups of the antibody; in the second one to oxidized carbohydrate moieties. The latter conjugate was a somewhat more effective inhibitor of dihydrofolate reductase in vitro and of colony formation by human renal cancer (Caki-1) cells than control nonregiospecific conjugates.

b) F_{ab} Antibody Fragments

As already mentioned, there is a considerable pool of murine monoclonal antibodies available against human tumors (BALDWIN and BYERS 1986). However, there are several problems associated with the use of whole antibody molecules as targeting moieties, some of which may be attributed to the Fc portion of the antibody molecule (HURWITZ et al. 1976). Anti-tumor antibodies may still be toxic to normal cells. This toxicity is complement mediated. Binding of complement occurs via the F_c portion of the immunoglobulin. However, not all drug-antibody molecules reach the target tissue and react with tumor cells. It is desired that the portion of the conjugate which does not interact with the target cell antigen be removed from the circulation as quickly as possible. Since the half-life of $(F_{ab})_2$ in the blood circulation is much shorter than that of the intact immunoglobulin, the former should be superior in this respect. The F_c fragment is the most immunocompetent region of an immunoglobulin and its removal decreases the immunogenicity of the resulting $(F_{ab})_2$. Antibodies bearing the F_c portion may interact with F_c receptors on a number of tissues and thus increase nonspecific toxicity.

Using this concept, HURWITZ et al. (1976) attached DNM to $(F_{ab})_2$ prepared from the imunoglobulin fraction of a rabbit antiserum towards Yac

Moloney virus lymphoma cells. The conjugates containing $(F_{ab})_2$ exerted pharmacologic activity and specificity toward Yac target cells similar to that obtained with conjugates of intact anti-Yac lgG. The activity was manifested both in vitro by inhibition of RNA synthesis and by reduction of the growth of the tumor cells in vivo.

VITETTA et al. (1986) treated BCL_1 leukemia with conjugates of ricin A chain and the F_{ab} against the normal B cell antigen (slgD). It appears that this conjugate is effective in delivering the ricin A chain to tumor cells in vivo and in achieving therapeutic activity.

c) Boron-Neutron Capture Therapy

Boron-neutron capture therapy is based on the nuclear reaction of non-radioactive boron-10 with low energy thermal neutrons. The result is boron-11, an unstable intermediate, which leads to instantaneous fission and the formation of lithium-7 and α particles. This application is attractive because low energy reactants can be converted to cytotoxic agents inside of the cancer cell. Therefore it is necessary that the boron be targeted to tumor tissue for effective therapy. Different boron compounds have been produced containing functional moieties capable of antibody binding without causing protein denaturation. A problem to overcome is the ability to bind sufficient boron atoms to the antibody and still retain immunoreactivity. ALAM et al. (1985) have incorporated 10^3 boron atoms per molecule of monoclonal antibody (17-1A against colorectal carcinoma) via the heterobifunctional cross-linking reagent dicesium N-succinimidyl 3-(undecahydro-*closo*-dodecaboranyldithio)propionate. However, they observed a 90% reduction in antibody activity. To circumvent this problem, ALAM et al. (1989) synthesized isocyanatoundecahydro-*closo*-dodecaborate and isocyanato (trimethylamino)octahydro-*closo*-decaborate, two cross-lingking reagents to link boronated polylysine to antibody molecules. The 3-(2-pyridyldithio) propionic acid N-hydroxysuccinimide ester (SPDP) method was used to modify the boronated polylysine, incorporating a thiol group. Then, the antibody was modified with m-maleimido-benzoyl sulfosuccinimide ester incorporating a free maleimido group. The two modified substances were mixed. With this method, an average of 2700 boron atoms were incorporated into IB 16-6 antibodies against B16 melanoma and 58% immunoreactivity was retained. Other antibodies modified by this method retained 40%–90% immunoreactivity.

d) Targeting Radionuclides

Radiopharmaceuticals are used to study the structure and function of organs. They are also useful for tumor diagnostics as well as internal radiation therapy. As with other drugs, the major problem with radiopharmaceuticals is nonspecific uptake in normal tissue. Therefore, steroid and polypeptide hormones, neurotransmitters, desialated serum glycoproteins, and antibodies are being considered as targeting moieties for radiopharmaceuticals. In the future it may even be possible to detect quantitiative changes in receptor expression with this method. For example, normal breast tissue is low in estradiol receptor content whereas two-thirds of breast cancers contain variable yet higher amounts (CARROLL and ZALUTSKY 1984).

Antibodies and antibody fragments have been investigated for the delivery of radiopharmaceuticals by receptor-mediated pinocytosis. However, many of the methods for attachment of the radioisotope result in unstable conjugates. ROBERTS et al. (1987) labeled a host of immunoglobulins with copper-67 using the metal chelating agent, N-benzyl-5,10,15,20-tetrakis(4-carboxyphenyl)porphine (N-bzHTCPP). The N-benzyl group allows the incorporation of metal ions quickly and easily under mild aqueous conditions suitable for antibodies. Two different coupling methods were studied. First, the chelating agent was activated with either 1-ethyl-3-(3-dimethylaminopropyl)carbodiimide hydrochloride and N-hydroxysuccinimide or 1,1'-carbonyldiimidazole. At best, two porphyrin molecules could be coupled per antibody molecule nonspecifically for either binding strategy. The samples were metalated in a ratio of one copper to one porphyrin molecule. The conjugates were found to be stable because of the tight hold the porphyrin has on the copper and immunoreactivity was retained. There is, however, a problem in using N-bzHTCPP as a metal chelator for binding to antibodies. N-bzHTCPP contains four carboxylate groups which cause antibody cross-linking. For this reason, conjugates were synthesized (ROBERTS et al. 1989) in the same manner using N-4-nitrobenzyl-5-(4-carboxyphenyl)-10,15,20-tris (4-sulfophenyl)porphine (N-bzHCS3P) as a ^{64}Cu or ^{67}Cu metal chelator which only contains one carboxyl group. Again, approximately two porphyrin molecules were coupled per antibody molecule with little or no loss in antibody activity (for the ^{67}Cu conjugate). These conjugates, especially the ^{67}Cu derivatives, have potential for cancer therapy and γ-imaging, particularly if an intermediate polymer carrier will be incorporated in the conjugate.

2. Antibody-Synthetic Polymer-Drug Conjugates

Antibodies usually retain more activity when a water soluble polymer serves as a link between it and the drug. This also makes it possible to bind more drug molecules per antibody without altering solubility. To this end polyclonal and monoclonal anti-Thy 1.2, anti-la^{κ}, or anti-CD3 antibodies were attached to HPMA copolymer-DNM conjugates and the applicability of targeting therapy intervention in lymphatic tissue was studied (ŘÍHOVÁ and KOPEČEK 1985; ŘÍHOVÁ et al., 1986, 1988, 1989a, 1990, 1991). The effect was measured as the inhibition of anti-sheep red blood cell antibody response expressed in plaque-forming cells (Table 8). Targetable HPMA copolymer-DNM (or ADR) conjugates with degradable oligopeptide side chains (Gly-Phe-Leu-Gly) decreased the antibody reaction by 60%–85% in vivo. A comparable amount of free antibody was without a significant effect. The toxicity of the

Table 8. In vivo suppression of anti-sheep red blood cell antibody response by free daunomycin or daunomycin bound to *N*-(2-hydroxypropyl)methacrylamide copolymers with targeting anti Thy 1.2 antibodies. (From Říhová et al. 1988)

Polymer structure	Total dose of		IgM PFC/10^8 spleen cells $\times 10^3$ (mean ± SE)	Suppression (%)
	Immunoglobulin (mg)	DNM (mg)		
P-Gly-Gly-DNM	–	0.33	82 ± 8.3	0
P-Gly-Phe-Leu-Gly-DNM	–	0.33	38 ± 7.6	53.1
P-Gly-Gly-anti-Thy 1.2	4	–	80 ± 13.5	0
P-Gly-Phe-Leu-Gly-anti Thy 1.2	4	–	73 ± 16.2	9.9
P⟨Gly-Gly-DNM / Gly-Gly-anti-Thy 1.2	4	0.44	89 ± 14.3	0
P⟨Gly-Phe-Leu-Gly-DNM / Gly-Phe-Leu-Gly-anti-Thy 1.2	4	0.33	12 ± 3.7	85.2
anti-Thy 1.2	4	–	36 ± 10.8	55.6
DNM	–	0.4	29 ± 8.1	64.2
DNM	–	0.04	45 ± 13.4	44.5
Control	–	–	81 ± 10.3	

The differences between the experimental groups and controls was calculated according to the multiple comparison method and was found significant at the level of 0.05. PFC, plaque-forming cells.

polymeric conjugates against bone marrow, liver, and heart was considerably lower than that of free drug (Říhová et al. 1988). Specificity of targeting with these conjugates was proven in vitro on mouse splenocytes and human peripheral blood lymphocytes and in vivo on inbred strains of mice. Only T cell proliferation and thymus-dependent antibody response was decreased by the polymeric conjugates targeted either with anti-CD3 or anti-Thy 1.2 antibodies (Říhová et al. 1990).

In another study, monoclonal B3/25 antibody against the transferrin receptor was conjugated with HPMA. The uptake of the conjugate in human skin fibroblasts was up to nine fold greater than the uptake of the parent HPMA copolymer (FLANAGAN et al. 1989).

YOKOYAMA et al. (1988, 1989, 1990) prepared a new micelle-forming polymeric drug carrier based on a polyethylene glycol block-polyaspartic acid copolymer (Fig. 77). ADR was bound to this carrier by amido group formation between the amino group of ADR and carboxyl groups of the polyaspartic acid block. This carrier permits a large amount of ADR to be bound. Since the drug is buried in the micellar core, its binding affinity to serum albumin is eliminated. The conjugate of ADR and this carrier was highly active against P388 mouse leukemia in vivo.

An attempt has been made (YOKOYAMA et al. 1988) to bind immunoglobulin to these conjugates. However, as the authors pointed out, binding of

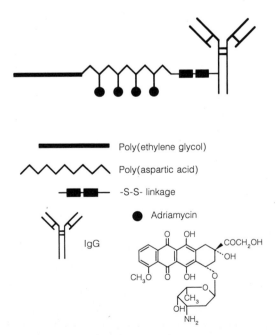

Poly(ethylene glycol)

Poly(aspartic acid)

-S-S- linkage

● Adriamycin

IgG

Fig. 11. A polyethylene glycol-block-polyaspartic acid copolymer containing adriamycin and IgG. (From YOKOYAMA et al. 1989)

IgG to the polyaspartic acid block is not advantageous, since the IgG molecules can be buried inside the micelles. Work is under way to attach IgG molecules to the polyethylene glycol portion of the conjugate. Such conjugates would have great potential in cancer chemotherapy.

3. Antibody-Natural Polymer-Drug Conjugates

Dextran was used to carry DNM to an α-fetoprotein (AFP) producing tumor. An anti-AFP antibody (produced in horse) was used to target the conjugate to rat hepatoma (rat ascites AH66 cell line) in vitro and in vivo. The biological activity of the DNM-dextran-antibody conjugate was measured in vitro by the inhibition of DNA synthesis (inhibition of [³H]thymidine uptake) and the trypan blue exclusion assay. In vivo, animals were injected with hepatoma cells (10^4) and then treated with conjugate on the 3rd, 5th, and 7th day following inoculation. The longest survivors were those treated with the conjugate. In all cases, the conjugate was more effective than free drug, a mixture of free drug and antibody, and antibody-DNM conjugate. It was also found that incorporation of polymer decreased drug toxicity (TSUKADA et al. 1982).

In similar studies (TSUKADA et al. 1987) polyclonal horse or monoclonal mouse antibodies against rat AFP were conjugated to dextran containing DNM. The conjugates were tested in Donryu rats bearing an AFP producing subcutaneous solid hepatoma with metastasis in the lungs. After surgical resection of the tumor (day 14), the conjugate (and appropriate controls) was administered once every other day for five doses beginning on the day of resection. Survival of the conjugate treated animals was substantially pro-longed compared with controls and 60% of them were tumor free on day 100, at which time they were sacrificed. There was a corresponding decrease in serum AFP levels in the circulation of treated animals throughout the treat-ment period. This is an interesting model, because it tests the conjugate against residual tumor burden after resection, which could clinically be important after surgery, as well as targeting to metastatic foci in locations such as in the lungs. Figure 12 illustrates the serum AFP levels for the various combination therapies.

MANABE et al. (1983) linked bleomycin (an anticancer glycopeptide antibiotic) to a murine monoclonal anti-HLA IgG antibody (H-1) through a dextran carrier. An indirect membrane immunofluorescent test was used to observe that the conjugate was approximately 15-fold more toxic in vitro against a B cell line (BALL-1 cells) than free drug.

The properties of a human serum albumin (HSA)-MTX monoclonal antibody (791T/3b) conjugate were studied in order to determine optimal activity with respect to binding activity. Osteogenic sarcoma cell lines were used and the conjugate was evaluated based on its cell binding ability and cytotoxicity using a chronic selenomethionine uptake assay. The conjugate achieved a good balance between cytotoxicity and discrimination. Experi-

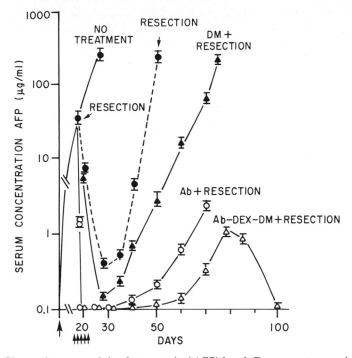

Fig. 12. Change in serum alpha-fetoprotein (*AFP*) level. Donryu rats were inoculated s.c. with 1×10^6 AFP-producing rat hepatoma cells (AH66 cells) in the right thigh. By day 14, solid tumors were present and all animals had micrometastases in their lungs. Tumors were resected on the same day. Treatment was initiated on the same day and every other day for 5 doses; 60% of the animals treated with monoclonal AFP antibody-dextran-daunomycin conjugates survived 100 days after tumor inoculation at which time they were sacrificed. *Resection*, resection only; *DM + resection*, daunomycin + resection; *Ab-DEX-DX + resection*, antibody-dextran-daunomycin conjugate + resection (From TSUKADA et al. 1987)

ments in the presence of cysteine proteinase inhibitors proved the involvement of these enzymes in the mechanism of action of these targetable drug carriers (GARNETT et al. 1985).

SHEN and RYSER (1984) studied an Fc receptor-mediated drug delivery system. These receptors are found mostly in cells of the immune system; they are also present in certain tumor tissues and cultured tumor cells. A conjugate of MTX with HSA was synthesized. Two Fc receptor positive cell lines, WEHI-3 and M5076, were exposed to the conjugate in the presence or absence of anti-HSA antiserum. Both cell types were killed by a low dose (30 nM) of MTX when the conjugate was given in the presence of antiserum but were totally unaffected in the absence of antiserum.

In a follow-up study (SHEN et al. 1989) MTX was conjugated to trinitrophenyl (TNP)-labeled poly-D-lysine, either directly or through a disulfide or triglycine spacer. Conjugates were complexed with heparin and anti-TNP antiserum and tested for their growth inhibitory effects on WEHI-3 cells. The positive results obtained suggest that hapten-polymer conjugates can be used as drug carriers for targeting F_c receptor bearing cells when given with an antihapten antibody.

a) Enzyme Conjugates

Approximately 30 lysosomal storage disorders have been found in humans. (For details see VON FIGURA et al. 1984). Attempts have been made to replace missing enzymes by exploiting natural enzyme specific uptake mechanisms. However, there are problems associated with administering free enzymes alone. For one, repeated doses are needed to overcome protein degradation and turnover. The enzymes can be highly immunogenic especially with the second and following doses. Also targeting and permeability barriers must be taken into account. To try and overcome these problems, enzyme-albumin conjugates were synthesized (POZNANSKY 1984). The reasons for choosing albumin as a polymeric carrier were that it is natural and abundant, it has a relatively long circulation time, and its normal function is probably the transport of fatty acids, steroids, and polypeptide hormones. It is also fairly stable. Uricase, superoxide dismutase, catalase, and L-asparaginase were bound to albumin using glutaraldehyde, water soluble carbodiimides, sodium periodate, and other bifunctional reagents. The enzymes retained approximately 90% activity. To achieve selectivity, polyclonal antibodies against rat hepatocytes were incorporated into the α-1,4 glucosidase-albumin conjugate. Whereas the conjugate in the absence of specific antibodies was directed primarily to Kupffer cells, the presence of a conjugated antibody (specific for hepatoctes) resulted in a redirection of the enzyme to hepatocytes, the cells which exhibit severe glycogen storage and dysfunction in Pompe's disease (POZNANSKY 1984).

POZNANSKY et al. (1982) studied conjugates for other enzyme therapies and found that L-asparaginase-albumin conjugates were about 20 times more effective against 6C3HED lymphosarcoma in C3H/He mice than free enzyme. The increased effectiveness of the polymer bound L-asparaginase was attributed to its resistance to enzymatic degradation. To obtain a higher tumor/ normal cell ratio, monoclonal antibodies were introduced into these polymer conjugates (POZNANSKY 1986).

V. Hormones

Peptide hormones enter cells by receptor-mediated endocytosis. Cell entry is by the same mechanism as for transport proteins. Receptors are located in clathrin-coated pits or aggregate there upon hormone binding. The pit invaginates and pinches off intracellularly forming a clathrin-coated vesicle. Once the clathrin coat is shed, the fate of the hormone, receptor, or hormone-receptor complex is determined. Either the endosome containing hormone and receptor fuses with lysosomes, the receptor recycles or is sequestered, or a combination of the two takes place. Nevertheless, the fate of the hormone is degradation in the lysosome. There is ongoing controversy over whether or not the internalized and/or degraded hormone triggers a cellular response; however, most experiments to date imply that internalization causes the action of the hormone to cease. Details of hormone receptor-mediated endocytosis may be found in SEGALOFF and ASCOLI (1988).

Hormones can be used as targeting vectors because they have corresponding specific receptors. The advantages of using hormones as opposed to other targeting moieties are that they are relatively easy to obtain in pure form, they are not bound by Fc receptors recognized by macrophages, and no allergic reactions are anticipated. However, in vitro results are more promising than in vivo. One problem is that receptors are multispecific. There could be a number of possible places within the binding site capable of binding structurally unrelated compounds (VARGA and ASATO 1983).

Cancer cells often have receptors for hormones. Melanotropin (MSH) binds to specific receptors on the plasma membrane of murine melanoma cells, especially those in the G-2 phase of the cell cycle. It is then internalized into the cell via receptor-mediated endocytosis (VARGA et al. 1977). A β-melanotropin-DNM conjugate was synthesized and its effect studied on MSH responsive murine melanoma cells in vitro and in vivo. The conclusion drawn was that the conjugate enters the cell lysosome where free drug is liberated by hydrolysis. In another study, VARGA (1985) synthesized an MSH-DNM conjugate which was found to be more deadly to murine melanoma than free DNM. Since addition of large quantities of MSH had an inhibitory effect and since lysosomotropic amines had no protecting effect on the cells compared to the conjugate, it was concluded that the hormone-drug conjugate must be processed in the lysosome to be effective against melanoma. It is not possible for DNM that is hormone bound to bind to DNA. Therefore, DNM is cleaved from the hormone carrier inside of the lysosome or cell kill is via another mechanism. Similarly, an MSH-ouabain conjugate was synthesized. However, in this case, free ouabain was toxic to melanoma cells whereas the conjugate was not. In fact, the conjugate was stimulating during the early stages of cell growth. This was explained by the possibility that the receptor for MSH and the Na/K pump may be close to each other on the plasma membrane and may interfere with the other's processes. Also, importantly, some hormone activity is lost in binding.

VI. Other Targeting Systems

Another method of enhancing the concentration of carriers in target tissue is by virtue of charge. Although this is not as specific a method as using a targeting moiety, it is a good in vitro method to study uptake mechanisms and drug release. For instance, SHEN and RYSER (1986) studied the degradation of MTX-polylysine conjugates. This type of polymer, due to its positive charge, is taken up by cells by adsorptive endocytosis. The MTX was bound to the polymer by a disulfide linkage which was cleaved intracellularly releasing MTX. Neither an acid environment nor proteolytic enzymes are needed for drug release in this case, and it is thought that the compartment responsible for drug release is prelysosomal. This would be a system to consider if the drug itself is rendered inactive by lysosomal enzymes. An MTX-polylysine conjugate linked via a triglycyl spacer was also studied and showed comparable cytotoxic effects as the disulfide linked conjugate. However, lysosomal cathepsins are probably responsible for drug liberation of the triglycyl linked conjugate because leupeptin, a lysosomal protease inhibitor, caused this conjugate to be inactive i.e., did not affect the disulfide linked conjugate). Both wild-type CHO cells and transport-defective mutants were used as in vitro systems.

As discussed, pharmacokinetics are a major obstacle in in vivo drug systems compared with testing in vitro. MAEDA et al. (1988) have been working with the anticancer protein drug neocarzinostatin (NCS). Protein drugs are antigenic and are not very biocompatible. Since metastasizing cancer cells follow the lymphatic drainage route, this group decided to design their drug to follow the same route. They did this by binding NCS to a styrene-co-maleic acid/anhydride copolymer. This increased the lipophilicity of the drug and changed its body distribution. Accumulation of drug in the tumor was enhanced along with enhanced lymphotropism and prolonged plasma half-life. Also, protein antigenicity was eliminated. MAEDA et al. (1988) contend that conjugates of this type are more promising than monoclonal antibodies as targeting moieties.

An interesting combination was discussed by MATTES (1987). Ovarian cancer is usually confined to the peritoneal cavity, although it often spreads before it is detected. Monoclonal antibodies were conjugated with sugars and injected intraperitoneally. By using carbohydrates, the conjugate enters the bloodstream and is rapidly cleared from the circulation. It would be useful to come up with conjugates that could be confined to the peritioneal cavity and that, once they left the cavity, could rapidly cleared.

A new strategy for the delivery of cytostatic agents to solid tumors was recently proposed (BAGSHAWE 1989; SENTER 1990). Monoclonal antibodies are used as carriers for enzymes to tumor cell surfaces. The enzymes are chosen for their abilities to convert relatively noncytotoxic prodrugs into active anticancer drugs. The drug thus formed can penetrate into nearby tumor cells, resulting in cell death.

F. Photosensitization: Activation by Light

The combination of light and certain light absorbing molecules, called photosensitizers, in the presence of oxygen, can lead to rapid cell destruction. It is most widely believed that the generation of singlet oxygen, a reactive species, is ultimately responsible for the majority of devastating effects, although other reactions do indeed occur. There is also another class of photosensitizer which does not require oxygen (in some cases oxygen is even inhibitory), however, photosensitization effected by this type of photosensitizer is beyond the scope of this discussion. (For informative reviews see SPIKES 1988 and STRAIGHT 1990).

I. Photodynamic Therapy

Porphyrins are photosensitizers that are activated with visible light, which itself is not detrimental to biomolecules. In recent years, porphyrin research has progressed enormously due to the use of porphyrins in diagnostic medicine and for the treatment of tumors. This is a result of the discovery that some porphyrins, for example hematoporphyrin derivative (Hpd), are selectively retained in tumor tissue in vivo. However, there is no steadfast evidence that the tumor cells themselves actually take up porphyrins or are sensitized to a greater extent than normal cells in vivo or in vitro. Therefore, the precise mechanism of selective uptake and tumor destruction following light treatment remains as speculation (SPIKES and STRAIGHT 1985). Also, it has been shown that little prophyrin is internalized into tumor cells; most porphyrin retention is located in interstitial regions of the tumor. There is also little evidence that tumor destruction in vivo results from the direct photosensitization of the tumor cells. HENDERSON et al. (1984) studied EMT6 tumor photodestruction with Hpd photodynamic therapy (PDT) and results indicated that, instead, tumor destruction was probably a result of vascular damage. Explanted tumor tissue immediately following PDT was found to grow; however, tumor clonogenicity of tissue remaining in situ was reduced 100-fold for tumor excised 10 h post irradiation. Blood deprivation and consequent anoxia are implicated in tumor death as a result of vasculature collapse. This mechanism is suported in another study (HENDERSON and FARRELL 1989), in which a number of different photosensitizers were compared for their effect on vascular damage.

Even though porphyrins are effective photosensitizers for PDT, they are not optimal due to their relatively poor spectral properties. Deeper tissue penetration can be obtained with longer wavelengths in the red region of the spectrum where porphyrins do not absorb intensely. In addition, Hpd, which is the only photosensitizer used clinically at this time, is actually a mixture of components. Side effects including light ultrasensitivity requires patients to remain out of direct sunlight for 6–8 weeks following treatment. This is due to the uptake of the porphyrin in tissue other than tumor tissue. Current research efforts are aimed at developing new photosensitizers in pure form with superior spectral and tumor localizing properties to those of Hpd. Phthalocyanines absorb strongly in the red region of the spectrum and a number have been found to selectively localize in tumors. Zinc phthalocyanine, for example, absorbs at 677 nm and has been studied under aqueous conditions for its sensitization properties on biomolecules including lysozyme (SPIKES and BOMMER 1986). Several chlorins (derivatives of chlorphyll) also absorb at longer wavelengths and are effective photosensitizers (SPIKES and BOMMER 1991; SPIKES 1990). BRASSEUR et al. (1987) experimented with water soluble sulfonated phthalocyanines and three metal chelate derivatives to determine their effect against EMT6 mammary tumors in mice. It is known that some metal chelates of photosensitizers have increased uptake compared to the parent potosensitizer. The ability to induce tumor necrosis and cure was best for Ga and Al phthalocyanine derivatives without dark toxicity (the metal free photosensitizer had no activity in vivo). Nevertheless, uptake is still not specific enough and there is a need to devise more efficient ways of delivering porphyrins to tumor tissue. This may be accomplished by targeting porphyrins to tumor tissue using polymeric carriers.

1. Double Targeting

In order to achieve a double targeting effect, site specificity of the drug, by virtue of a targeting moiety, and light specificity, photosensitizers have been linked to antibodies. This was originally pursued by MEW et al. (1983) in which hematoporphyrin (Hp) was covalently bound to anti-M-1 antibodies and injected into animals bearing DBA/2J myosarcoma M-1. Animals were subjected to incandescent light following treatment, which had an effect on tumor suppression. The conjugate was more effective in tumor suppression than either drug or antibody alone. In another study, Hp-monoclonal antibody conjugates against a leukemia associated antigen was shown to have selective phototoxicity (MEW et al. 1985). However, these conjugates have the same disadvantages as do other conjugates in which the drug is bound directly to the antibody. To circumvent some of these problems, OSEROFF et al. (1986) conjugated an anti-T cell monoclonal antibody to chlorin e_6 through a dextran spacer, which enabled the coupling of more chlorin molecules per antibody molecule than antibody alone. The conjugate was investigated against HBP-ALL human T cells in vitro. Selective photodestruction was attained. The conjugate was more effective than drug alone or antibody-chlorin conjugates.

Conjugates with high photosensitizer to monoclonal antibody ratios were prepared (HASAN et al. 1989). Chlorin e_6 monoethylene diamine monoamide was bound via polyglutamic acid to the monoclonal anti-T cell (anti-Leu-1) antibody. When anti-Leu-1 target cells, HPB-ALL T leukemia cells treated with the conjugate, were exposed to broad band, long wavelength irradiation a radiant exposure-dependent cytotoxicity was observed. Cells treated similarly with free drug or antibody were unaffected.

a) Synthetic Targetable Polymer Bound Photosensitizers

In our laboratory, HPMA conjugates containing chlorin e_6 and anti-Thy 1.2 antibodies were tested for immune suppression on splenocytes (isolated from

A/J mice) in vitro (KRINICK et al. 1990). Two conjugates were synthesized differing only in their method of antibody attachment. The conjugate synthesized by a specific orientation through antibody carbohydrate oxidation, which leaves the antibody binding sites free for targeting, was significantly more active than the other, in which antibody was bound through N^{ε}-amino groups of lysine residues. In the latter case the antibody activity may have been partially reduced due to binding of the HPMA copolymer near or at the binding site. This indicates the importance of the chemistry of antibody binding. Only the conjugate containing antibody bound via the F_c fragment (carbohydrate groups) was a more efficient sensitizer than free drug.

Similarly, we have synthesized an HPMA copolymer containing side chains terminating in chlorin e_6 and galactosamine residues. This conjugate was tested in vitro against a human hepatoma cell line, PLC/PRF/5 (Alexander cells), which contains asialoglycoprotein receptors. It was found that the targeted conjugate was more biologically active than a nontargeted one (not containing galactosamine) (KRINICK et al. 1988).

In both systems, i.e. in anti-Thy 1.2 or galactosamine targeted HPMA copolymers containing chlorin e_6 it was proven that: (a) more than 1 h of incubation of target cells with the conjugates is necessary to obtain a significant pharmacological effect; (b) photosensitized cytotoxicity depends on incubation temperature. A pinocytosis nonpermissive temperature (4°C) gave only a marginal effect when compared with experiments performed at a pinocytosis permissive temperature (37°C) (ŘÍHOVÁ et al. 1991).

STEELE et al. (1988, 1989) have taken a new approach in cancer photochemotherapy. Using a P815 mastocytoma (solid) tumor model in DBA/2 mice they tried to achieve tumor cure via immune modulation of the host. It has been established that the growth of P815 mastocytoma cells in mice stimulates the development of T suppressor (Ts) cells specific for the tumor and capable of abrogating the development of cytotoxic T lymphocytes with specificity for P815. A monoclonal antibody (B16G) has been generated which recognizes a constant epitope on Ts cells and their soluble factors in DBA/2 mice.

The results of treatment of DBA/2 mice bearing P815 mastocytoma with B16G-Hp conjugates and appropriate controls is shown in Table 9. A significant number of mice treated with B16G-Hp conjugate underwent tumor regression, slowed tumor growth, or complete regression. Control animals treated with Hp alone or with a (unconjugated) mixture of B16G and Hp did not display any differences in the rate of tumor growth or in survival times in comparison to animals injected with phosphate buffered saline (PBS). The results support their hypothesis that B16G-Hp acts via suppressor cell deletion rather than through other mechanisms associated directly with the tumor. To overcome the problem of drug loading on the antibody molecules, new conjugates containing polymeric carriers (modified polyvinyl alcohol) have been synthesized (STEELE et al. 1988, 1989).

Table 9. Treatment of mice bearing P815 mastocytoma by targetable hematoporphyrin conjugates. (From STEELE et al. 1989)

Treatment	Mean survival time days ± SEM	p[a]	Number of cures	% Tumor free after 100 days
PBS	25 ± 1.1		0/7	0
B16G-Hp	41.3 ± 6.4[b]	<0.001	3/9	33
PBS	23.5 ± 2.4		0/6	0
Hp	21.0 ± 2.3	NS	0/8	0
B16G-Hp	24.2 ± 3.8	NS	3/8	37.5
PBS	25.2 ± 2.8		0/8	0
B16G	28.3 ± 4.6	NS	0/8	0
Hp	24.2 ± 1.9	NS	0/8	0
B16G + Hp	24.6 ± 2.1	NS	0/7	0
B16G-Hp	36.7 ± 2.5	<0.01	3/7	43

All animals received 10^4 P815 cells on days 0 and various i.v. injections on day 8. Mice received a total dose of 10 µg of Hp and 100 µg of MAb.
Hp, hematoporphyrin; Mab, monoclonal antibody; PBS, phosphate buffered saline.
[a] p values are based on the Student's t test in which survival times in individual groups were compared to values for PBS controls.
[b] Averaged survival times in B16G-Hp treated animals utilized data taken only from animals which died from their tumors (long-term survivors were not included).

2. Uptake of Photosensitizer Conjugates

Much work is necessary concerning the cellular uptake and subcellular trafficking of polymeric conjugates containing photosensitizers. PORETZ et al. (1989) have studied the intracellular distribution of chlorophyll derivatives in EJ human bladder tumor cells in vitro. The free drugs were found to localize in the plasma membrane of the cells. This reinforces the need for creating polymeric conjugates bearing photosensitizers that can be internalized by fluid phase pinocytosis. Direct photodynamic killing of the cancer cells could intensify the indirect vasculature effects seen with free photosensitizers.

It is important that the conjugate be removed from the body following treatment. Even if the conjugate becomes trapped in the lysosome of the target cancer cell, upon cell death it can be removed from the body via glomerular filtration. However, a forseen problem is that a conjugate of low or middle MW may be recaptured by kidney tubules upon reabsorption. This is especially true for polymers containing hydrophobic side chains, and most of the photosensitizers have hydrophobic properties. If the polymer is non-degradable, it will be trapped in the lysosomes of kidney epithelial cells through pinocytic entry (DROBNÍK and RYPÁČEK 1984) and will elicit lysosomal storage disorders. Lysosomal storage is particularly a problem if the conjugate becomes trapped in lysosomes of tissue, as a result of some nonspecific uptake, which may be exposed to light. The problem might be avoided by synthesizing conjugates containing enzymatically degradable bonds. Theoretically, the free drug would be quickly eliminated after cleavage in the lysosomes of nontarget tissue. The level of free drug circulating would be substantially lower than if the free drug was administered, because non-specific uptake should be reduced by using a targeting system. Consequently, the main side effect, skin photosensitivity after treatment, can be reduced.

G. Decreased Toxicity and Immunogenicity of Drug-Polymer Conjugates

I. Toxicity of Drug – Polymer Conjugates

Decreased toxicity and immunogenicity are other major advantages associated with targetable polymer-drug conjugates. Binding drugs to polymeric carriers changes not only the mechanism of cellular uptake and subcellular trafficking, but also the body distribution of the drug. Consequently, uptake in tissues where the major side effects occur may decrease. In the following paragraphs we shall demonstrate the decreased toxicity of polymer bound drugs, compared to free drugs, with examples of the anthracycline antibiotics, DNM and ADR.

Irreversible cardiac damage caused by anthracycline antibiotics is the major dose-limiting factor (LENAZ and PAGE 1976). PRATESI et al. (1985) found that, in comparison to free drug, administration of ADR covalently linked to poly-L-aspartic acid resulted in reduced toxicity in mice and rats after single and multiple administrations. ŘÍHOVÁ et al. (1989a) studied the body distribution and T cell accumulation of HPMA copolymers containing oligopeptide side chains terminated in ^{125}I-daunomycin and anti-Thy 1.2 antibodies. After i.v. administration in inbred mice (C57L/J) the level of polymer bound drug in the blood was 5–20 times higher than the free drug. The organs of maximum accumulation of the polymer bound drug were the spleen, thymus, and liver 2h after administration. These results are in accordance with the observed lower toxicity of anthracyclines bound to targetable HPMA copolymers (ŘÍHOVÁ et al. 1988, 1989b). SEYMOUR et al. (1990) studied the pharmacokinetics of ADR bound to HPMA copolymers in DBA mice. The circulating half-life of the HPMA copolymer-ADR conjugate was approximately 15 times longer than that of the free drug. The initial peak level of free ADR in the heart was reduced 100-fold following administration of the copolymer conjugate. Approximately ten times more HPMA copolymer bound ADR (compared to free ADR) can be administered to mice bearing L1210 leukemia without overt signs of toxicity (DUNCAN et al. 1989). YOKOHAMA et al. (1990) bound ADR to polyethylene glycol-polyaspartic acid block copolymers. In experiments on CDF$_1$ mice bearing P388 leukemia, they were able to administer i.p. tenfold higher doses of the polymer bound drug without signs of toxicity.

CASSIDY et al. (1989) studied the activity of HPMA copolymer-ADR conjugates against Walker 256 tumor in Wistar rats. It was found that the concentration of polymer bound drug in solid tumor was greater for all time points (24 h period) than free drug. Tumor AUC (area unde the curve) was increased approximately four fold in 24 h. There was also a substantial decrease in the cardiac concentration with HPMA copolymer – ADR conjugate suggesting an improved therapeutic index in this model system.

The other major site of toxicity of anthracyclines is bone marrow. ŘÍHOVÁ et al. (1988) studied the toxicity of free DNM and DNM bound to HPMA copolymers bearing anti-Thy 1.2 antibodies or anti-Ia^k antibodies as targeting residues against hematopoietic stem cells in bone marrow and against the liver and heart. Free DNM was highly toxic when given i.v. (total dose 150–600 µg); it eliminated most of the hematopoietic precursors in bone marrow. Moreover, significant irritation of Kupffer cells in liver and damage of myocardium were observed. By contrast, no signs of hepatotoxicity and heart toxicity were seen after the administration of the DNM-HPMA copolymer-anti-Thy 1.2 antibody conjugated with the same drug concentration. Toxicity against hematopoietic precursors in bone marrow was considerably reduced as measured by enumeration of spleen colony-forming units (CFU-s) (Table 10). Similar results were obtained with HPMA copolymer-ADR conjugates (ŘÍHOVÁ et al. 1989b).

II. Immunogenicity of Polymer-Drug Conjugates

It is generally known that attachment of soluble polymers to proteins increases their intravascular half-life and reduces the immunogenicity of the proteins. Methoxy polyethylene glycol was attached to bovine serum albumin

Table 10. Bone marrow stem cells detected in vivo as spleen colony-forming units after injection of free daunomycin or daunomycin bound to N-(2-hydroxypropyl)-methacrylamide copolymers with targeting antibodies. (From ŘÍHOVÁ et al. 1988)

Polymer structure	Total doses of		Number of CFUs per spleen (mean ± SE)
	Immunoglobulin (mg)	DNM (mg)	
P-Gly-Gly-DNM	–	0.25	32 ± 3
P-Gly-Phe-Leu-Gly-DNM	–	0.25	34 ± 4
P⟨Gly-Gly-DNM / Gly-Gly-anti-Thy 1.2*	3.0	0.33	20 ± 2
P⟨Gly-Phe-Leu-Gly-DNM / Gly-Phe-Leu-Gly-anti-Thy 1.2*	3.0	0.25	20 ± 4
P⟨Gly-Phe-Leu-Gly-DNM / Gly-Phe-Leu-Gly-anti-Thy 1.2**	2.5	0.23	21 ± 3
Anti Thy 1.2*	3.0	–	15 ± 3
Anti Thy 1.2**	3.0	–	10 ± 3
P-Gly-Phe-Leu-Gly-anti Thy 1.2	3.0	–	25 ± 6
DNM	–	0.3	8 ± 3
Controls	–	–	26 ± 6

CFU, colony-forming unit; DNM, daunomycin; * polyclonal; ** monoclonal.

(ABUCHOWSKI et al. 1977) and after i.m. or i.v. injection, the conjugate did not elicit antibodies against itself. Moreover, it did not react with antibodies raised against native BSA. FUERTGES and ABUCHOWSKI (1990) used this method for other proteins. Modification of recombinant interleukin-2 by polyethylene glycol increased its water solubility and its potency in the murine Meth A sarcoma model (KATRE et al. 1987). Considerable attention was devoted to the evaluation of the immunogenicity of HPMA copolymers (ŘÍHOVÁ et al. 1983, 1984, 1985). A study in five different inbred strains of mice (A/J; Balb/c; C57B10; C3H/Di; and C57L/J) indicates that the HPMA homopolymer is not recognized as a foreign macromolecule, and no detectable antibodies against it are formed. Attachment of oligopeptide side chains give rise to a thymus-independent antigen which induces a weak lgM antibody response. Its intensity depends both on the structure of the oligopeptide sequence and on the genetic background of the mice. On the average, the titers of antibodies against HPMA copolymers were lower by four orders of magnitude than those of antibodies against bovine gamma globulin (ŘÍHOVÁ et al. 1984), which indicates a very low immunogenicity of these compounds. ADR bound to HPMA copolymers does not behave as a hapten (ŘÍHOVÁ et al. 1989b). LÄÄNE et al. (1985) increased the intravascular half-life and decreased the immunogenicity of acetylcholinesterase by modifying it with HPMA copolymer. ŘÍHOVÁ and KOPEČEK (1985) studied the immunogenicity of anti-Thy 1.2 antibodies bound to HPMA copolymers after administration to A/J mice. HPMA copolymer bound anti-Thy 1.2 showed lower immunogenicity than free antibody. FLANAGAN et al. (1990) conjugated human immunoglobulin and human transferrin to HPMA copolymers. The copolymers were administered in A/J and B10 mice and the antibody elicited against them was compared to that elicited against the free protein. The antibody titers decreased up to 250-fold compared to free protein. HPMA copolymers also reduce the immunogenicity of monoclonal antitumor antibodies A5B7 or B72.3.

Experiments testing the interaction of HPMA copolymers with complement showed that they only activate complement at very high concentrations (20 mg/ml) which would never be used therapeutically. Lower concentrations (2 mg/ml or 0.2 mg/ml) did not activate either the classical or alternate complement pathway (ŠIMEČKOVÁ et al. 1986).

H. Soluble Polymers for Site Specific Oral Drug Delivery

I. Enzyme Controlled Site Specific Drug Release

The approaches outlined above for the design of parenterally administered polymer bound drugs can be modified for use in oral drug delivery. Enzymes present in only certain parts of the gastrointestinal tract (GIT) can be used for site specific drug release. The specific activity of colonic microflora is the target of tailor-made low MW or macromolecular prodrugs. BROWN et al. (1983) synthesized water soluble copolymers which contained salicylic acid bound via an aromatic azobond for treatment of inflammatory bowel disease. Upon arrival in the large bowel bacteria cleave (reduce) the azobond, releasing 5-aminosalicylic acid at this site only. FRIEND and CHANG (1984) described a colon delivery system of steroid glycosides using the unique glycosidase activity of colonic microflora. LANCASTER and WHEATLEY (1989) evaluated the susceptibility to colonic degradation of a number of poly-saccharides and determined the levels of glycosidase activity in rat colon. The results have shown that polysaccharides have a potential in the develop-ment of colon specific drug carriers. Recently, naproxene was bound to dextran carriers and the release of drug in the pig colon was attributed to the action of dextranases secreted from colonic bacteria (LARSEN et al. 1989). For both systems mentioned, the glycoside-based system and the azo-based system rely on enzymes unique to the lower GIT of humans and many other mammals (HOAG et al. 1989).

It is possible to use the activity of intestinal peptidases (FLEISHER et al. 1985) or brush border membrane enzymes (LONGER et al. 1989; KOPEČKOVÁ et al. 1991a) for site specific oral delivery. However, the feasibility of these approaches must be evaluated after more experimental data are available.

II. Bioadhesion of Polymeric Carriers

There are limitations in using the oral route for site specific oral delivery due to the rapid transit time of soluble macromolecules through the GIT. To modify the transit time of polymeric drugs the use of bioadhesives has been proposed (PARK and ROBINSON 1984, 1985), and attempts have been made to understand the relationship between their physicochemical properties and bioadhesion (PEPPAS and BURI 1985; LEUNG and ROBINSON 1988). The present concepts of bioadhesion are based on electrostatic interaction, hydrogen bonding, hydrophobic interactions, and simple mechanical interlocking (LONGER and ROBINSON 1986). These approaches may lead to partial success, as was shown in the studies with copolymers of polyacrylic acid (PARK and ROBINSON 1984). However, the future of tailor-made bioadhesive polymeric carriers lies in the discovery of specific recognition systems which have developed during evolution and are an implicit part of human and animal physiology. The specificity of such bioadhesive systems would have greater potential.

There are reports which indicate that there are physiological mechanisms operating in the GIT which are site specific. It was shown that some bacteria, e.g. *Shigella flexneri*, adhere to the colon (IZHAR et al. 1982). The colonic epithelial cells of guinea pigs were found to have an intestinal lectin active in binding and specific for glucose and fucose (MIRELMAN et al. 1982). The existence of this carbohydrate binding glycoprotein on the colonic cells was also proven with a strain of *Escherichia coli* 0124. The adherence process was found to be inhibited by glucose, fucose, and mannose (ASHKENAZI 1986). It was shown that HPMA copolymers which contain side chains terminating in

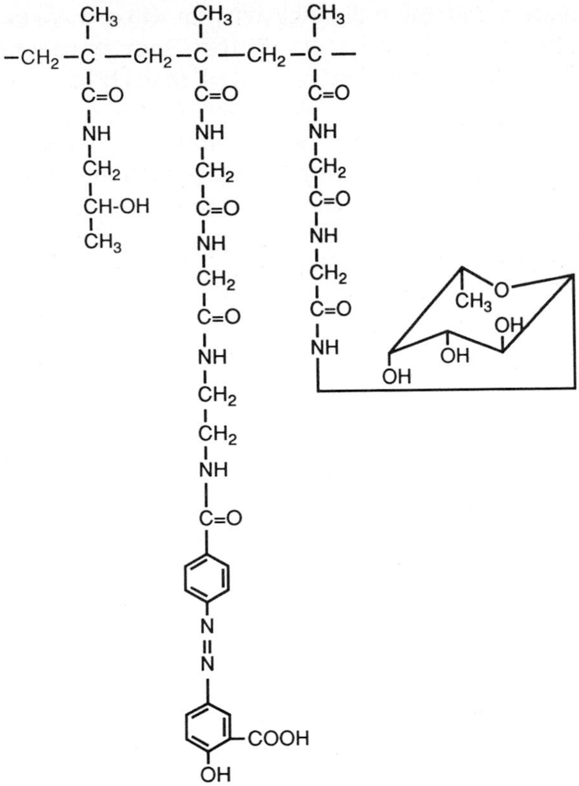

Fig. 13. Structure of HPMA copolymer containing 5-aminosalicylic acid bound via azoaromatic bonds and a bioadhesive moiety

sugar residues have a slightly greater affinity for rat small intestine in vitro than neutral control HPMA copolymers without bound sugar moieties (BRIDGES et al. 1988). Recently, it was shown that HPMA copolymers containing side-chains terminated in fucosylamine residues adhere to the colonic tissue of guinea pigs in vitro (RATHI et al. 1991).

III. Two Fold Specificity in Oral Drug Delivery

It appears that there is potential for the synthesis of copolymers which would have a twofold specificity: in bioadhesion and drug release. To verify the feasibility of this concept we are currently studying HPMA copolymers which contain 5-aminosalicylic acid (5-ASA) bound via azoaromatic bonds and a bioadhesive sugar moiety (Fig. 13).

We have shown that 5-ASA is released from these copolymers when incubated with *Streptococcum faecium*, a strain of bacteria commonly found in the colon (GRIM and KOPEČEK 1989, 1991) and in rat cecal extracts (KOPEČKOVÁ and KOPEČEK 1990). The relationship between the structure of

HPMA copolymers and their bioadhesivity in vitro was studied in detail (RATHI et al. 1991, KOPEČKOVÁ et al. 1991b). Body distribution analysis in guinea pigs after oral administration showed that HPMA copolymers containing fucosylamine as a bioadhesive moiety had an increased association with the colon (FORNŮSEK et al. 1989) compared to HPMA copolymers without carbohydrate moieties or with bound galactosamine, glucosamine, or mannosamine. The results obtained so far are encouraging, however, much more work is necessary to verify the therapeutic potential of these new polymeric drugs for colon specific delivery.

There are other avenues for site specific oral delivery: lectin-mediated endocytosis, interaction with M cells in Peyer's patches (PUSZTAI 1989), and the vitamin B12 transport system (RUSSELL-JONES and DE AIZPURUA 1988). Increased interest in using polymeric carriers which are soluble, branched (SAFFRAN et al. 1986), or cross-linked (BRONDSTED and KOPEČEK 1991) in site specific oral drug delivery indicates the rapid development of this extremely interesting and promising area of drug delivery.

I. Concluding Remarks

Results obtained so far with targetable, water soluble, polymeric drug carriers show their great potential in efficient treatment of disease. It is well-accepted that conjugates can be synthesized which are nontoxic, non-immunogenic and, if desired, biodegradable. However, many problems are still unsolved, eg., their extravasation, nonspecific interactions of targeting moieties (antibodies) in vivo, and the acquired resistance of cells due to drug exposure. Clinical evaluation of these conjugates in the near future will show if the current enthusiasm of experimental scientists will be translated into important clinical applications.

Acknowledgement. We thank Dr. B. ŘÍHOVÁ for valuable discussions.

References

Abuchowski A, van Es T, Palczuk NC, Davis FF (1977) Alteration of immunological properties of bovine serum albumin by covalent attachment of polyethylene glycol. J Biol Chem 252:3578–3581
Ajioka RS (1987) The biochemistry and physiology of endocytic apparatus. Thesis, University of Utah
Alam F, Soloway, McGuire JE, Barth RF, Carey WE, Adams DM (1985) Dicesium *N*-succinimidyl 3-(undecahydro-closo-dodecaboranyldithio) propionate, a novel heterobifunctional boronating agent. J Med Chem 28:522–525
Alam F, Soloway AH, Barth RF, Mafune N, Adams DM, Knoth WH (1989) Boron neutron capture therapy: linkage of a boronated macromolecule to monoclonal antibodies directed against tumor-associated antigens. J Med Chem 32:2326–2330

Alvarez VL, Wen M-L, Lee C, Lopes AW, Rodwell JD, McKearn TJ (1986) Site specifically modified ^{111}In labelled antibodies give low liver background and improved radioimmunoscintigraphy. Nucl Med Biol 13:347–352

Ammon R (1963) The occurrence of dextranase in human tissues (in German). Enzymologia 25:245–251

Anghileri LJ, Heidbreder M, Mathas R (1976) Accumulation of [57]Co-poly-L-lysine by tumors: an effect of the tumor electrical charge. J Nucl Biol Med 20:79–80

Armstrong BK, Smith Q, Rapoport SI, Strohalm J, Kopeček J, Duncan R (1989) Osmotic opening of the blood-brain barrier permeability to N-(2-hydroxy-propyl)methacrylamide copolymers. Effect of polymer M_w, charge and hydro-phobicity. J Control Release 10:27–35

Artursson P, O'Mullane J (1989) Cellular and biological interaction of macromolecular drug delivery systems. Adv Drug Delivery Rev 3:165–189

Ashkenazi S (1986) Adherence of non-fimbriate entero-invasive *Escherichia coli 0124* to guinea pig intestinal tract in vitro and in vivo. J Med Microbiol 21:117–123

Ashwell G, Harford J (1982) Carbohydrate specific receptors of targeting of the liver. Annu Rev Biochem 51:531–554

Ashwell G, Morell AG (1974) The role of surface carbohydrates in the hepatic recognition and transport of circulating glycoproteins. Adv Enzymol 41:99–128

Bader H, Ringsdorf H, Schmidt B (1984) Water soluble polymers in medicine. Makromol Chem 123/124:457–485

Bagshawe KD (1989) Towards generating cytotoxic agents at cancer sites. Br J Cancer 60:275–281

Baldwin RW, Byers VS (1986) Monoclonal antibody targeting of anti-cancer cells. Springer Semin Immunopathol 9:39–50

Banks W, Greenwood CT, Muir DD (1972) Hydroxyethylstarch.I. Review of the chemistry of hydroxyethylstarch with reference to its use as a blood plasma volume expander. Staerke 24:181–187

Basu SK, Goldstein JL, Anderson RGW, Brown MS (1981) Monesin interrupts the recycling of low density lipoprotein receptors in human fibroblasts. Cell 24:493–502

Blättler WA, Kuenzi BS, Lambert JM, Senter PD (1985) New heterobifunctional protein cross-linking reagent that forms an acid-labile link. Biochemistry 24:1517–1524

Blow DM (1974) Stereochemistry of substrate binding and hydrolysis in the trypsin family of enzymes. Bayer Symp 5:473

Brasseur N, Ali H, Langlois R, Wagner JR, Rosseau J, van Lier JE (1987) Biological activities of phthalocyanines V. Photodynamic therapy of EMT-6 mammary tumors in mice with sulfonated phthalocyanines. Photochem Photobiol 45:581–586

Bridges JF, Woodley JF, Duncan R, Kopeček J (1988) Soluble N-(2-hydroxypropyl)-methacrylamide copolymers as potential oral, controlled release, drug delivery system. I. Bioadhesion to the rat intestine in vitro. Int J Pharm 44:213–223

Brodsky FM (1988) Living with clathrin: its role in intracellular membrane traffic. Science 242:1396–1402

Brondsted H, Kopeček J (1991) Hydrogels for site-specific oral delivery. Synthesis and characterization. Biomaterials (in press)

Brown JP, McGarraugh GV, Parkinson TM, Wingard RE Jr, Onderdonk AB (1983) A polymeric drug for treatment of inflammatory bowel disease. J Med Chem 26:1300–1307

Byers VS, Pawluczyk I, Berry N, Durrant L, Robins RA, Garnett MC, Price MR, Baldwin RW (1988) Potentiation of anti-carcinoembryonic antigen immunotoxin cytotoxicity by monoclonal antibodies reacting with co-expressed carcino-embryonic antigen epitopes. J Immunol 140:4050–4055

Carroll AM, Zalutsky MR (1984) Receptor mediated pharmaceuticals. In: Lamble JW, Abbott AC (eds) Receptors again. Elsevier, New York, pp 39–45

Cartlidge SA, Duncan R, Lloyd JB, Kopečková-Rejmanová P, Kopeček J (1987) Soluble, crosslinked N-(2-hydroxypropyl)methacrylamide copolymers as potential drug carriers. III. Targeting by incorporation of galactosamine residues. Effect of route of administration. J Control Release 4:265–278

Cassidy J, Duncan R, Morrison GJ, Strohalm J, Plocová D, Kopeček J, Kaye SB (1989) Activity of N-(2-hydroxypropyl)methacrylamide copolymers containing daunomycin against a rat tumor model. Biochem Pharmacol 38:875–879

Cawley DB, Simpson DL, Herschman HR (1981) Asialoglycoprotein receptor mediates the toxic effects of and asialofetuin-diphtheria toxin fragment A conjugate on cultured rat hepatocytes. Proc Natl Acad Sci USA 78:3383–3387

Chakraboty P, Bhaduri AN, Das PK (1990) Sugar receptor mediated drug delivery to macrophages in the therapy of experimental visceral leishmaniasis. Biochem Biophys Res Commun 166:404–410

Chaves MS, Arranz F (1985) Water-insoluble dextrans by grafting. II. Reaction of dextrans with N-alkyl chloroformates. Chemical and enzymatic hydrolysis. Makromol Chem 186:17–29

Chin DJ, Straubinger RM, Acton S, Nathke I, Brodsky FM (1989) 100-kDa polypeptides in peripheral clathrin-coated vesicles are required for receptor-mediated endocytosis. Proc Natl Acad Sci USA 86:9289–9293

Courtoy PJ, Quintart J, Baudhuin P (1984) Shift of equilibrium density induced by 3,3'-diaminobenzidine cytochemistry: a new procedure for the analysis and purification of peroxidase containing organelles. J Cell Biol 98:870–876

Crepon B, Chytrý V, Říhová, B, Kopeček J, Jozefonvicz J (1991) Enzymatic degradation and immunogenic properties of substituted dextrans. Biomaterials (in press)

De Duve C (1983) Lysosomes revisited. Eur J Biochem 137:391–397

De Duve C, de Barsy T, Poole B, Trouet A, Tulkens P, van Hoof F (1974) Lysosomotropic agents. Biochem Pharmacol 23:2495–2531

Diaz R, Mayorga LS, Weidman PJ, Rothman JE, Stahl PD (1989) Vesicle fusion following receptor-mediated endocytosis requires a protein active in Golgi transport. Nature 339:398–400

Dorn K, Hörpel G, Ringsdorf H (1985) Polymeric antitumor agents on a molecular and cellullar level. In: Gebelein CG, Carraher CE (eds) Bioactive polymeric systems. Plenum, New York, pp 531–585

Drobník J (1989) Biodegradable soluble macromolecules as drug carriers. Adv Drug Delivery Res 3:229–245

Drobník J, Rypáček F (1984) Soluble synthetic polymers in biological systems. Adv Polym Sci 57:1–50

Duncan R (1986) Lysosomal degradation of polymers used as drug carriers. CRC Crit Rev Biocomp 2:127–145

Duncan D, Kopeček J (1984) Soluble synthetic polymers as potential drug carriers. Adv Polym Sci 57:51–101

Duncan R, Starling D, Rypáček F, Drobník J, Lloyd JB (1982a) Pinocytosis of poly(α,β-(N-2-hydroxyethyl))-DL-aspartamide and a tyramine derivative by rat visceral yolk sac cultured in vitro. Ability of hydrophobic residues to enhance the rate of pinocytic capture of a macromolecule. Biochim Biophys Acta 717:248–254

Duncan R, Cable HC, Lloyd JB, Rejmanová, P, Kopeček J (1982b) Degradation of side-chains of N-(2-hydroxypropyl)methacrylamide copolymers by lysosomal thiol-proteinases. Biosci Rep 2:1041–1046

Duncan R, Cable HC, Lloyd JB, Rejmanová P, Kopeček J (1983) Polymers containing enzymatically degradable bonds. VII. Design of oligopeptide side-chains in poly[N-(2-hydroxypropyl)methacrylamide] copolymers to promote efficient degradation by lysosomal enzymes. Makromol Chem 184:1997–2008

Duncan R, Cable HC, Rejmanová P, Kopeček J, Lloyd JB (1984) Tyrosinamide residues enhance pinocytic capture of N-(2-hydroxypropyl)methacrylamide copolymers. Biochim Biophys Acta 799:1–8

Duncan R, Seymour LCW, Scarlett L, Lloyd JB, Rejmanová P, Kopeček J (1986) Fate of N-(2-hydroxypropyl)methacrylamide copolymers with pendent galactosamine residues after intravenous administration to rats. Biochim Biophys Acta 880:62–71

Duncan R, Kopečková-Rejmanová, P, Strohalm J, Hume I, Cable HC, Pohl J, Lloyd JB, Kopeček J (1987) Anticancer agents coupled to N-(2-hydroxypropyl)-methacrylamide copolymers. I. Evaluation of daunomycin and puromycin con-jugates in vitro. Br J Cancer 55:165–174

Duncan R, Kopečková, P, Strohalm J, Hume IC, Lloyd JB, Kopeček J (1988) Anticancer agents coupled to N-(2-hydroxypropyl)methacrylamide copolymers. II. Evaluation of daunomycin conjugates in vivo against L1210 leukemia. Br J Cancer 57:147–156

Duncan R, Hume IC, Kopečková P, Ulbrich K, Strohalm J, Kopeček J (1989) Anticancer agents coupled to N-(2-hydroxypropyl)methacrylamide copolymers. III. Evaluation of adriamycin conjugates against mouse leukemia L1210 in vivo. J Control Release 10:51–63

Durrant LG, Garnett MC, Gallego J, Armitage NC, Ballantyne KC, Marksman RA, Hardcastle JD, Baldwin RW (1987) Sensitivity of newly established colorectal cell lines to cytotoxic drugs and monoclonal antibody drug conjugated. Br J Cancer 56:722–726

Feizi T (1984) Monoclonal antibodies reveal saccharide structures of glycoproteins and glycolipids as differentiation and tumour-associated antigens. Biochem Soc Trans 12:545–549

Ferrutti P, Tanzi MC (1986) New polymeric and oligomeric matrices as drug carriers. CRC Crit Rev Ther Drug Carrier Syst 2:175–244

Fersht A (1985) Enzyme structure and mechanism, 2nd edn. Freeman, New York

Fischer E, Stein E (1960) Dextranases. In: Boyer PD, Lardy H, Myrback K (eds) The enzymes, vol 4A. Academic, New York, p 304

Fiume L, Busi C, Mattioli A (1982) Lactosaminated human serum albumin as hepatropic drug carrier. Rate of uptake by mouse liver. FEBS Lett 146:42–46

Fiume L, Busi C, Mattioli A (1983) Targeting of antiviral drugs by coupling with protein carriers. FEBS Lett 153:6–9

Fiume L, Busi C Mattioli A, Spinoza G (1988) Targeting of antiviral drugs bound to protein carriers. CRC Crit Rev Ther Drug Carrier Syst 4:265–284

Flanagan PA, Kopečková P, Kopeček J, Duncan R (1989) Evaluation of protein-N-(2-hydroxypropyl)methacrylamide copolymer conjugates as targetable drug-carriers. I. Binding, pinocytic uptake and intracellular distribution of transferrin and anti-transferrin receptor antibody conjugates. Biochim Biophys Acta 993:83–91

Flanagan PA, Duncan R, Říhová B, Šubr V, Kopeček J, (1990) Immunogenicity of protein–N-(2-hydroxypropyl)methacrylamide copolymer conjugates in A/J and B10 mice. J Bioact Compat Polym 5:151–166

Fleisher D, Stewart BH, Amidon GL (1985) Design of prodrugs for improved gastrointestinal absorption by intestinal enzyme targeting. Methods Enzymol 112:360–381

Fornůsek L, Grim Y, Duncan R, Woodley JF, Kopeček J (1989) Bioadhesive water-soluble polymeric drug carriers for site-specific oral delivery. II. Body distribution after oral administration. Proc Int Symp Control Release Bioact Mater 16:398–399

Forster S, Lloyd JB (1988) Solute translocation across the mammalian lysosome membrane. Biochim Biophys Acta 947:465–491

Friend DR, Chang GW (1984) A colon-specific drug-delivery system based on drug glycosides and the glycosidases of colon bacteria. J Med Chem 27:261–266

Fuertges F, Abuchowski A (1990) The clinical efficacy of poly(ethylene glycol)-modified proteins. J Control Release 11:139–148

Garnett MC, Embleton MJ, Jacobs E, Baldwin RW (1985) Studies on the mechanism of action of an antibody-targeted drug-carrier conjugate. Anticancer Drug Design 1:3–12

Geisow J, Evans WH (1984) pH in the endosome. Exp Cell Res 150:36–46

Geuze HJ, Slot JW, Strous GJAM, Lodish HF, Schwartz AL (1983) Intracellular site of asialoglycoprotein receptor-ligand uncoupling: double label immunoelectron microscopy during receptor-mediated endocytosis. Cell 32:277–287

Geuze HJ, Slot JW, Strous JAM, Peppard J, von Figura K, Haslik A, Schwartz AL (1984) Intracellular receptor sorting during endocytosis: comparative immuno-electron microscopy of multiple receptors in rat liver. Cell 37:195–204

Glenney JR Jr, Chen WS, Lazar CS, Walton GM, Zokas LM, Rosenfeld MG, Gill GN (1988) Ligand-induced endocytosis of the EGF receptor is blocked by mutational inactivation and by microinjection of antiphosphotyrosine antibodies. Cell 52:675–684

Goddard P, Petrak K (1989) Biodegradation of drug-modified polymers in drug delivery — a critical analysis. J Bioact Compat Polym 4:372–402

Grim Y, Kopeček J (1989) Bioadhesive water-soluble polymeric drug carriers for site-specific oral delivery. I. Synthesis, characterization and 5-aminosalicylic acid release in vitro. Proc Int Symp Control Release Bioact Mater 16:211–212

Grim Y, Kopeček J (1991) Bioadhesive water-soluble polymeric drug carriers for site-specific oral delivery. Synthesis, characterization and 5-aminosalicylic acid release in vitro. New Polym Mater (in press)

Hagan PL, Halpern SE, Dillman RO, Shawler DL, Johnson DE, Chen A, Krishnan K, Frincke J, Bartholomew RM, David GS, Carlo D (1986) Tumor size: effect on monoclonal antibody uptake in tumor models. J Nucl Med 27: 422–427

Hanover JA, Beguinot L, Willingham MC, Pastan IH (1985) Transit of receptors for epidermal growth factor and transferrin through clathrin-coated pits. J Biol Chem 260:15938–15945

Hasan T, Lin A, Yarmush D, Oseroff A, Yarmush M (1989) Monoclonal antibody-chromophore conjugates as selective phototoxins. J Control Release 10:107–117

Haylett T, Thilo L (1986) Limited and selective transfer of plasma membrane glycoproteins to membrane of secondary lysosome. J Cell Biol 103:1249–1256

Helenius A, Mellman I, Wall D, Hubbard A (1983) Endosomes. TIBS 8:245–250

Henderson BW, Farrell G (1989) Possible implications of vascular damage for tumor cell inactivation in vivo: comparison of different photosensitizers. Proc SPIE 1065:2–10

Henderson BW, Dougherty TJ, Malone PB (1984) Studies on the mechanism of tumor destruction by photoradiation therapy. In: Doiron DR, Gomer CJ (eds) Porphyrin localization and treatment of tumors. Liss, New York, pp 601–612

Hespe W, Meier AM, Blankwater YJ (1977) Excretion and distribution studies in rats with two forms of ^{14}C-labelled polyvinylpyrrolidone with a relatively low mean molecular weight after intraveneous administration. Drug Res 27:1158–1162

Heuser JE, Anderson RGW (1989) Hypertonic media inhibit receptor-mediated endocytosis by blocking clathrin-coated pit formation. J Cell Biol 108:389–400

Heuser JE, Kirchhausen T (1985) Deep-etch views of clathrin assemblies. J Ultrastruct Res 92:1–27

Hoag K, Rigod J, Gungon R, Tozer TN, Friend DR (1989) Colonic drug delivery: glycoside produgs in the guinea pig. Proc Int Symp Control Release Bioact Mater 16:54–55

Hoes CJT, Feijen J (1989) The application of drug-polymer conjugates in chemotherapy. In: Roerdink FG, Kroo AM (eds) Drug carrier systems. Wiley, New York, pp 57–109

Hoes CJT, Potman W, van Heeswijk WAR, Mud J, de Grooth BG, Greve J, Feijen J (1985) Optimization of macromolecular prodrugs of the antitumor antibiotic adriamycin. J Control Release 2:205–213

Hoes CJT, Potman W, de Grooth BG, Greve J, Feijen J (1986) Chemical control of drug delivery. In: Harms AF (ed) Innovative approaches in drug research. Elsevier, Amsterdam, pp 267–283

Hörpel G, Klesse W, Ringsdorf H, Schmidt B (1982) Micelle forming co- and block copolymers for sustained drug release. IUPAC Int Symp on Macromolecules, Amherst, p 346

Hurwitz E, Levy R, Maron R, Wilchek M, Arnon R, Sela M (1975) The covalent binding of daunomycin and adriamycin to antibodies with retention of both drug and antibody activities. Cancer Res 35:1175–1181

Hurwitz E, Maron R, Arnon R, Sela M (1976) F$_{ab}$ dimers of antitumor immunoglobulins as covalent carriers of daunomycin. Cancer Biochem Biophys 1:197–202

Iacopetta BJ, Rothenberger S, Kuhn LC (1988) A role for the cytoplasmic domain in transferrin receptor sorting and coated pit formation during endocytosis. Cell 54:485–489

Iveson GP, Bird SJ, Lloyd JB (1989) Passive diffusion of non-electrolytes across the lysosome membrane. Biochem J 261:451–456

Izhar M, Nuchamowitz Y, Mirelman D (1982) Adherence of *Shigella flexneri* to guinea pig intestinal cells is mediated by mucosal adhesin. Infect Immun 35:1110–1118

Kasafírek E, Frič P, Slabý J, Mališ F (1976) p-Nitroanilides of 3-carboxypropionyl-peptides. Their cleavage by elastase, trypsin and chymotrypsin. Eur J Biochem 69:1–13

Katchalski E, Levin Y, Neumann H, Riesel E, Sharon N (1961) Studies on the enzymatic hydrolysis of poly-α-amino acids. Bull Res Counc Isr [A] 10:159–171

Katre NV, Knauf MJ, Laird WJ (1987) Chemical modification of recombinant interleukin-2 by polyethylene glycol increases its potency in the murine Meth A sarcoma model. Proc Natl Acad Sci USA 84:1487–1491

Kopeček J (1981) Soluble polymers in medicine. In: Williams DF (ed) Systemic aspects of biocompatibility, vol 2. CRC, Boca Raton, pp 159–180

Kopeček J (1982) Biodegradation of polymers for biomedical use. In: Benoit H, Rempp P (eds) IUPAC macromolecules. Pergamon, Oxford, pp 305–320

Kopeček J (1984a) Synthesis of tailor-made soluble polymeric drug carriers. In: Anderson JM, Kim SW (eds) Recent advances in drug delivery systems. Plenum, New York, pp 41–62

Kopeček J (1984b) Controlled biodegradability of polymers – a key to drug delivery systems. Biomaterials 5:19–25

Kopeček J (1988) Development of tailor-made polymeric prodrugs for systemic and oral delivery. J Bioact Compat Polym 3:16–26

Kopeček J (1990) The potential of water-soluble polymeric carriers in targeted and site-specific drug delivery. J Control Release 11:279–290

Kopeček J (1991) Targetable polymeric anticancer drugs: temporal control of drug activity. Ann NY Acad Sci 618:335–344

Kopeček J, Duncan R (1987) Targetable polymeric drugs. J Control Release 6:315–327

Kopeček J, Rejmanová P (1979) Reactive copolymers of N-(2-hydroxypropyl)-methacrylamide with N-methacryloylated derivatives of L-leucine and L-phenylalanine. II. Reaction with the polymeric amine and stability of crosslinks towards chymotrypsin in vitro. J Polym Sci Polym Symp 66:209–219

Kopeček J, Rejmanová P (1983) Enzymatically degradable bonds in synthetic polymers. In: Bruck SD (ed) Controlled drug delivery, vol 1. CRC, Boca Raton, pp 81–124

Kopeček J, Rejmanová P, Chytrý V (1981) Polymers containing enzymatically degradable bonds. I. Chymotrypsin catalyzed hydrolysis of p-nitroanilides of phenylalanine and tyrosine attached to side-chains of copolymers of N-(2-hydroxypropyl)methacrylamide. Makromol Chem 182:799–809

Kopeček J, Rejmanová P, Strohalm J, Ulbrich K, Říhová B, Chytrý V, Duncan R, Lloyd JB (1985) Synthetic polymeric drugs. Br Pat Appl 8 500 209 (4.1 1985)

Kopečková P, Kopeček J (1990) Release of 5-aminosalicylic acid from bioadhesive N-(2-hydroxypropyl)methacrylamide copolymers by azoreductases in vitro. Makromol Chem 191:2037–2045

Kopečková P, Longer MA, Woodley JF, Duncan R, Kopeček J (1991a) Release of p-nitroaniline from oligopeptide side-chains attached to N-(2-hydroxyproply) methacrylamide copolymers by rat intestinal brush border membrane enzymes. Makromol Chem Rapid Commun 12:601–606

Kopečková P, Říhová B, Rathi R, Kopeček J (1991b) Bioadhesive polymers for colon specific drug delivery. Proc Int Symp Control Release Bioact Mater 18:341–342

Kornfeld S (1987) Trafficking of lysosomal enzymes. FASEB J 1:462–468

Kralovec J, Spencer G, Blair AH, Mammen M, Singh M, Ghose T (1989) Synthesis of methotrexate-antibody conjugates by regiospecific coupling and assessment of drug and antitumor activities. J Med Chem 32:2426–2431

Krinick NL, Říhová B, Ulbrich K, Andrade JD, Kopeček J (1988) Targetable photoactivatable drugs: synthesis of water soluble galactosamine containing polymeric carriers of chlorin e$_6$ and their photodynamic effect on PLC cells in vitro. Proc SPIE 997:70–83

Krinick NL, Říhová B, Ulbrich K, Strohalm J, Kopeček J (1990) Targetable photo-activatable drugs. II. Synthesis of N-(2-hydroxypropyl)methacrylamide copolymer-anti-Thy 1.2 antibody-chlorin e$_6$ conjugates and a preliminary study of their photodynamic effect on mouse splenocytes in vitro. Makromol Chem 191:839–856

Krolick K, Yuan D, Vitetta E (1981) Specific killing of a human breast carcinoma cell line by a monoclonal antibody coupled to the A-chain of ricin. Cancer Immunol Immunother 12:39–41

Lääne A, Aaviksaar A, Haga M, Chytrý V, Kopeček J (1985) Preparation of polymer-modified enzymes of prolonged circulation times. Poly[N-(2-hydroxypropyl)-methacrylamide]–bound acetylcholinesterase. Makromol Chem [Suppl] 9:35–42

Lagueux J, Pagé M, Delorme F (1984) Daunorubicin-albumin copolymer targeting to leukemic cells in vitro and in vivo. Semin Oncol [Suppl 3] 2(4):59–63

Lancaster CM, Wheatley MA (1989) Drug delivery to the colon: polymer susceptibilty to degradation by colon contents. Polym Preprints 30:480–481

Larsen C, Harboe E, Johansen M, Olesen HP (1989) Macromolecular prodrugs. XVI. Colon-targeted delivery – comparison of the rate of release of naproxen from dextran ester prodrugs in homogenates of various segments of the pig gastrointestinal tract. Pharm Res 6:995–999

Lee YC, Lee RT (1982) Neoglycoproteins as probes for binding and cellular uptake of glycoconjugates. In: Horowitz MI (ed) Glycoproteins, glycolipids and proteoglycans. Plenum, New York, pp 57–83 (The glycoconjugates, vol 43)

Lefrak EA, Pitha J, Rosenheim S, Gottlieb JA (1973) A clinicopathologic analysis of adriamycin cardiotoxicity. Cancer 32:302–314

Lenaz L, Page JA (1976) Cardiotoxicity of adriamycin and related anthracyclines. Cancer Treat Rev 3:111–120

Leung SHS, Robinson JR (1988) The contribution of anionic polymer structural features to mucoadhesion. J Control Release 5:223–231

Limet JN, Quintart J, Schneider Y-J, Courtoy PJ (1985) Receptor mediated endocytosis of polymeric IgA and galactosylated serum albumin in rat liver. Evidence for intracellular ligand sorting and identification of distinct endosomal compartments. Eur J Biochem 146:539–548

Ling V (1987) Multidrug resistance and P-glycoprotein expression. Ann NY Acad Sci 507:7–8

Ling V, Juranka P, Endicott JA, Deuchars KL, Gerlach JH (1988) Multidrug resistance and P-glycoprotein expression. In: Woolen PV 3rd, Tew KD (eds) Mechanism of drug resistance in neoplastic cells. Academic, New York, pp 197–209

Lloyd JB (1985) Macromolecules as vehicles for intracellular drug delivery. Pharm Int 6:252–255

Lloyd JB (1986) Endocytosis and lysosomes: recent progress in intracellular traffic. In: Gregoriadis G, Senior J, Poste G (eds) Targeting of drugs with synthetic systems. Plenum, New York, pp 57–63

Lloyd JB (1989) Explorations in cell biology and pharmacology using synthetic polymers. Angew Makromol Chem 166/167:191–200

Lloyd JB, Forster S (1986) The lysosome membrane. TIBS 11:365–368

Lobel P, Fujimoto K, Ye RD, Griffiths G, Kornfeld S (1989) Mutations in the cytoplasmic domain of the 275 kd mannose 6-phosphate receptor differentially alter lysosomal enzyme sorting and endocytosis. Cell 57:787–796

Longer MA, Robinson JR (1986) Fundamental aspects of bioadhesion. Pharm Int 7:114–117

Longer MA, Woodley JF, Duncan R (1989) Comparison of the activities of rat small intestine and colon brush border membrane peptidases. Proc Int Symp Control Release Bioact Mater 16:54–55

Maeda H, Oda T, Matsumura Y, Kimura M (1988) Improvement of pharmacological properties of protein-drugs by tailoring with synthetic polymers. J Bioact Compat Polym 3:27–43

Manabe Y, Tsubota T, Haruta Y, Okazaki M, Haisa S, Nakamura K, Kimura I (1983) Production of a monoclonal antibody-bleomycin conjugate utilizing dextran T-40 and the antigen-targeting cytotoxicity of the conjugate. Biochem Biophys Res Commun 115:1009–1014

Masquelier M, Baurain R, Trouet A (1980) Amino acid and dipeptide derivatives of daunorubicin. Synthesis, physicochemical properties and lysosomal digestion. J Med Chem 23:1166–1170

Mattes J (1987) Biodistribution of antibodies after intraperitoneal or intravenous injection and effect of carbohydrate modifications. JNCI 79:855–864

Maxfield FR (1985) Acidification of endosomic vesicles and lysosomes. In: Pastan I, Willingham MC (eds) Endocytosis. Plenum, New York, pp 235–257

McCormick LA, Seymour LCW, Duncan R, Kopeček J (1986) Interaction of a cationic N-(2-hydroxypropyl)methacrylamide copolymer with rat visceral yolk sac cultured in vitro and rat liver in vivo. J Bioact Compat Polym 1:4–9

Meijer AEFH, Willinghagen RGJ (1963) The activity of glucose-6-phosphatase, adenosine triphosphatase, succinic dehydrogenase, and acid phosphatase after dextran or polyvinylpyrrolidone uptake by liver in vivo. Biochem Pharmacol 12:973–980

Messmer K (1988) Characteristics, effects and side-effects of plasma substitutes. In: Lowe KC (ed) Blood substitutes. VCH, Weinheim, pp 51–70

Mew D, Wat C-K, Towers GHN, Levy J (1983) Photoimmunotherapy: treatment of animal tumors with tumor-specific monoclonal antibody-hematoporphyrin conjugates. J Immunol 130:1473–1477

Mew D, Lum V, Wat C-K, Towers GHN, Sun C, Oh C, Walter RJ, Wright W, Berns MW, Levy JG (1985) Ability of specific monoclonal antibodies and conventional antisera conjugated to hematoporphyrin to label and kill selected cell lines subsequent to light activation. Cancer Res 45:4380–4386

Miller WG (1961) Degradation of poly-α-L-glutamic acid. I. Degradation on high-molecular weight polyglutamic acid by papain. J Am Chem Soc 83:259–265

Miller WG (1964a) Degradation of synthetic polypeptides. II. Degradation of poly-α-L-glutamic acid by proteolytic enzymes in 0.20 M sodium chloride. J Am Chem Soc 86:3913–3918

Miller WG (1964b) Degradation of poly-α-L-lysine by proteolytic enzymes in 0.2 M sodium chloride. J Am Chem Soc 86:3918–3922

Miller WG, Monroe J (1968) Enzymatic hydrolysis of synthetic polypeptides under high helical content. Biochemistry 7:253–261

Mirelman D, Izhar M, Eshdat Y (1982) Carbohydrate recognition mechanisms which mediate microbial adherence to mammalian mucosal surfaces. Tokai J Exp Clin Med [Suppl] 7:177–183

Monsigny M, Kieda C, Roche A-C (1983) Membrane glycoproteins, glycolipids and membrane lectins as recognition signals in normal and malignant cells. Biol Cell 47:95–110

Moore MS, Mahaffey DT, Brodsky FM, Anderson RGW (1987) Assembly of clathrin-coated pits onto purified plasma membranes. Science 236:558–563

Neufeld EF, Ashwell G (1980) Carbohydrate recognition systems for receptor mediated pinocytosis. In: Lennarz WJ (ed) The biochemistry of glycoproteins and proteoglycans. Plenum, New York, pp 241–266

Ohno H, Abe K, Tsuchida E (1981) Interaction of human serum proteins with synthetic polymers in homogeneous systems. Makromol Chem 182:1253–1262

Oseroff AR, Ohuoha D, Hasan T, Bommer JC, Yarmush ML (1986) Antibody-targeted photolysis: selective photodestruction of human T-cell leukemia cells using monoclonal antibody-chlorin e_6 conjugates. Proc Natl Acad Sci USA 83:8744–8748

Page M, Emond JP (1983) Daunomycin targeting using carrier monoclonal antibodies. In: Mathe G, Marl R, Dejager R (eds) Anthracyclines: current status and future developments. Masson, New York, pp 105–108

Park K, Robinson JR (1984) Bioadhesive polymers as platforms for oral controlled drug delivery: methods to study bioadhesion. Int J Pharm 19:107–127

Park K, Robinson JR (1985) Physico-chemical properties of water insoluble polymers important to mucin/epithelial adhesion. J Control Release 2:47–57

Pastan I, Willingham MC (1983) Receptor mediated endocytosis: coated pits, receptosomes and the golgi, TIBS 8:250–254

Pastan I, Willingham MC (1985) The pathway of endocytosis. In: Pastan I, Willingham MC (eds) Endocytosis. Plenum, New York, pp 1–44

Peppas NA, Buri PA (1985) Surface, interfacial and molecular aspects of polymer bioadhesion on soft tissues. J Control Release 2:257–275

Petrak K, Goddard P (1989) Transport of macromolecules across the capillary walls. Adv Drug Delivery Rev 3:191–214

Pimm MV (1988) Drug-monoclonal antibody conjugates for cancer therapy: potentials and limitations. CRC Crit Rev Ther Drug Carrier Syst 5:189–227

Pitha J (1980) Nucleic acids and sulfate and phosphate polyanions. In: Donaruma IG, Ottenbrite RM, Vogl D (eds) Anionic polymeric drugs. Wiley, New York, p 277

Pitha J (1981) Effects of polyvinyl analogs of nucleic acids on cells, animals and their viral infections. In: Gebelein CG, Koblitz FF (eds) Biomedical and dental applications of polymers, Plenum, New York, pp 203–313

Poretz RD, Vucenik I, Bergstrom L, Segelman A, Sigel G Jr, Chernomorsky S (1989) Intracellular distribution of porphyrin-based photosensitizers in in vitro cultured human bladder tumor cells. SPIE 1065:197–203

Poznansky MJ (1984) Enzyme-albumin polymers. New approaches to the use of enzymes in medicine. Appl Biochem Biotechnol 10:41–56

Poznansky MJ (1986) Tailoring enzymes for more effective use as therapeutic agents. In: Feeny RE, Whitaker JR (eds) Protein Tailoring for Food and Medical Uses. Dekker, New York, pp 317–337

Poznansky MJ, Juliano RL (1984) Biological approaches to the controlled delivery of drugs: a critical review. Pharmacol Rev 36:277–336

Poznansky MJ, Shandling M, Salkie MA, Elliott J, Lau E (1982) Advances in the use of L-asparaginase-albumin polymer as an antitumor agent. Cancer Res 42:1020–1025

Pratesi G, Savi G, Pezzoni G, Bellini O, Penco S, Tinelli S, Zunino F (1985) Poly-L-aspartic acid as a carrier for doxorubicin: a comparative in vivo study of free and polymer-bound drug. Br J Cancer 52:841–848

Pusztai A (1989) Transport of proteins through the membranes of the adult gastrointestinal tract–a potential for drug delivery. Adv Drug Delivery Rev 3:215–228

Pytela J, Saudek V, Drobník J, Rypáček F (1989) Poly(N-hydroxyalkylglutamines). IV. Enzymatic degradation of N-(2-hydroxyethyl)-L-glutamine homopolymers and copolymers. J Control Release 10:17–25

Rathi RC, Kopečková P, Ríhová B, Kopeček J (1991) N-(2-Hydroxypropyl)methacrylamide copolymers containing pendant saccharide moieties. Synthesis and bioadhesive properties. J Polym Sci, A: Polym Chem (in press)

Reichner JS, Whiteheart SW, Hart GW (1988) Intracellular trafficking of cell surface sialoglycoconjugates. J Biol Chem 263:16316–16326

Rejmanová P, Kopeček J, Pohl J, Baudyš M, Kostka V (1983) Polymers containing enzymatically degradable bonds. VIII. Degradation of oligopeptide sequences in N-(2-hydroxypropyl)methacrylamide copolymers by bovine spleen cathepsin B. Makromol Chem 184:2009–2020

Rennke HG, Venkatachalam MA, Patel Y (1979) Glomerular permeability of macromolecules. Effect of molecular configuration on the fractional clearance of uncharged dextran and neutral horseradish peroxidase in the rat. J Clin Invest 63:713–717

Říhová B, Kopeček J (1985) Biological properties of targetable poly[N-(2-hydroxypropyl)methacrylamide]-antibody conjugates. J Control Release 2: 289–310

Říhová B, Ulbrich K, Kopeček J, Mančal P (1983) Immunogenicity of N-(2-hydroxypropyl)methacrylamide copolymers–potential hapten or drug carriers. Folia Microbiol (Praha) 28:217–227

Říhová B, Kopeček J, Ulbrich K, Pospíšil M, Mančal P (1984) Effect of the chemical structure of N-(2-hydroxypropyl)methacrylamide copolymers on their ability to induce antibody formation in inbred strains of mice. Biomaterials 5:143–148

Říhová B, Kopeček J, Ulbrich K, Chytrý V (1985) Immunogenicity of N-(2-hydroxypropyl)methacrylamide copolymers. Makromol Chem [Suppl] 9:13–24

Říhová B, Kopeček J, Kopečková-Rejmanová P, Strohalm J, Plocová D, Semorádová H (1986) Bioaffinity therapy with antibodies and drugs bound to soluble synthetic polymers. J Chromatogr Biomed Appl 376:221–233

Říhová B, Kopečková P, Strohalm J, Rossmann P, Větvička V, Kopeček J (1988) Antibody-directed affinity therapy applied to the immune system: in vivo effectiveness and limited toxicity of daunomycin conjugated to HPMA copolymers and targeting antibody. Clin Immunol Immunopathol 46:100–114

Říhová B, Vereš K, Fornůsek L, Ulbrich K, Strohalm J, Bilej M, Kopeček J (1989a) Action of polymeric prodrugs based on N-(2-hydroxypropyl)-methacrylamide copolymers. II. Body distribution and T-cell accumulation of free and polymer bound [^{125}I] daunomycin. J Control Release 10:37–49

Říhová B, Bilej M, Větvička V, Ulbrich K, Strohalm J, Kopeček J, Duncan R (1989b) Biocompatibility of N-(2-hydroxypropyl)methacrylamide copolymers containing adriamycin. Biomaterials 10:335–342

Říhová B, Krinick NL, Kopeček J (1991) Targetable photoactivatable polymeric drugs. III. Specific in vitro photodestruction of mouse splenocytes or a human hepatoma cell line PLC/PRF/5 by polymer bound chlorin e6 targeted by anti-Thy 1.2 antibodies or galactosamine, respectively. J Control Release (submitted)

Říhová B, Strohalm J, Plocová D, Ulbrich K (1990) Selectivity of antibody-targeted anthracycline antibiotics on T lymphocytes. J Bioact Compat Polym 5:249–266

Ringsdorf H (1975) Structures and properties of pharmacologically active polymers. J Polym Sci Polym Symp 51:135–153

Riordan JR, Ling V (1985) Genetic and biochemical characterization of multidrug resistance. Pharmacol Ther 28:51–75

Roberts JC, Figard SD, Mercer-Smith JA, Svitra ZV, Anderson WL, Lavallee DK (1987) Preparation and characterization of copper-67 porphyrin-antibody conjugates. J Immunol Methods 105:153–164

Roberts JC, Newmyer SL, Mercer-Smith JA, Schreyer SA, Lavellee DK (1989) Labeling antibodies with copper radionuclides using N-4-nitrobenzyl-5-(4-carboxyphenyl)-10,15,20-tris (4-sulfophenyl) porphine. Appl Radiat Isotopes 40:775–780

Rodwell JD, Alvarez VL, Lee C, Lopes AD, Goers JWF, King HD, Powsner HJ, McKearn TJ (1986) Site-specific covalent modification of monoclonal antibodies: in vitro and in vivo evaluations. Proc Natl Acad Sci USA 83:2632–2636

Rosemeyer H, Sela F (1984) Polymer-linked acycloguanosine. Makromol Chem 185: 687–695

Rozenfeld EL, Lukomskaya IS, Rudakova NK, Shubina AI (1959) α-1,4- and α-1,6-

polyglucosidases of animal tissues. Biokhimiia [Engl] 24:965–970

Russell-Jones GJ, de Aizpurua HJ (1988) Vitamin B12: a novel carrier for orally presented antigens. Proc Int Symp ontrol Release Bioact Mater 15:142–143

Rypáček F, Drobník J, Chmelař V, Kálal J (1982) The renal excretion and retention of macromolecules: the chemical structure effect. Pflugers Arch 392:211–217

Saffran M, Kumar GS, Savariar C, Burnham JC, Williams F, Neckers DC (1986) A new approach to the oral administration of insulin and other peptide drugs. Science 233:1081–1084

Schacht E (1987a) Polysaccharide macromolecules as drug carriers. In: Illum L, Davis SS (eds) Polymers in controlled drug delivery. Wright, Bristol, pp 131–151

Schacht E (1987b) Modification of dextran and application in prodrug design. In: Yalpani M (ed) Industrial polysaccharides: genetic engineering, structure/property relations and applications. Elsevier, Amsterdam, pp 389–400

Schacht E, Vercauteren R, Vansteenkiste S (1988) Some aspects of the application dextran in prodrug design. J Bioact Compat Polym 3:72–80

Schechter I, Berger A (1967) On the size of active site in proteases. I. Papain. Biochem Biophys Res Commun 27:157–162

Schneider YJ (1983) The role of endocytosis and lysosomes in cell physiology. PhD thesis, Catholic University of Louvain

Schneider Y-J, Abarca J, Pirak EA, Baurain R, Ceulemans F, Deprez-de Campeneere D, Lesur B, Masquelier M, Otte-Slachmuylder C, Rolin-van Swieten D, Trouet A (1984) Drug targeting in cancer chemotherapy. In: Gregoriadis G, Poste G, Senior J, Trouet A (eds) Receptor-mediated targeting of drugs. Plenum, New York, pp 1–25

Segaloff D, Ascoli M (1988) Internalization of peptide hormones and hormone receptors. In: Cooke BA, King RJB, van der Molen HJ (eds) Hormones and their actions, part I. Elsevier, Amsterdam, pp 133–149

Senter PD (1990) Activation of prodrugs by antibody-enzyme conjugates: a new approach to cancer therapy. FASEB J 4:188–193

Serry TW, Hehre EJ (1956) Degradation of dextrans by enzymes of intestinal bacteria. J Bacteriol 71:373–380

Seymour LW, Duncan R, Strohalm J, Kopeček J (1987) Effect of molecular weight of N-(2-hydroxypropyl)methacrylamide copolymers on body distribution and rate of excretion after subcutaneous, intraperitoneal and intravenous administration to rats. J Biomed Mater Res 21:1341–1358

Seymour LW, Ulbrich K, Strohalm J, Kopeček J, Duncan R (1990) The pharmacokinetics of polymer-bound adriamycin. Biochem Pharmacol 39:1125–1131

Sezaki H, Takamura Y, Hashida M (1989) Soluble macromolecular carriers for the delivery of antitumor drugs. Adv Drug Delivery Rev 3:247–266

Shen W-C, Ryser HJ-P (1981) Cis-aconityl spacer between daunomycin and macromolecular carriers: a model of pH-sensitive linkage releasing drug from a lysosomotropic conjugate. Biochem Biophys Res Commun 102:1048–1054

Shen WC, Ryser HJ-P (1984) Selective killing of F_c-receptor-bearing tumor cells through endocytosis of drug-carrying immune complex. Proc Natl Acad Sci USA 81:1445–1447

Shen W-C, Ryser HJ-P (1986) Disulfide and other spacers for the intracellular release of drugs from polymeric carriers. Polym Prepr (Am Chem Soc Div Polym Chem) 27:9–10

Shen W-C, Ryser HJ-P, LaManna L (1985) Disulfide spacer between methotrexate and poly(D-lysine). Biol Chem 260:10905–10908

Shen W-C, Ballou B, Ryser HJ-P, Hakala TR (1986) Targeting, internalization and cytotoxicity of methotrexate-monoclonal anti-stage-specific embryonic antigen-1 antibody conjugates in cultured F-9 teratocarcinoma cells. Cancer Res 46:3912–3916

Shen WC, Du X, Feener EP, Ryser HJ-P (1989) The intracellular release of methotrexate from a synthetic drug carrier system targeted to Fc receptor-bearing cells. J Control Release 10:89–96

Shepherd VL (1989) Intracellular pathways and mechanisms of sorting in receptor-mediated endocytosis. Trends Pharmacol Sci 10:458–462

Shepherd VL, Lee YC, Schlesinger PH, Stahl PD (1981) L-fucose-terminated glycoconjugates are recognized by pinocytosis receptors on macrophages. Proc Natl Acad Sci USA 78:1019–1022

Šimečková J, Říhová B, Plocová D, Kopeček J (1986) The activity of complement in the presence of N-(2-hydroxypropyl)methacrylamide copolymers. J Bioact Compat Polym 1:20–31

Sinkula AA (1987) Drug delivery systems research from an industrial perspective. In: Roche EB (ed) Bioreversible carriers in drug design. Theory and application. Pergamon, Oxford, pp 262–280

Snider MD, Rogers OC (1986) Membrane traffick in animal cells: cellular glycoproteins return to the site of Golgi mannosidase. J Cell Biol 103:265–275

Spikes JD (1988) Photosensitization. In: Smith KC (ed) The science of photobiology, 2nd edn. Plenum, New York, pp 79–110

Spikes JD (1990) Chlorins as photosensitizers in biology and medicine. J Photochem Photobiol B6:259–274

Spikes JD, Bommer JC (1986) Zinc tetrasulphophthalocyanine as a photodynamic sensitizer for biomolecules. Int J Radiat Biol 50:41–45

Spikes JD, Bommer JC (1991) Chlorophyll and related pigments as photosensitizers in biology and medicine. In: Sheer H (ed) The chlorophylls. CRC, Boca Raton pp 1181–1204

Spikes JD, Straight RC (1985) Photodynamic behavior of porphyrins in model cell, tissue and tumor systems. In: Jori G, Perria C (eds) Photodynamic therapy of tumors and other diseases. Progetto, Padova, pp 46–53

Stahl PD, Rodman JS, Miller MJ, Schlesinger PH (1978) Evidence for receptor-mediated binding of glycoproteins, glycoconjugates, and lysosomal glycosidases by alveolar macrophages. Proc Natl Acad Sci USA 75:1399–1403

Steele JK, Liu D, Stammers AT, Whitney S, Levy JG (1988) Suppressor deletion therapy: selective elimination of T suppressor cells in vivo using a hematoporphyrin conjugated monoclonal antibody permits animals to reject syngeneic tumor cells. Cancer Immunol Immunother 26:125–131

Steele KJ, Liu D, Davis N, Deal H, Levy JG (1989) The preparation and application of porphyrin-monoclonal antibodies for cancer therapy. Proc SPIE 1065:73–79

Straight RC (1990) Photodynamic laser therapy. In: Keye WR (ed) Laser surgery in gynecology and obstetrics. Year Book Medical Publishers, Chicago (in press)

Šubr V (1986) N-(2-hydroxypropyl)methacrylamide copolymers containing enzymatically degradable sequences as carriers of biologically active molecules (in Czech), (PhD thesis). Institute of Macromolecular Chemistry, Czechoslovak Academy of Sciences, Prague

Šubr V, Rejmanová P, Pohl J, Baudyš M, Kostka V, Kopeček J (1984) Degradation of oligopeptide-poly[N-(2-hydroxypropyl)methacrylamide] conjugates by cathepsins L and H (Abstr 69). 26th Microsymposium Polymers in Medicine and Biology, Prague

Šubr V, Kopeček J, Pohl J, Baudyš M, Kostka V (1988) Cleavage of oligopeptide side-chains in N-(2-hydroxypropyl)methacrylamide copolymers by mixture of lysosomal enzymes. J Control Release 8:133–140

Tartakoff AM (1987) The secretory and endocytic paths. Wiley, New York

Tomlinson E (1987) Theory and practice of site-specific drug delivery. Adv Drug Delivery Rev 1:87–198

Trouet A, Jollés G (1984) Targeting of daunorubicin by association with DNA or proteins: a review. Semin Oncol (4)[Suppl 3] 11:64–72

Trouet A, Masquelier M, Baurain R, Deprez-de Campeneere D (1982a) A covalent linkage between daunorubicin and proteins that is stable in serum and reversible by lysosomal hydrolases, as required for a lysosomotropic drug-carrier conjugate. In vitro and in vivo studies. Proc Natl Acad Sci USA 79:626–629

Trouet A, Baurain R, Deprez-deCampeneere D, Masqelier M, Pirson P (1982b)

Targeting of antitumor and antiprotozoal drugs by covalent linkage to protein carriers. In: Gregoriadis G, Senior J, Trouet A (eds) Targeting of drugs. Plenum, New York, pp 19–30

Tsukada Y, Bischof WK-D, Hibi N, Hirai H, Hurwitz E, Sela M (1982) Effect of a conjugate of daunomycin and antibodies to rat α-fetoprotein on the growth of α-fetoprotein-producing tumor cells. Proc Natl Acad Sci USA 79:621–625

Tsukada Y, Ohkawa K, Hibi N (1987) Therapeutic effect of treatment with polyclonal or monoclonal antibodies to α-fetoprotein that have been conjugated to daunomycin via a dextran bridge: studies with α-fetoprotein producing rat hepatoma tumor model. Cancer Res 47:4293–4295

Tycko B, Maxfield FR (1982) Rapid acidification of endocytic vesicles containing alpha₂-macroglobulin. Cell 28:643–651

Ulbrich K, Koňák Č, Tuzar Z, Kopeček J (1987) Solution properties of drug carriers based on poly[N-(2-hydroxypropyl)methacrylamide] containing biodegradable bonds. Makromol Chem 188:1261–1272

Van Heeswijk WAR, Stoffer T, Eenink MJD, Potman W, van der Vijgh WJF, van der Poort J, Pinedo HM, Lelieveld P, Feijen J (1984) Synthesis, characterization and antitumor activity of macromolecular prodrugs of adriamycin. In: Anderson JM, Kim SW (eds) Recent advances in drug delivery systems. Plenum, New York, pp 77–100

Varga JM (1985) Hormone-drug conjugates. Methods Enzymol 112:259–269

Varga JM, Asato N (1983) Hormones as drug carriers. Polym Biol Med 2:73–88

Varga JM, Asato N, Lande S, Lerner AB (1977) Melanotropin-daunomycin conjugate shows receptor-mediated cytotoxicity in cultured murine melanoma cells. Nature 267:56–58

Vercauteren R, Bruneel D, Schacht E, Duncan R (1990) Effect of the chemical modification of dextran on the degradation by dextranase. J Bioact Compat Polym 5:4–15

Vitetta ES, Fulton RJ, Uhr JW (1986) Immunotoxins: the development of new strategies for treating B cell tumours. In: Tomlinson E, Davis SS (eds) Site specific drug delivery. Wiley, New York, pp 69–80

Von Figura K, Hasilik A, Steckel F (1984) Lysosomal storage disorders caused by instability of the missing enzymes. In: Barranger JA, Brady RO (eds) Molecular basis of lysosomal storage disorders. Academic, New York, pp 133–143

Waley SG, Watson J (1953) The action of trypsin on polylysine. Biochem J 55: 328–337

Wileman T, Boshans RL, Schlesinger P, Stahl P (1984) Monesin inhibits recycling of macrophage mannose-glycoprotein receptors and ligand delivery to lysosomes. Biochem J 220:665–675

Wileman, T, Harding C, Stahl P (1985) Receptor-mediated endocytosis. Biochem J 232:1–14

Willingham M, Pastan I (1982) The transit of epidermal growth factor through coated pits of the golgi system. J Cell Biol 94:207–212

Willingham MC, Hanover JA, Dickson RB, Pastan I (1984) Morphologic characterization of the pathway of transferrin endocytosis and recycling in KB cells. Proc Natl Acad Sci USA 81:175–179

Woodman PG, Warren G (1988) Fusion between vesicles from the pathway of receptor-mediated endocytosis in a cell-free system. Eur J Biochem 173:101–108

Woods JW, Doriaux M, Farquhar MG (1986) Transferrin receptors recycle to cis and middle as well as trans Golgi cisternae in Ig-secreting myeloma cells. J Cell Biol 103:277–286

Worrell NR, Cumber AJ, Parnell GD, Mirza A, Forrester JA, Ross WCJ (1986) Effect of linkage variation on pharmacokinetics of ricin A chain-antibody conjugates in normal rats. Anticancer Drug Design 1:179–188

Yaacobi Y, Sideman S, Lotan N (1985) A mechanistic model for the enzymic degradation of synthetic biopolymers. Life Support Syst 3:313–326

Yamamoto I, Izumiya N (1966) Action of chymotrypsin on synthetic substrates. VI. The action of α-chymotrypsin on glycyl-amino-acyl-L-tyrosine ethyl esters. Arch Biochem Biophys 114:459–464

Yokoyama M, Maeda M, Inoue S, Kataoka K, Yui N, Sakurai Y (1988) Molecular design of missile drug: synthesis of poly(ethylene glycol)-poly(aspartic acid) block copolymer binding adriamycin. Proc The Third World Biomat Cong 4D-14:229

Yokoyama M, Inoue S, Kataoka K, Yui N, Okano T, Sakurai Y (1989) Molecular design for missile drug: Synthesis of adriamycin conjugated with immunoglobulin G using poly(ethylene glycol)-block-poly(aspartic acid) as intermediate carrier. Makromol Chem 190:2041–2054

Yokoyama M, Miyauchi M, Yamada N, Okano T, Sakurai Y, Kataoka K, Inoue S (1990) Characterization and anticancer activity of the micelle-forming polymeric anticancer drug adriamycin conjugated poly(ethylene glycol)-poly(aspartic acid) block copolymer. Cancer Res 50:1693–1700

Young RC, Ozols RF, Myers CE (1981) Medical progress. The anthracycline antineoplastic drugs. N Engl J Med 305:139–153

CHAPTER 6

Systemic Delivery of Pharmacologically Active Molecules Across the Skin

Y.W. CHIEN

A. Biomedical Logic of Transdermal Drug Delivery

I. Introduction

Continuous intravenous infusion of a systemically active drug at a programmed rate has been recognized as a superior mode of drug delivery not only to bypass hepatogastrointestinal "first-pass" elimination, but also to maintain a constant and prolonged plasma drug level within the therapeutically effective range. A closely monitored intravenous infusion can provide both the advantages of direct entry of drug into the systemic circulation and also the control of circulating drug levels. However, this mode of drug delivery entails certain potential risks and, therefore, necessitates hospitalization of the patient and close medical supervision of the drug administration.

Recently, it has been recognized that the benefits of intravenous drug infusion can be closely duplicated by continuous administration of drug through the intact skin without using a hypodermic needle and the potential hazards associated with its use (SHAW et al. 1976b).

In response to this new idea, several transdermal drug delivery (TDD) systems have been recently developed, aiming to achieve the objective of systemic medication of the drug at a specific site on the intact skin with a controlled area of medication. This is exemplified by the marketing of a scopolamine-releasing TDD system (Transderm-Scop System) for 72 h prophylaxis or treatment of motion sickness and nausea (SHAW and CHANDRASEKARAN 1978), the successful marketing of several nitroglycerin-releasing TDD systems (Transderm-Nitro, Nitrodisc, Nitro-Dur, and Deponit) as well as an isosorbide dinitrate-releasing TDD system (Frandol tape) for once-a-day medication of angina pectoris (RUTGERS 1982; WORLD CONGRESS 1984); and most recently, by the regulatory approval of both a clonidine-releasing TDD system (Catapres-TTS) for weekly therapy of hypertension (GOLDMAN 1984) and an estradiol-releasing TDD system (Estraderm) for twice-a-week treatment of postmenopausal symptoms (GOOD et al. 1985).

This chapter intends to review the biomedical logic behind the systemic delivery of pharmacologically active agents via the transdermal route of delivery.

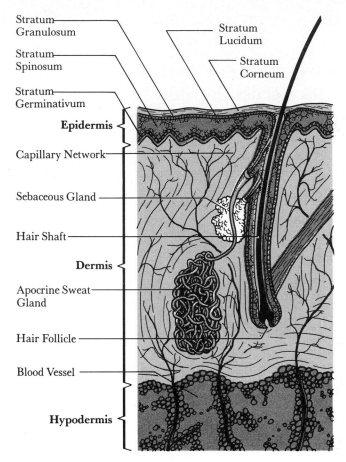

Fig. 1. Cross-sectional view of human skin showing various skin tissue layers and appendages. (From ZANOWIAK and JACOBS 1982)

II. The Skin Site for Percutaneous or Transdermal Drug Delivery

The skin of an average adult body covers a surface area of approximately $2\,m^2$ (or 3000 in.^{2}) and receives about one-third of the blood circulating through the body (JACOB and FRANCONE 1970). It is one of the most readily accessible organs on the human body. Microscopically, the skin is a multilayered organ composed of many histological layers: the epidermal, dermal, and hypodermal (subcutaneous) tissues (Fig. 1). The epidermis is further divided into five anatomical layers with the stratum corneum forming the outermost layer and thus exposed to the external environment.

The stratum corneum consists of several layers of compacted, flattened, dehydrated, and keratinized cells. These cells are physiologically rather inactive and are continuously shed with constant replacement from the underlying viable epidermal tissue (ZANOWIAK and JACOB 1982). The stratum corneum has a water content of around 20% as compared to 70% in a physiologically active tissue, such as the stratum germinativum (which is the regenerative layer of the epidermis).

An average human skin surface is known to contain, on the average, 40–70 hair follicles and 200–250 sweat ducts on every square centimeter of the skin. These skin appendages, however, actually occupy grossly only one-tenth of 1% (0.1%) of the total human skin surface. Even though foreign agents, especially the water soluble type, may be able to penetrate into the skin via these skin appendages at a rate which is faster than through the interfollicular region (undamaged area) of the stratum corneum, this trans-appendageal route of percutaneous absorption has provided only a very limited contribution to the overall kinetic profile of transdermal permeation. Therefore, the transdermal permeation of most neutral molecules at steady state can thus be considered as primarily a process of passive diffusion through the intact stratum corneum in the interfollicular region. So, for a fundamental understanding of TDD (CHIEN 1983), the structure of the skin can be represented by a simplified multilayer model (Fig. 2).

For many decades, the skin has often been used as the site for topical administration of dermatological drugs to achieve a localized pharmacologic action in the skin tissues, such as the use of hydrocortisone for dermatitis (KASTRIP and BOYD 1983). In this case, the drug molecule is considered to diffuse to a target tissue in the vicinity of drug application to produce its therapeutic effect prior to its systemic distribution for elimination (Fig. 2).

In the case where the skin serves as the port of administration for systemically active drugs, the drug applied topically is distributed, following

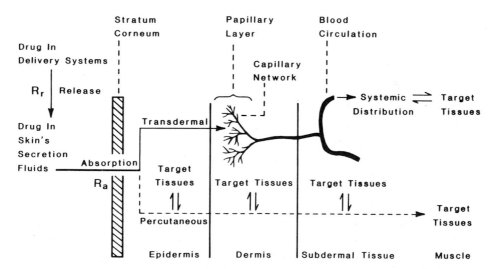

Fig. 2. Drug release from a topical drug delivery system and absorption across the skin for localized therapeutic action in tissues lying directly underneath or for systemic medication in remote tissues

percutaneous absorption, first into the systemic circulation and then into the target tissues (which can be relatively remote from the site of drug application) to achieve its therapeutic action (Fig. 2). This new mode of drug delivery is exemplified by the transdermal controlled delivery of nitroglycerin to the myocardium for the treatment of angina pectoris, of scopolamine to the vomiting center for the prevention of motion-induced sickness, and of estradiol to various estradiol receptor sites for the relief of postmenopausal syndromes (SHAW et al. 1976b; ARMSTRONG et al. 1980; SITRUCK-WARE et al. 1980).

III. Mechanisms and Kinetics of TDD

For a pharmacologically active molecule applied topically on the skin surface to reach a target tissue which is rather remote from the site of drug application, some understanding of the mechanisms and kinetics involved in transdermal delivery are critically important. Thus, the fundamental aspects of drug delivery will be briefly discussed in this section. For more in-depth analysis, interested readers are referred to review articles in this field (CHIEN 1987).

For transdermal delivery to proceed, the pharmacologically active molecule has to possess some physicochemical properties which will facilitate its sorption by the stratum corneum, its penetration through the viable epidermis, and its uptake by the microcirculation in the dermal papillary layer (Fig. 2). The rate of permeation, dQ/dt, across various layers of skin tissues in the course of transdermal permeation can be expressed mathematically (CHIEN 1982) as:

$$\frac{dQ}{dt} = P_s \left(C_d - C_r \right) \tag{1}$$

where C_d and C_r are, respectively, the concentrations of a pharmacologically active molecule in the donor phase, e.g., its concentration on the stratum corneum surface, and in the receptor phase, e.g., its concentration in the systemic circulation; and P_s is the overall permeability coefficient of the skin tissues to the penetrating pharmacologically active molecule, which is called the penetrant, and is defined by:

$$P_s = \frac{K_s D_s}{h_s} \tag{2}$$

where K_s is the partition coefficient for the interfacial partitioning of the penetrant molecule from a TDD system onto the stratum corneum; D_s is the apparent diffusivity for the steady state diffusion of penetrant molecule through the skin tissues; and h_s is the overall thickness of the skin tissues. The permeability coefficient (P_s) for a skin penetrant can be considered as an invariant value if K_s, D_s and h_s in Eq. 2 are maintained at constant values under a given set of conditions.

Analysis of Eq. 1 suggests that, to achieve a constant rate of transdermal permeation, one needs to maintain a condition in which the drug concentration on the surface of stratum corneum (C_d) is consistently and/or substantially greater than the drug concentration in the body (C_r), i.e., $C_d > C_r$; under such a condition Eq. 1 can be reduced to:

$$\frac{dQ}{dt} = P_sC_d \tag{3}$$

and the rate of transdermal permeation (dQ/dt) should be a constant, as the magnitude of C_d remains fairly constant throughout the course of skin permeation. To maintain the C_d at a constant value, it is necessary to deliver the drug to the skin surface at a rate (R_d) that is either constant or always greater than the rate of skin absorption (R_a), i.e., $R_d > R_a$ (Fig. 3). By making R_d greater than R_a, the drug concentration on the skin surface (C_d) will soon achieve a drug level which is equal to or greater than the equilibrium (or saturation) solubility of the drug in the stratum corneum (C_s^e), i.e., $C_d \geq C_s^e$; and the maximum rate of transdermal permeation, $(dQ/dt)_m$, as expressed by Eq. 4, is thus reached:

$$\left(\frac{dQ}{dt}\right)_m = P_sC_s^e \tag{4}$$

In such a case, the magnitude of $(dQ/dt)_m$ is determined by the inherent permeability coefficient (P_s) of the skin to the drug and the equilibrium solubility of the drug in the stratum corneum (C_s^e). This concept of a stratum corneum-limited rate of transdermal permeation was investigated by depositing various doses of pure nitroglycerin, in a radiolabeled form dissolved in a volatile organic solvent, onto a controlled skin surface area of rhesus monkeys (SANVORDEKER et al. 1982). Analysis of the urinary recovery data suggested that the rate of transdermal permeation (dQ/dt) increases as the nitroglycerin dose (C_d) applied on a unit surface area of the skin increases (Fig. 4). It appears that the maximum rate of transdermal permeation ($1.585\ mg/cm^2/day$) is achieved for nitroglycerin in rhesus monkeys when the applied dose reaches the level of $4.786\ mg/cm^2$ or higher.

The kinetics of skin permeation can be assessed more precisely by studying drug permeation profiles across a freshly excised skin specimen mounted on a two-compartment diffusion cell, such as the Franz diffusion cell (Fig. 5). A typical skin permeation profile is shown in Fig. 6 for nitroglycerin. Results indicated that nitroglycerin penetrates through the freshly excised abdominal skin of a hairless mouse at a zero-order rate of $0.476\ (\pm0.041)$ $mg/cm^2/day$ when the pure nitroglycerin, which is an oily liquid, is directly deposited on the surface of stratum corneum (in this case the skin permeation of drug is under no influence from either an organic solvent or a rate-controlled drug delivery system) (KESHARY and CHIEN et al. 1984). Using a hydrodynamically well-calibrated horizontal skin permeation cell, the same

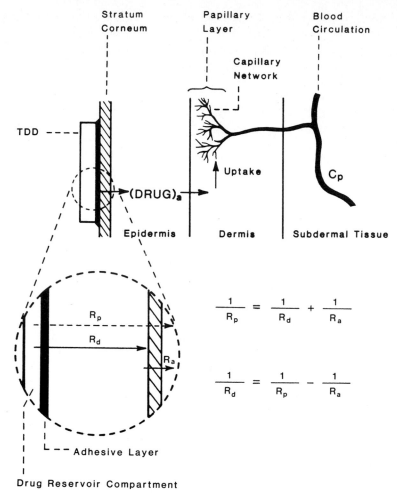

Fig. 3. The relationship among the rate of skin permeation (R_p) of a drug, the rate of drug delivery (R_d) from a TDD system, and the rate of drug absorption (R_a) by the skin

observations were also made in a series of long-term skin permeation kinetic studies for estradiol (VALIA and CHIEN 1984a). These studies provide kinetic data required for a critical analysis of the relationships among skin permeation rate, permeability coefficient, partition coefficient, diffusivity, and solubility. The effects of the kinetics of skin uptake, binding, and metabolism on the skin permeation rate profiles of estradiol and its esters were also evaluated and illustrated (VALIA and CHIEN 1984b; VALIA et al. 1985a,b).

To gain a fundamental understanding of the skin permeation kinetics for a drug and/or to assist the research and formulation development of TDD systems, in vitro skin permeation studies, using a freshly excised skin

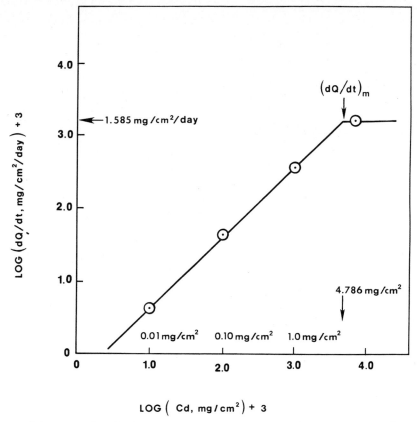

Fig. 4. Linear relationship between the skin permeation rate of nitroglycerin (dQ/dt), determined from daily urinary recovery data, and the nitroglycerin dose applied to rhesus monkey skin (C_d). (Plotted from the data by SANVORDEKER et al. 1982)

specimen mounted in a hydrodynamically well-calibrated skin permeation cell, are considered to be a must before one conducts costly in vivo evaluations in human volunteers.

B. Historic Development of TDD

The potential of using the intact skin as the port for drug delivery has been recognized for over several decades, as evidenced by the development and popularity of medicated plasters. By definition, the plaster is also a drug delivery system developed for external applications. It is prepared by dispersing drugs in natural adhesive materials, such as gum rubber. With proper balance of cohesive strengths, the adhesive is bonded to the backing support, providing both good bonding to the skin as the plaster is applied and a

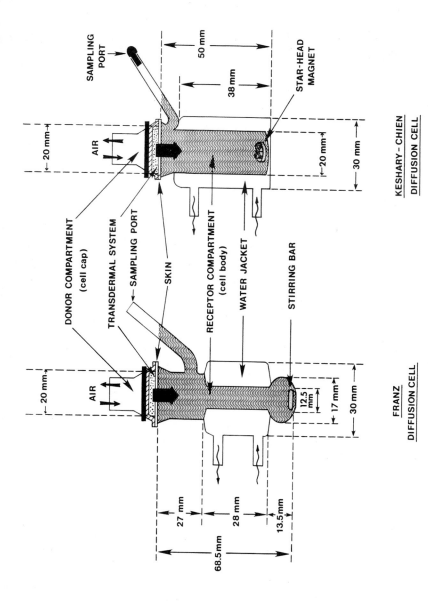

Fig. 5. Two typical vertical type in vitro skin permeation systems, the Franz and Keshary-Chien diffusion cells. The transdermal system is mounted and in intimate contact with the skin

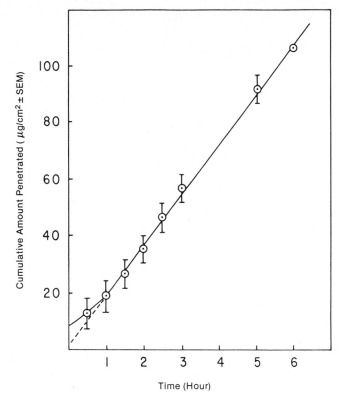

Fig. 6. Permeation profile of pure nitroglycerin across hairless mouse abdominal skin mounted on a Franz diffusion cell at 37°. A constant skin permeation profile was obtained with a permeation rate of 19.85 (±1.71) mcg/cm²/h

clean adhesive break from the skin surface when the plaster is removed. Historically, the medicated plaster could be viewed as the first development of TDD, bringing medication into close contact with the skin so that drug can be delivered transdermally (OSLO et al. 1980).

To date, the historic development of medicated plasters has not been well-documented. However, the use of medicated plasters can be traced several hundred years back to ancient China. One representative Chinese medicated plaster, which is still available for medical use, is shown in Fig. 7. As shown in Table 1, these early generations of medicated plasters tend to contain several herbal drugs and are indicated for localized medication of the tissues directly underneath the site of application.

Medicated plasters have also been very popular in Japan and are available as over-the-counter doses commonly called cataplasms. Salonpas is a typical example and is formulated to contain multiple ingredients, including six therapeutically active agents (Table 2). The formulation has been improved to consist of only the purified drugs.

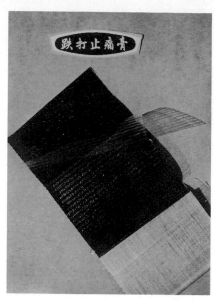

Fig. 7. A representative Chinese medicated plaster (Yang-Cheng; United Pharmaceutical Manufactory, Kwangchow, China). Its composition is outlined in Table 1

Medicated plasters have also been used in Western medicine for several decades. There are several brands of medicated plasters still available in European pharmacies such as Allcock's Pflaster (Table 3). In the United States, three medicated plasters have been listed in the official compendia for more than 40 years (NATIONAL FORMULARY 1946; UNITED STATES PHARMACOPEIA 1950):

1. *Belladonna plaster* which contains belladonna root extract (0.275%) and is indicated for local analgesia
2. *Mustard plaster* which contains black mustard powder and generates allyl isothiocyanate after moistening with warm water; used as a local irritant
3. *Salicylic acid plaster* which contains salicylic acid (10%–40%) and has been used as a keratolytic agent

It is interesting to note that these American medicated plasters are rather simple in formula and all contain only a single active ingredient, which is in great contrast to the European and Oriental medicated plasters (Tables 1–3). However, like the Oriental plasters, the Western medicated plasters have also been developed mainly for local medication.

C. Transdermal Delivery of Pharmacologically Active Organic Molecules

The potential of using intact skin as the port for continuous transdermal infusion of drug has been recently recognized beyond the boundary of topical

Table 1. Chinese medicated plaster

Main ingredients	Content (%)
Menthol	20.00
Fossilia Ossis Mastodi	10.42
Eupolyphagasinensis Walker	10.42
Flos Carthami	9.17
Rhizoma Rhei	8.33
Herba Taraxaci	8.33
Methyl salicylate	8.32
Catechu	6.25
Myrrh	6.25
Sanguis Draconis	4.17
Rhizoma Drynariae	4.17
Radix Dipsaci	4.17

Description and Action: This plaster is prepared on the basis of the dialectic therapeutics of traditional Chinese medicine. The elements of various drugs and herbs, when applied to the skin, will penetrate into the subcutaneous tissues to stimulate circulation and produce a local analgesic effect. The plaster helps to cure inflammation in the muscles and promotes healing of bone fractures.
Indications: Bruises, fractures, sprains, swelling and pain, poor blood circulation, injuries and wounds, rheumatic arthritis, neuralgia, limb languor, etc.
Directions: Cut a piece of desired size from the roll, remove the cellophane, and apply it to the affected part. Medicinal effect lasts 24 h.

medication. The development of female syndromes in males working in manufacturing areas for estrogen-containing pharmaceutical products has challenged the traditional belief that the skin is a perfectly impermeable barrier and triggered the research curiosity of biomedical scientists to evaluate the feasibility of transdermal delivery of drugs for systemic medication. The findings accumulated over the years have practically revolutionized the old theory of the impermeable skin barrier and have also motivated a number of pharmaceutical scientists to develop controlled-release drug delivery systems for rate-controlled transdermal delivery of drugs for systemic medication (MICHAELS et al. 1975; SHAW et al. 1976a,b; SHAW and CHANDRASEKARAN 1978).

Over a decade of intensive research and development efforts, several controlled-release TDD systems have been successfully developed and commercialized (Fig. 8). These TDD systems can be classified, according to the technological basis of their approach, into the following three basic types: (1) *Membrane permeation-controlled drug reservoir type TDD systems*, (2) *Matrix diffusion-controlled drug dispersion type TDD systems*, and (3) *Interfacial partitioning-controlled microreservoir type TDD systems*.

Table 2. Salonpas medicated plaster

Active ingredients	Content (mg/250 cm^2)
Methyl salicylate	330
l-Menthol	300
dl-Camphor	65
Glycol salicylate	50
Thymol	42
Tocopheral acetate	6

Directions: Clean and dry affected area. Remove Salonpas plaster from the cellophane film and apply to affected area. Change plaster once or twice a day. Salonpas plaster is more effective if used after a hot bath. Keep unused portions in a cool place.

So far, eleven TDD systems have been successfully developed and marketed on the worldwide prescription drug market: Transderm-Scop (Ciba), Transderm-Nitro (Ciba), Catapres-TTS (Boehringer-Ingelheim), Estraderm (Ciba), Minitran (3M Riker) Nitro-Dur (Key) and Nitrodisc (Searle), Deponit (Pharma-Schwarz/Lohmann), NTS (Bolar/Horcon), Duragesic (Janssen) and Frandol tape (Toaeiyo-Yamanouchi) (Fig. 8). These TDD systems are discussed individually in the following sections on the basis of the pharmacologically active organic molecules delivered.

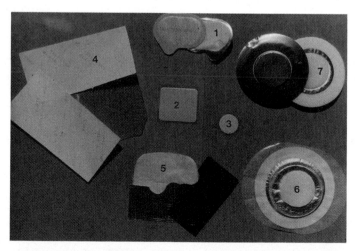

Fig. 8. Some representative TDD systems: *1* Transderm-Nitro; *2* Catapres-TTS; *3* Transderm-Scop; *4* Frandol tape; *5* Deponit; *6* Nitro-Dur; and *7* Nitrodisc

Table 3. Allcock's pflaster

Main ingredients	Content (%)
Cautchuc	43.39
Pix Brugundica	27.14
Gummi-resina Olibanum	20.25
Rhizoma Iridis	8.70
Fructus Capsici	0.27
Cera Flava	0.18
Camphor	0.04
Elemi	0.02
Gummi-resina Myrrba	0.01

I. Nitroglycerin-Releasing TDD System

Nitroglycerin is the best known organic nitrate and its antianginal activity has been documented for over a century. By oral administration, it is extensively metabolized by hepatic first-pass metabolism (Fig. 9). This can be bypasssed by sublingual administration, but the duration of action is extremely short as a result of the drug's inherent biological half-life (<5 min). By topical administration in ointment formulation the duration is extended to 3–4 h. Several technologies have been successfully developed to provide rate control over the release of nitroglycerin and its subsequent permeation across the skin. The three basic types of technologies outlined above have been applied in the controlled release of nitroglycerin. The nitroglycerin-release TDD systems currently available will be the first examples to be discussed in order to illustrate the technical approaches used in formulation development and system design of rate-controlled TDD. They will also serve as the foundation for discussion of other TDD systems.

1. Membrane Permeation-Controlled Drug Delivery

In this approach, the drug reservoir is sandwiched between a rate-controlling polymeric membrane and a drug-impermeable metallic plastic laminate (Fig. 10). In the single reservoir compartment, the nitroglycerin/lactose triturate solids are homogeneously suspended in an unleachable, viscous, liquid medium (e.g., silicone fluid) to form a paste-like suspension. The rate-controlling membrane is a microporous membrane of ethylene-vinyl acetate copolymer with its pores filled with lipophilic mineral oil to act as the channels for drug transport. The nitroglycerin molecules are permitted to release only through the rate-controlling polymeric membrane. The external surface of the polymeric membrane is further coated with a thin layer of a drug-compatible, hypoallergenic, pressure-sensitive, silicone-based, adhesive polymer to maintain intimate contact between the TDD system and the skin surface. The rate of drug release from this TDD system can be tailored by varying the composition of drug reservoir formulation, the permeability co-

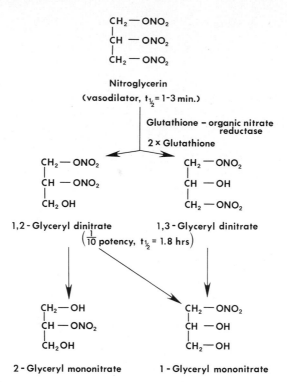

Fig. 9. Biotransformation and metabolism of oral nitroglycerin by hepatic enzymes and change in vasodilation potency and plasma half-life

efficient, and/or the thickness of the rate-controlling membrane. Transderm-Nitro is the TDD system which has been successfully developed from this technology and has received regulatory approval for marketing for once-a-day medication of angina pectoris (GERARDIN et al. 1981; GOOD 1983).

The intrinsic rate of drug release from this type of drug delivery system is defined by:

$$\frac{dQ}{dt} = \frac{K_m/_r K_a/_m \cdot D_a \cdot D_m}{K_m/_r D_m h_a + K_a/_m D_a h_m} C_R \tag{5}$$

where C_R is the drug concentration in the reservoir compartment; $K_m/_r$ and $K_a/_m$ are, respectively, the partition coefficients for the interfacial partitioning of drug from the reservoir formulation to the rate-controlling polymeric membrane and from the polymeric membrane to the adhesive layer; D_m and D_a are the respective diffusion coefficients in the rate-controlling membrane with thickness of h_m and in the adhesive layer with thickness of h_a. Since this TDD system consists of a microporous membrane as the rate-controlling barrier, the porosity and tortuosity of the membrane should also be taken into consideration for determination of D_m and h_m values.

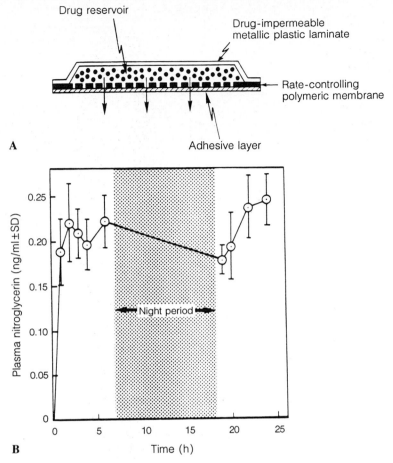

Fig. 10. A Cross-sectional view showing various major structural components of a membrane permeation-controlled reservoir type TDD system such as Transderm-Nitro. **B** Plasma nitroglycerin concentration profiles in 14 healthy human volunteers; each received one unit of the Transderm-Nitro system ($20\,cm^2$) for 24 h. A $(C_p)_{ss}$ value of 209.8 ($\pm$ 22.8) pg/ml was yielded. (Plotted from the data by GERARDIN et al. 1981)

This membrane permeation-controlled TDD technology has also been applied to the development of TDD systems for the rate-controlled transdermal permeation of scopolamine, clonidine, estradiol, testosterone, fentanyl, and prostaglandin derivative. Some of these TDD systems have already received regulatory approval for marketing, e.g., Transderm-Scop, Catapres-TTS, and Estraderm, and will be discussed later in this chapter.

2. Matrix Diffusion-Controlled Drug Delivery

In this approach, the drug reservoir is formed by homogeneously dispersing the nitroglycerin/lactose triturate solids in a gel type hydrophilic polymer

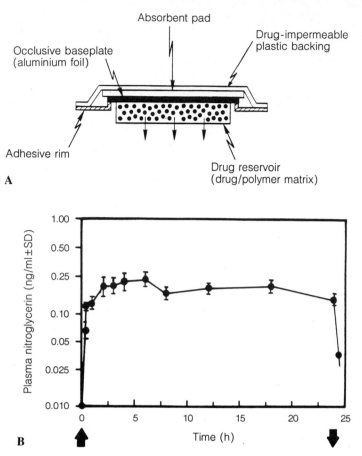

Fig. 11. A Cross-sectional view showing various major structural components of a polymer diffusion-controlled matrix type TDD system such as Nitro-Dur. **B** Plasma nitroglycerin concentration profiles in 24 healthy male volunteers; each received one unit of the Nitro-Dur system (20 cm²) over the chest for 24 h. A $(C_p)_{ss}$ value of 182 (±114) pg/ml was achieved. (Plotted from the data by Noonan et al. 1986) (↑), application of patch; (↓), removal of patch

matrix. The medicated polymer formed is molded and then sliced into medicated discs with a defined surface area and controlled thickness. This nitroglycerin-containing polymer disc is then mounted onto an occlusive baseplate in a compartment fabricated from a drug-impermeable plastic backing (Fig. 11). Instead of applying the adhesive polymer directly onto the drug-releasing surface of the medicated disc, as in the membrane permeation-controlled TDD systems, the adhesive polymer is spread along the circumference of the patch to form a strip of adhesive rim surrounding the medicated disc. The instantaneous rate of nitroglycerin release from this drug dispersion type TDD system is defined as:

$$\frac{dQ}{dt} = \left(\frac{ACpDp}{2t}\right)^{1/2} \qquad (6)$$

where A is the loading dose of nitroglycerin initially dispersed in the polymer matrix; and Cp and Dp are, respectively, the solubility and diffusivity of the nitroglycerin in the polymer. In view of the fact that only the nitroglycerin solute dissolved in the polymer can release, Cp is practically equal to C_R.

At steady state, a Q vs $t^{1/2}$ drug release profile is obtained (CHIEN 1982, 1987) as defined by:

$$\frac{Q}{t^{1/2}} = \left[\left(2A - C_R\right)C_R Dp\right]^{1/2} \qquad (7)$$

Nitro-Dur (KEITH 1983) is the TDD system which has been successfully developed from this technology and has received regulatory approval for marketing for once-a-day medication of angina pectoris. A similar system design has been applied to the development of NTS (KYDONIUS 1986). Instead of the hydrophilic polymer used in the Nitro-Dur system, lipophilic polyvinyl chloride is utilized as the polymer matrix.

Instead of using a nonadhesive hydrophilic polymer, as illustrated by the Nitro-Dur system, an adhesive polymer, e.g., a polyacrylate based adhesive, can also be used as the polymer matrix. In this case, the drug reservoir is formulated by directly dispersing the nitroglycerin in the adhesive polymer and then coating the medicated adhesive, by solvent casting, onto a flat sheet of drug-impermeable backing support to form a single layer of drug reservoir (Fig. 12). The release of nitroglycerin from this type of TDD system is expected also to follow the matrix diffusion process (Eq. 7). Nitro-Dur II is the TDD system which has been successfully developed from this technology and has recently received regulatory approval for once-a-day medication of angina pectoris (NOONAN et al. 1986). It results in a TDD system which has a surface adhesive and is smaller and thinner. Similar system design has been applied to the development of Frandol tape for the transdermal delivery of isosorbide dinitrate and of a new generation of Salonpas medicated plasters with active ingredients similar to those shown in Table 2.

To overcome the nonconstant drug release profiles, this matrix type TDD system can be modified to have the loading level of nitroglycerin varied incrementally to form a gradient of drug reservoir along the multilaminate adhesive layers (Fig. 13). The instantaneous rate of drug release from this drug reservoir gradient-controlled TDD system can be expressed by:

$$\frac{dQ}{dt} = \left(\frac{K_{a/r}D_a}{h_a(t)}\right) A\ (h_a) \qquad (8)$$

In Eq. (8), the thickness of the adhesive layer for drug molecules to diffuse through increases with time [$h_a(t)$], which is a special feature of the matrix-type TDD system. To compensate for this time-dependent increase in

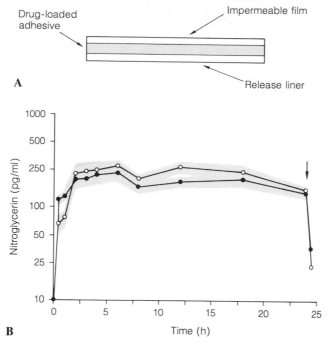

Fig. 12. A Cross-sectional view showing the various major structural components of an adhesive polymer drug dispersion type TDD system such as Nitro-Dur II. **B** Plasma profiles of nitroglycerin in 24 healthy male volunteers; each received one unit of the Nitro-Dur II system (○) (20 cm²) over the chest for 24 h. A $(C_p)_{ss}$ value of 224 (±172) pg/ml was achieved as compared to 182 (± 114) pg/ml for Nitro-Dur I (●). (Plotted from the data by NOONAN et al. 1986)

diffusional path as a result of drug depletion by release, the loading level of nitroglycerin is also increased proportionally $[A(h_a)]$. A near constant drug release profile is thus produced. This type of TDD system is best illustrated by Deponit (WOLFF et al. 1985), which has recently received regulatory approval for once-a-day medication of angina pectoris.

3. Interfacial Partitioning-Controlled Drug Delivery

This approach to drug delivery can be viewed as a hybrid of the reservoir and matrix type drug delivery systems. In this nitroglycerin-releasing TDD system, the drug reservoir is first formed by suspending the nitroglycerin/lactose triturate solids in a solution of a water soluble polymer, e.g., polyethylene glycol. The drug suspension formed is then dispersed homogeneously in a lipophilic polymer, by high-shear mechanical force, to form thousands of tiny unleachable drug microreservoirs (Fig. 14). This thermodynamically unstable dispersion is quickly stabilized by immediately crosslinking the polymer chains in situ, which produces a medicated polymer disc with a constant surface area and a fixed thickness. A nitroglycerin-releasing TDD

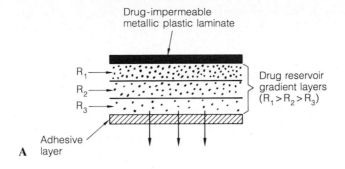

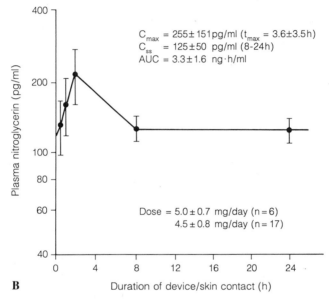

Fig. 13. A Cross-sectional view showing the various major structural components of a drug reservoir gradient-controlled matrix-type TDD system such as Deponit. R's drug concentration in various drug reservior layers. **B** Plasma profiles of nitroglycerin in six healthy male volunteers; each received one unit of the Deponit system ($16\,cm^2$) over the chest for 24 h. A $(C_p)_{ss}$ value of 125 (± 50) pg/ml was obtained. (Plotted from the data by WOLFF et al. 1985). C_{max}, Maximum plasma drug concentration C_{ss}, steady-state plasma drug concentration; AUC, area under plasma concentration

system is then produced by forming the medicated disc at the center of an adhesive pad. This technology has been successfully utilized in the development and marketing of Nitrodisc, which has received regulatory approval for once-a-day treatment of angina pectoris (CHIEN and LAMBERT 1976a,b, 1977; SANVORDEKER et al. 1982; KARIM 1983; CHIEN 1984a, 1985a).

The intrinsic rate of nitroglycerin release from the microreservoir type drug delivery system is defined (CHIEN 1982, 1984a) by:

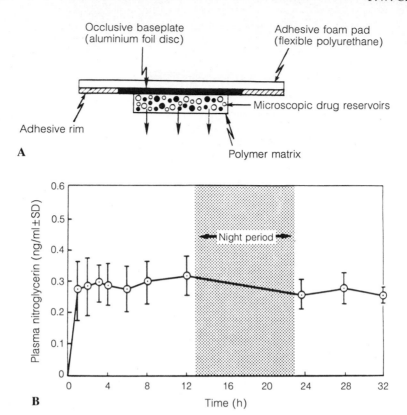

Fig. 14. A Cross-sectional view showing the various major structural components of an interfacial partitioning-controlled microreservoir type TDD system such as Nitrodisc. **B** Plasma profiles of nitroglycerin in 14 healthy male volunteers; each received one unit of the Nitrodisc system ($16\,cm^2$) on the chest for 32 h. A $(C_p)_{ss}$ value of 280.6 (±18.7) pg/ml was obtained (Plotted from the data by KARIM 1983)

$$\frac{dQ}{dt} = \frac{D_p D_s m K_p}{D_p h_d + D_s h_p m K_p}\left[nS_p - \frac{D_1 S_1(1-n)}{h_1}\left(\frac{1}{K_1} + \frac{1}{K_m}\right)\right] \qquad (9)$$

where $m = \dfrac{a}{b}$, in which a is the ratio of drug concentration in the bulk of the elution solution to drug solubility in the same medium and b is the ratio of drug concentration at the outer edge of the coating polymer membrane to drug solubility in the same polymer composition; n is the ratio of drug concentration at the inner edge of the interfacial barrier to drug solubility in the polymer matrix. K_1, K_m and K_p are, respectively, the partition coefficients for the interfacial partitioning of drug from the liquid compartment to the polymer matrix, from the polymer matrix to the coating polymer membrane, and from the coating polymer membrane to the elution solution (or skin); D_1, D_p and D_s are, respectively, the drug diffusivities in the liquid compartment, coating polymer membrane, and elution solution (or skin); S_1 and S_p are, respectively, the solubilities of the drug in the liquid compartment and in the polymer matrix; h_1, h_p and h_d are, respectively, the thicknesses of the liquid layer surrounding the drug particles, the coating polymer membrane around the polymer matrix, and the hydrodynamic diffusion layer surrounding the coating polymer membrane. Release of drugs from the microreservoir type TDD system can follow either a partition control or matrix diffusion control process depending upon the relative magnitude of S_1 and S_p (CHIEN 1984a). So, a Q vs t or Q vs t½ release profile could result (CHIEN 1984b; CHIEN et al. 1983).

Currently, there are six major nitroglycerin-releasing TDD systems on the market. They have been the most successful TDD systems with 1988 sales of approximately 500 million dollars.

II. Scopolamine-Releasing TDD System

A scopolamine-releasing TDD system, the Transderm-Scop transdermal therapeutic system, was the first TDD system to receive regulatory approval (SHAW and CHANDRASEKARAN 1978) and was marketed approximately 2 years before the regulatory approval of nitroglycerin-releasing TDD systems (Transderm-Nitro, Nitro-Dur, and Nitrodisc). There is a slight difference in system design from the Transderm-Nitro system, in which the drug reservoir is a paste-like suspension of nitroglycerin/triturate in silicone fluid; in the Transderm-Scop system the scopolamine solids are dispersed homogeneously in a solid polymer matrix prepared from a polyisobutylene based adhesive polymer. A priming does of scopolamine, which is released at the beginning of topical application to saturate the binding sites in the skin tissue on contact, is also incorporated into the surface adhesive coating on the microporous polypropylene membrane. Judging from pharmacology and toxicology standpoints, scopolamine is an excellent drug candidate for transdermal delivery. If administered by conventional parenteral route (i.m.), a patient will experience a number of cardiovascular adverse effects before the beneficial antinausea action can be realized (Fig. 15).

III. Clonidine-Releasing TDD System

From the standpoint of system design, the clonidine-releasing TDD system, Catapres-TTS, has a structural similarity to Transderm-Scop. It is also constructed from a matrix dispersion type solid state drug reservoir with clonidine solids dispersed homogeneously in a polyisobutylene based adhesive polymer. A microporous polypropylene membrane is added to the surface of the drug-releasing area as the rate-limiting barrier onto which a surface adhesive coating is applied to maintain intimate contact with the skin for a duration of up to 1 week. Three sizes, 3.5, 7.0, and 10.5 cm^2, are available which deliver, respectively, 0.1, 0.2, and 0.3 mg/day of clonidine throughout the course of 7 day treatment.

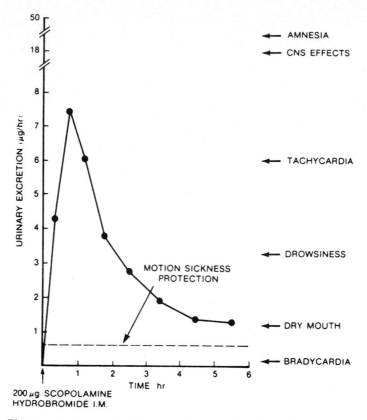

Fig. 15. Pharmacologic effects of scopolamine as a function of systemic drug levels, expressed by urinary excretion profiles, following intramuscular administration of scopolamine hydrobromide. For beneficial motion sickness protection only a very low level of scopolamine is needed. (From Shaw 1983)

After application of Catapres-TTS, plasma levels of clonidine gradually increased and attained an average steady state value of approximately 400 pg/ml during day 3; this average value remained constant throughout the duration of application until the system was removed on day 7 (Fig. 16). On the other hand, the plasma levels of clonidine following twice-a-day oral administration of Catapres tablets assumed a "peak-and-trough" profile with an average ratio of peak to trough concentration of approximately 2 (Shaw 1984). Both 7 day Catapres-TTS and twice-a-day oral Catapres treatments achieved equivalent hypotensive effects (Fig. 17).

IV. Estradiol-Releasing TDD System

Estraderm, the first estradiol-releasing TDD system, is designed to release 17α-estradiol, the natural estrogenic hormone secreted by the human ovary for the development and maintenance of the female reproductive system and

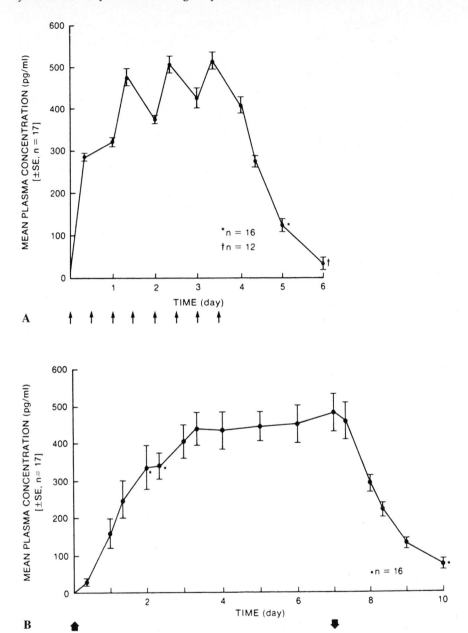

Fig. 16. Comparison of plasma concentration profiles of clonidine during and after **A** twice-a-day oral administration of Catapres tablets and **B** once-a-week transdermal delivery by Catapres-TTS in 17 subjects. (From Shaw 1984) (↑), time for oral administration; (◆), time for patch application; (▼), removal

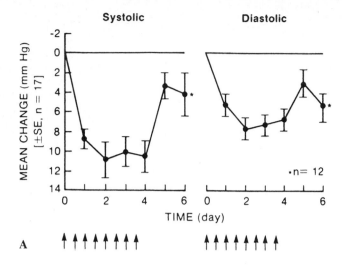

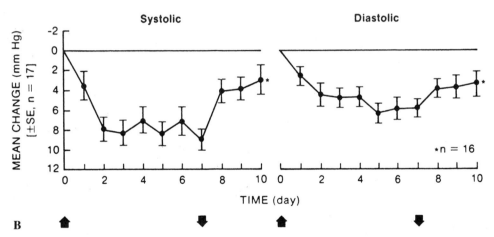

Fig. 17. Comparison of pharmacodynamic profiles, systolic and diastolic blood pressure, during and after **A** twice-a-day oral administration of Catapres tablets and **B** once-a-week transdermal delivery by Catapres-TTS in 17 subjects. (From Shaw 1984) (↑), time for oral administration; (▲), time for patch application; (▼), removal

of secondary sexual characteristics. The system consists of a drug reservoir of estradiol USP in ethanolic solution gelled with hydroxypropyl cellulose, which is sandwiched between a drug-impermeable transparent polyester film and a drug-permeable polyisobutylene adhesive-coated ethylene-vinyl acetate copolymer membrane. The ethylene-vinyl acetate copolymer membrane acts as the rate-limiting membrane which controls the release of estradiol for a duration of up to 72 h. Two sizes, 10 and 20 cm^2, are available to provide nominal in vivo delivery of 0.05 or 0.1 mg/day, respectively, of estradiol via skin of average permeability.

In bypassing the hepatic first-pass metabolism, transdermal delivery of estradiol by the Estraderm system produces mean serum concentrations of estradiol comparable to those produced by a daily oral dose of estradiol at about 20 times the daily transdermal dose. In single-dose studies in 14 postmenopausal women using an Estraderm system that delivers 0.1 mg/day of estradiol, the system produced increased blood levels of estradiol within 4 h and maintained mean serum concentrations of 67 and 27 pg/ml, respectively, of estradiol (E_2) and estrone (E_1), its major metabolite, above the baseline over the course of the application period (Fig. 18). Serum concentrations of estradiol and estrone returned to pretreatment levels within 24 h after removal of the system.

By comparison, oral administration of estradiol from Estrace (2 mg/day) to postmenopausal women resulted in an increase in mean serum concentration of 59 pg/ml of estradiol and 302 pg/ml of estrone above baseline on the third consecutive day of dosing. It yielded an unphysiological ratio of estradiol/estrone as compared to transdermal estradiol delivery by Estraderm. Similar situations also occur with Premarin (Fig. 18).

V. Determination of TDD Kinetics

The release and skin permeation kinetics of drug from various TDD systems developed from different rate-controlled drug release technologies can be evaluated, under identical conditions, using a two-compartment diffusion cell assembly. This is carried out by individually mounting a skin specimen, which has been freshly excised from either a human cadaver or an animal model (DURRHEIM et al. 1980), on a diffusion cell, such as a Franz diffusion cell (Fig. 5). Each TDD system is then applied onto the skin with its drug-releasing area in intimate contact with the stratum corneum surface (CHIEN et al. 1983). The drug permeation profile across the skin is followed by sampling the receptor chamber solution at regular intervals and assaying drug concentrations in the samples by a sensitive analytical method, such as high-performance liquid chromatography (HPLC), until the steady-state skin permeation profile is established. The release profiles of drug from these TDD systems can also be investigated in the same experimental setup without a skin specimen.

In actual measurements of drug release and skin permeation kinetics, the rate profiles obtained could be somewhat below the intrinsic rates estimated from Eqs. 5 and 7–9 due to the effect of mass transfer across the hydrodynamic diffusion layer on the surface of a TDD system or the dermis. The magnitude of reduction is related to the thickness of the hydrodynamic diffusion layer and the physicochemical properties of the drugs (TOJO et al. 1985a,b). It is rather important to take these effects into consideration, so

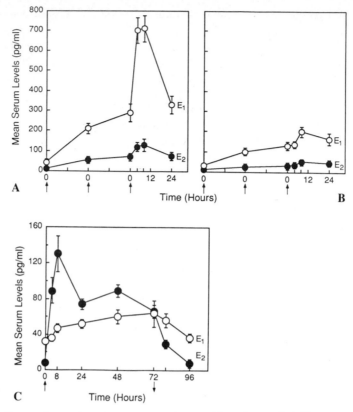

Fig. 18. Comparison of serum concentration profiles of estradiol (E_2; a mg/day) and estrone (E_1), its major metabolite, during and after **A** once-a-day oral administration of Estrace tablets (E_2; 2 mg/day) or **B** Premarin tablets (1.25 mg/day) and **C** 3-day transdermal administration of estradiol (Estraderm; E_2, 0.10 mg/day). (From the data by SHAW personal communication). (↑) beginning of treatment; (↓) termination of treatment

that drug release and skin permeation rate profiles can be accurately determined (CHIEN 1987). All the controlled drug release technologies outlined in Sect. C.I.1 have been applied to the development of nitroglycerin-releasing TDD systems. Thus, these TDD systems will be discussed in this section in order to exemplify the effect of system design on both drug release and skin permeation kinetics as well as to demonstrate how one can optimize the formulation of TDD systems.

1. In Vitro Drug Release Kinetics

Using a Franz diffusion cell assembly, the mechanisms and rates of release of nitroglycerin from these technologically different TDD systems were evaluated and compared (CHIEN et al. 1983). The results indicated that nitroglycerin is released with a constant rate profile (Q vs t) from TDD

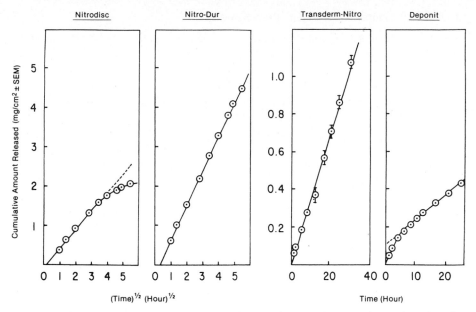

Fig. 19. Comparative release profiles of nitroglycerin from various nitroglycerin releasing TDD systems into saline solution under sink conditions (drug concentration is less than 10% of solubility) at 37°C. The release flux of nitroglycerin is: Nitrodisc $(2.443 \pm 0.136\,\text{mg/cm}^2/\text{day}^{1/2})$, Nitro-Dur $(4.124 \pm 0.047\,\text{mg/cm}^2/\text{day}^{1/2})$, Transderm-Nitro $(0.843 \pm 0.035\,\text{mg/cm}^2/\text{day})$, and Deponit $(0.324 \pm 0.011\,\text{mg/cm}^2/\text{day})$

systems such as Transderm-Nitro (a membrane permeation-controlled drug reservoir type TDD system) and Deponit (a drug reservoir gradient-controlled TDD system) (Fig. 19). The release rate of nitroglycerin from the Transderm-Nitro system $(0.843 \pm 0.035\,\text{mg/cm}^2/\text{day})$ is almost three times greater than that from the Deponit system $(0.324 \pm 0.011\,\text{mg/cm}^2/\text{day})$. It suggests that diffusion through the rate-controlling adhesive multilaminate in the Deponit system plays a greater rate-limiting role over the release of nitroglycerin than does permeation across the rate-controlling membrane in the Transderm-Nitro system.

On the other hand, the release profiles of nitroglycerin from the Nitrodisc and Nitro-Dur systems are not constant, but follow a linear Q vs t½ pattern as expected from matrix diffusion-controlled drug release kinetics (CHIEN 1982, 1987). The release flux of nitroglycerin from Nitro-Dur (a matrix diffusion-controlled TDD system) is almost twice that from Nitrodisc (an interfacial partitioning-controlled microreservoir type TDD system; 4.124 ± 0.047 vs. $2.443 \pm 0.136\,\text{mg/cm}^2/\text{day}^{1/2}$). Apparently, the mechanisms and/or the rates of nitroglycerin release from these four TDD systems are quite different from one another, as expected from Eqs. 5 and 7–9.

2. In Vitro Transdermal Permeation Kinetics

Skin permeation kinetics studies in a Franz diffusion cell using hairless mouse skin demonstrated that, as expected from Eq. 3, all four TDD systems give a constant rate of transdermal permeation (Fig. 20). The highest rate was observed with the Nitrodisc system (0.426 ± 0.024 mg/cm²/day), which was, however, statistically no different from the rate of skin permeation for pure nitroglycerin (0.476 ± 0.041 mg/cm²/day, Fig. 6). For the Nitro-Dur system, practically the same transdermal permeation rate (0.408 ± 0.024 mg/cm²/day) was obtained initially and 12 h later; however, the rate slowed down (0.248 ± 0.018 mg/cm²/day). On the other hand, the transdermal permeation rate of nitroglycerin delivered by the Transderm-Nitro system (0.338 ± 0.017 mg/cm²/day) was 30% lower than the rate achieved by pure nitroglycerin or 21% slower than that by the Nitrodisc system. The lowest rate of transdermal permeation was observed with the Deponit system (0.175 ± 0.016 mg/cm²/day), which achieved only one-third of the skin permeation rate of pure nitroglycerin.

Comparing the rate of skin permeation (Fig. 20) with the rate of release (Fig. 19) suggests that, under the sink conditions (drug concentration in the solution less than 10% of solubility), all TDD systems release nitroglycerin at a rate which is greater than its rate of permeation across the skin. For example, the Transderm-Nitro system, which is a membrane permeation-

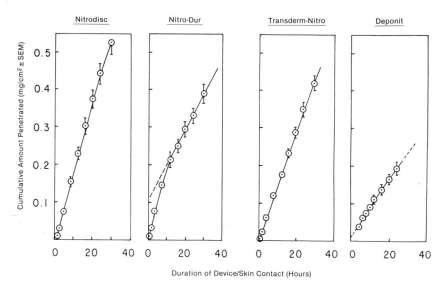

Fig. 20. Comparative permeation profiles of nitroglycerin from various nitroglycerin-releasing TDD systems through the freshly excised abdominal skin of the hairless mouse at 37°C. The rate of transdermal permeation is: Nitrodisc (0.426 ± 0.024) mg/cm²/day), Nitro-Dur (0.408 ± 0.024 mg/cm²/day, <12 h); 0.248 ± 0.018 mg/cm²/day, >12 h), Transderm-Nitro (0.338 ± 0.017 mg/cm²/day), and Deponit (0.175 ± 0.016 mg/cm²/day)

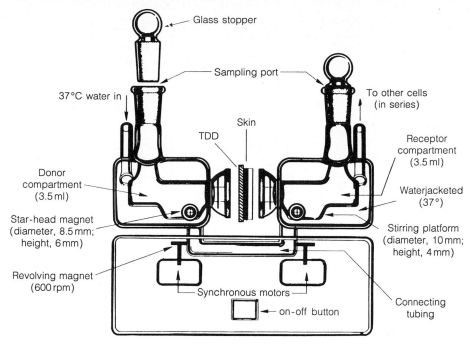

Fig. 21. A horizontal type in vitro skin permeation system (the Valia-Chien skin permeation cell). The TDD system is mounted and in intimate contact with the skin

controlled TDD system, releases nitroglycerin at a rate $(0.843\,mg/cm^2/day)$ which is 2.5 times greater than its rate of permeation across the skin $(0.338\,mg/cm^2/day)$; likewise, the rate of release of nitroglycerin from the Deponit system, whch is a drug reservoir gradient-controlled TDD system having the slowest release rate of nitroglycerin $(0.324\,mg/cm^2/day)$, was also almost twofold faster than the rate of transdermal permeation $(0.175\,mg/cm^2/day)$. The same observations were also true for Nitrodisc and Nitro-Dur. This phenomenon is an indication that the stratum corneum plays a rate-limiting role in the course of skin permeation as a result of its extremely low permeability to most penetrants, including nitroglycerin.

The permeation of nitroglycerin across the skin of a human cadaver was also investigated using a hydrodynamically well-calibrated Valia-Chien skin permeation cell (Fig. 21). The results (Fig. 22) indicated that the transdermal permeation of nitroglycerin through human cadaver skin also follows the same zero-order kinetic profile as observed with hairless mouse skin (Fig. 20). It is interesting to note that the transdermal permeation rates generated from the freshly excised skin specimen of hairless mouse agree fairly well with the data obtained from human cadaver skin not only for nitroglycerin, but also for estradiol and clonidine (Table 4). This agreement suggests that hairless mouse skin could be an acceptable skin model for transdermal permeation

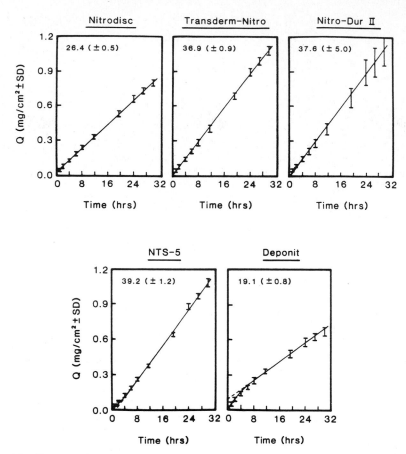

Fig. 22. Comparative permeation profiles of nitroglycerin from various nitroglycerin-releasing TDD systems across the dermatomed skin of a human cadaver as determined in the Valia-Chien skin permeation cell

kinetics studies. It has been noted that the difference in the type and the thickness of skin specimen and in the hydrodynamics of in vitro skin permeation cells could affect the interspecies correlation of skin permeation rates (T.Y. CHIEN et al. 1986, unpublished data). For a better correlation, a skin model with a controlled source and a skin permeation cell with well-calibrated hydrodynamics should be used in skin permeation kinetics studies (Fig. 23).

3. In Vivo Transdermal Permeation Kinetics

The plasma nitroglycerin profiles shown in Figs. 10–14 suggest that all the nitroglycerin-releasing TDD systems achieve a plateau plasma concentration of nitroglycerin within 1–2 h and maintain this steady state level for a duration of at least 24 h as a result of continuous transdermal infusion of drug,

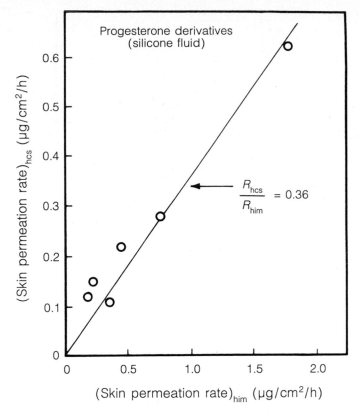

Fig. 23. Correlation of the permeation rates of progesterone and its hydroxyl derivatives across the dermatomed skin of a human cadaver (*hcs*) and the freshly excised skin of the hairless mouse (*hlm*) of approximately the same thickness

Table 4. Interspecies correlation of the in vitro transdermal controlled administration of drugs from TDD systems

Drug	TDD system	Permeation rate (mcg/cm²/h)	
		Human cadaver	Hairless mouse
Nitroglycerin	Transderm-Nitro	19.23	14.55[a]
	Nitro-Dur I	20.33	16.67[a]
Estradiol	Estraderm	0.27[b]	0.40[b]
Clonidine	Catapres-TTS	2.05[c]	3.62[c]

[a] Determined in Franz diffusion cells (Fig. 5) at 37°C (*haq* = 0.0338 cm) (CHIEN et al. 1983).
[b] Determined in Valia-Chien skin permeation cells (Fig. 21) at 37°C (*haq* = 0.0054) (T.Y. CHIEN et al. 1986, unpublished data).
[c] Determined in Valia-Chien skin permeation cells at 37°C (T.Y. CHIEN et al. 1986, unpublished data).

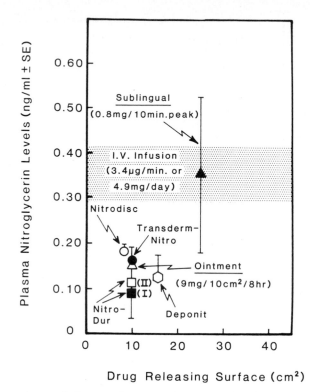

Fig. 24. Comparison of the steady state plasma levels of nitroglycerin achieved by various nitroglycerin-releasing TDD systems (5 mg/day patch) with that by i.v. infusion at practically the same daily dose. Also included for comparison is the plateau plasma level from the topical application of an ointment formulation over a $10 \, cm^2$ skin area (t.i.d.) and the peak plasma concentration from a sublingual administration. (Plotted from the data in Figs. 10–14 and ARMSTRONG et al. 1979, 1980)

at a controlled rate, from the TDD systems. A comparative systemic bioavailability study was conducted and the results demonstrated that there is no statistically significant difference among the plasma profiles of nitroglycerin delivered by Transderm-Nitro, Nitrodisc, and Nitro-Dur (SHAW 1984; KARIM 1986). The same results were also reported for Nitro-Dur I and II (Fig. 12) (NOONAN et al. 1986). The plasma levels obtained by transdermal controlled delivery of nitroglycerin were found to be only one-half to one-third of the levels achieved by either i.v. infusion or sublingual administration (Fig. 24).

The plasma level was found to be linearly proportional to the area of drug-releasing surface of the TDD systems in intimate contact with the skin (Fig. 25). Thus, the plasma level of nitroglycerin can be easily adjusted to reach a target in a therapeutically effective range by simply changing the size of the nitroglycerin-releasing surface applied to the skin.

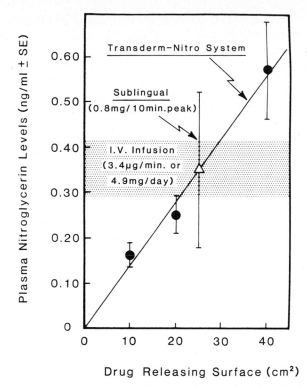

Fig. 25. Linear dependency of the steady state plasma nitroglycerin levels in humans on the drug-releasing surface of a Transderm-Nitro system in contact with the skin. A plasma nitroglycerin concentration of 14 pg/ml was achieved for every cm^2 of drug-releasing surface applied. The plasma levels achieved by i.v. infusion and sublingual administration can be easily duplicated by topical application of one unit of Transderm-Nitro with a drug-releasing surface of 25–30 cm^2 (Plotted from the data by GOOD 1983; ARMSTRONG et al. 1979, 1980). (●), transderm-Nitro system; (△) sublingual nitroglycerin

Further investigations demonstrated that the transdermal bioavailability of nitroglycerin released from TDD systems is independent of the site of application (GOOD 1983). The results of repeated daily applications also showed an excellent day-to-day reproducibility, whereas no drug accumulation was detected (GOOD 1983).

4. In Vitro and In Vivo Correlations of Transdermal Permeation Kinetics

The in vivo rate of skin permeation $(Q/t)_{i.v.}$ can be calculated from the steady state plasma level $(C_p)_{ss}$ data in Figs. 10–14, using the following relationship (CHIEN 1984a):

$$\left(\frac{Q}{t}\right)_{i.v.} = (C_p)_{ss} \cdot K_e \cdot V_d/A_s \qquad (10)$$

where K_e is the first-order rate constant for the plasma elimination of drug, V_d is the apparent volume of distribution for the drug, and A_s is the drug-releasing surface area in contact with the skin.

Results shown in Table 5 indicate that the in vivo transdermal permeation rates for various TDD systems, calculated from steady state plasma profiles using Eq. 10, show a reasonably good agreement with the in vitro data determined from either the dermatomed skin of human cadaver or the freshly excised full-thickness skin of hairless mouse. This agreement provides additional evidence that hairless mouse skin could be an acceptable model for studying the skin permeation kinetics of systemically active drugs in humans.

VI. Optimization of Transdermal Controlled Drug Delivery

To formulate a TDD system one should take into consideration the relationship between the rate of drug delivery (R_d) to the skin surface and the rate of skin absorption (R_a) of the drug (Fig. 3). It is particularly important since the stratum corneum has been known to be highly impermeable to most drugs. Ideally, a TDD system should be designed to have a transdermal permeation rate which is determined by the rate of drug delivery from the TDD system, not by the skin permeability to the drug to be delivered; in such a case, the transdermal bioavailability of a drug becomes less dependent upon the intra- and/or interpatient variabilities in skin permeability.

Table 5. Comparison of in vitro and in vivo transdermal permeation rates

Drug	Delivery system	Permeation rate (mcg/cm^2/day)		
		In vitro		In vivo[g]
		Hairless mouse	Human cadaver	
Nitroglycerin	Nitrodisc	435.6[a]	–	713.0
	Nitro-Dur I	400.1[a]	487.9[d]	371.9
	Transderm-Nitro	349.2[a]	461.5[d]	427.9
	Deponit	269.5[b]	–	282.5
Estradiol	Estraderm	9.6[c]	6.5[c,e]	5.0
Clonidine	Catapres-TTS	86.9[c]	49.2[c,f]	38.9

[a] Determined in Franz diffusion cells (Fig. 5) at 37°C ($h$aq = 0.0338 cm).
[b] Determined in Keshary-Chien diffusion cells (Fig. 5) at 37°C ($h$aq = 0.0108 cm).
[c] Determined in Valia-Chien diffusion cells (Fig. 21) at 37°C ($h$aq = 0.0054 cm).
[d] Determined from skin permeation studies at 37°C using epidermis isolated from human cadaver abdominal skin (MAGNUSON 1983, personal communication).
[e] Determined from skin permeation studies at 37°C using dermatomed human cadaver skin (male, 381 µm).
[f] Determined from skin permeation studies at 37°C using dermatomed human cadaver skin (female left anterior leg, 620 µm).
[g] Calculated from steady state plasma profiles using Eq. 10.

The rate of transdermal permeation of a drug at steady state, $(R_p)_{ss}$, is mathematically related both to the actual rate of drug delivery from a TDD system, $(R_d)_a$, to the skin surface and to the maximum achievable rate of skin absorption. $(R_a)_m$, by the following relationship (SHAW et al. 1975):

$$\frac{1}{(R_p)_{ss}} = \frac{1}{(R_d)_a} + \frac{1}{(R_a)_m} \tag{11}$$

The actual rate of drug delivery from a TDD system to the skin surface, which acts as the receptive medium in clinical applications, can thus be determined from:

$$\frac{1}{(R_d)_a} = \frac{1}{(R_p)_{ss}} - \frac{1}{(R_a)_m} \tag{12}$$

If the rate of skin permeation for pure nitroglycerin, which is freed from the rate-controlling effect of TDD systems, is considered as the value for $(R_a)_m$, the actual delivery rate of nitroglycerin from various TDD systems can be determined. The results are shown in Table 6 and indicate that the delivery rates of nitroglycerin from Nitrodisc, Nitro-Dur, Transderm-Nitro and Deponit are all greater than its maximum achievable rate of skin permeation ($0.621–4.058$ vs 0.476 mg/cm^2/day). The data suggest that the delivery rate of nitroglycerin from all four TDD systems has not been adequately optimized.

Table 6. Actual delivery rate of nitroglycerin from various TDD systems

TDD system	Delivery rate[a] (mg/cm^2/day)
Nitrodisc	4.058
Nitro-Dur I	2.857
Transderm-Nitro	1.166
Deponit	0.621

[a] Calculated from the hairless mouse data in Table 4 using Eq. 12, where $(R_a)_m = 0.476$ mg/cm^2/day.

Using a matrix diffusion-controlled TDD system, the relationship between the release rate of nitroglycerin from a TDD system and the transdermal permeation rate of nitroglycerin was established. The rate of transdermal permeation at steady state, $(R_p)_{ss}$, is related to the rate of release from the matrix type TDD system, $(Q/t^{1/2})$, by the following relationship (KESHARY et al. 1985):

$$(R_p)_{ss} = \frac{x\,(Q/t^{1/2})^2}{1 + y(Q/t^{1/2})^2} \tag{13}$$

in which x and y are composite constants and defined, respectively, as follows:

$$x = \frac{1}{2k} \tag{14}$$

$$y = \frac{R_{sc}}{2K_{sc/pm}kC_p}\left(1 + \frac{R_{vs}K_{rs/vs} + R_{aq}}{K_{vs/sc}K_{rs/vs}R_{sc}}\right) \tag{15}$$

where k is a constant; $K_{sc/pm}$, $K_{vs/sc}$, and $K_{rs/vs}$ are, respectively, the partition coefficients for the interfacial partitioning between stratum corneum and polymer matrix, between viable skin and stratum corneum, and between receptor solution and viable skin; C_p is the drug solubility in the polymer matrix; R_{sc}, R_{vs}, and R_{aq} are, respectively, the diffusional resistances for stratum corneum, viable skin, and receptive solution on the dermis side.

Equation 13 indicates that a hyperbolic relationship should exist between $(R_p)_{ss}$ and $(Q/t^{1/2})^2$. When the release flux of drug from the TDD system is low, the skin permeation rate of drug will be controlled by the delivery rate from the TDD system (Fig. 26). By increasing the release flux of drug, the rate of skin permeation will increase in a hyperbolic manner and then reach a plateau level at which the rate of skin permeation becomes rate-limited by the inherent permeability of stratum corneum to the drug species delivered. The same pattern of skin permeation rate vs drug release rate relationship may be expected for TDD systems delivering drugs at zero-order kinetics. Using Eq. 13, one can optimize the formulation and the design of a TDD system with

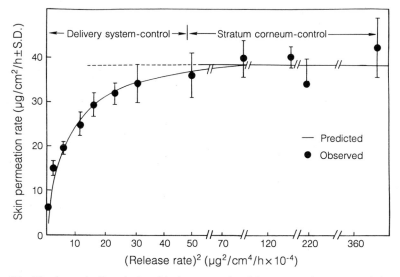

Fig. 26. The hyperbolic relationship between the skin permeation rate and the square of the release flux of nitroglycerin delivered by the polymer diffusion-controlled matrix type TDD system, as predicted by Eq. 13. When $(Q/t^{1/2})^2$ is equal to or less than $48\,\mu g^2/cm^4/h$, the skin permeation rate of nitroglycerin is controlled by the delivery system; when the $(Q/t^{1/2})^2$ is greater than $48\,\mu g^2/cm^4/h$, the skin permeation rate becomes limited by the stratum corneum. From the data by KESHARY et al. 1985)

Table 7. Pharmacologically active peptide/protein molecules and their biomedical applications (From CHIEN 1987; LEE 1987)

Peptide/protein drug	Functions/applications
Cardiovascular active peptide/proteins	
Angiotension II antagonist	Lowering blood pressure
Tissue plasminogen activator	Dissolution of blood clots
CNS active peptides/proteins	
Beta-endorphin	Relieving pain
Melanocyte-inhibiting factor-I	Improving the mood of depressed patients
GI active peptides/proteins	
Gastrin antagonist	Reducing secretion of gastric acid
Pancreatic enzymes	Digestive supplement
Somatostatin	Reducing bleeding of gastric ulcer
Immunomodulating peptides/proteins	
Cyclosporine	Prophylaxis of organ rejection in allogeneic transplants
Interferons	Enhancing activity of killer cells
Metabolism modulating peptide/proteins	
Human growth hormone	Treating hypopituitary dwarfism
Insulin	Treating diabetes mellitus
Vasopressins	Treating diabetes insipidus

the rate of skin permeation controlled by the rate of drug delivery from the TDD system.

D. Transdermal Delivery of Pharmacologically Active Peptide/Protein Molecules

Many petides/proteins are pharmacologically active macromolecules and their therapeutic importance has gained growing recognition in recent years. Many pharmacologically active peptides are increasingly used for the treatment of various diseases (Table 7). Each of the peptide/protein molecules consists of a unique genetically defined sequence of alpha-amino acids connected together by peptide linkage to form a specific molecular configuration, which often determines its physiological functions and therapeutic activities (HEY and JOHN 1973; DENCE 1980; MATHEWS 1975).

Since the inception of genetic engineering, a number of these pharmacologically active peptide/protein molecules, including human insulin (Fig. 27), have been produced commercially; as a result of the progress made in biotechnology, therapeutic application of these peptides/proteins has become both a reality and economical in recent years. A growing number of these peptide/protein drugs have received approval from the regulatory authorities for medical use (e.g., endocrine disorders, cardiovascular diseases, cancers, viral infections) or in preventive medicine (e.g., active and passive immunizations) and have emerged as very important therapeutic agents. Peptide drugs are very potent in activity and often require only a daily dose of micrograms or less.

Insulin

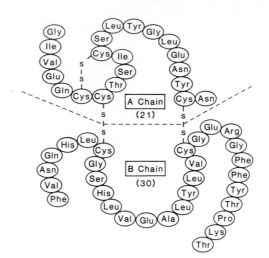

A

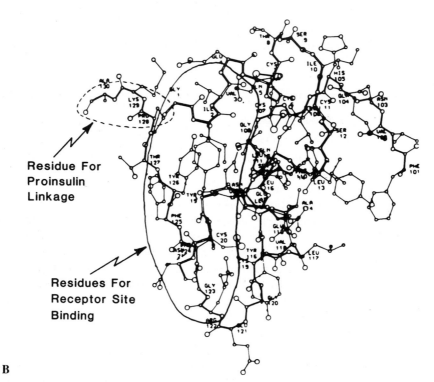

Residue For
Proinsulin
Linkage

Residues For
Receptor Site
Binding

B

Fig. 27. A Amino acid sequence of insulin and **B** its conformation in water. (Modified from BLUNDELL and WOOD 1975)

Although these molecules are highly potent and specific in their physiological functions and/or therapeutic activities, most of them are difficult to administer clinically for systemic medication, except by parenteral administration. Since peptide and protein molecules are highly susceptible to a strong acidic environment and to proteolytic enzymes in the gastrointestinal tract, they are generally not therapeutically active by oral delivery. Also, they are extremely short-acting when administered parenterally and repeated injections are required, often several times a day, to maintain the therapeutically effective levels needed. This treatment regimen has frequently subjected patients not only to constant pain, but also to some health hazards. These problems have often created many patient compliance issues.

Thus, the commercial success of peptide/protein drugs for medication will depend upon the successful establishment of alternative routes of delivery beyond parenteral administration, such as noninvasive routes of delivery, or on the successful development of other novel approaches, such as implantable long-acting delivery systems, to minimize the drawbacks associated with parenteral administration (BANGA and CHIEN 1988a). Over the years, much effort has been made to find nonparenteral routes of administration for effective delivery of peptide/protein drugs with fewer, adverse effects as well as better patient compliance (BANGA and CHIEN 1988a). The potential nonparenteral routes for the delivery of peptide/protein drugs include ocular, nasal pulmonary, buccal, rectal, vaginal, and transdermal routes. Although peptide/protein drugs are highly potent, there are a number of potential problems associated with their delivery through these nonparenteral routes. For instance, each of the potential mucosal routes outlined above will impose additional barriers for peptide/protein molecules to overcome, in addition to the constraints already existing, resulting from the unique biophysical and biochemical properties of peptide/protein molecules. The limitations inherent in these routes are very different from systemic delivery by parenteral administration (ROBINSON 1987).

Without the assistance of an absorption promoting adjuvant, drug delivery through these routes is generally much less efficient than parenteral administration. Incomplete absorption has often been noted, which could be due to a combined effect of poor permeability through these mucosal epithelia and metabolism by enzymes at the absorption site. It has been reported that protease activity in homogenates of the nasal, buccal, rectal, and vaginal mucosae of the albino rabbit is substantial, comparable to that in an ileal homogenate (LEE 1988). A recent study compared the absorption of insulin (Fig. 27), a protein molecule, via several nonparenteral routes of administration (AUNGUST et al. 1988). The results demonstrated that systemic delivery of insulin and its hypoglycemic activity vary from one mucosal site to another and is extremely low compared to intramuscular administration. However, with the coadministration of an absorption promotor, e.g., sodium glycocholate, the hypoglycemic effectiveness of insulin delivered by each mucosal route is substantially improved by as much as 100-fold. Nasal and

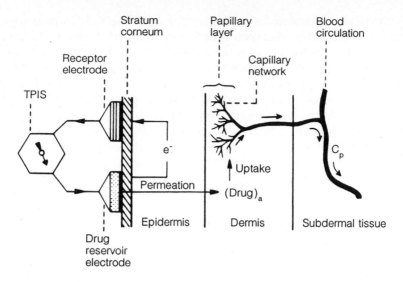

Inotophoresis-facilitated skin permeation flux of ionic species i can be expressed by:

$$J_i^{isp} = J^p + J^e + J^c$$

where

J^p = passive skin permeation flux

$\quad = K_s D_s \dfrac{dC}{h_s}$

J^e = electric current-driven skin permeation flux

$\quad = \dfrac{Z_i D_i F}{RT} C_i \dfrac{dE}{h_s}$

J^c = convective flow-driven skin permeation flux

$\quad = k C_s I_d$

in which:

K_s = Interficial partition from donor solution to stratum corneum
D_i = Diffusivity of ionic species i in the skin
C_i = Donor concentration of ionic species i
$\dfrac{dC}{h_s}$ = Concentration gradient across the skin
I_d = Current density applied
F = Faraday constant
T = Absolute temperature

D_s = Diffusivity across the skin
Z_i = Electric valence of ionic species i
C_s = Concentration in the skin tissue
$\dfrac{dE}{h_s}$ = Electric potential gradient across the skin
K = Proportionality constant
R = Gas constant

Fig. 28. Iontophoretic transdermal delivery of charged drug molecules and the various components defining the mathematical expression of iontophoresis-facilitated skin permeation flux. *TPIS*, transdermal periodic iontotherapeutic system

rectal delivery of insulin achieved roughly half of the systemic efficacy attained by intramuscular insulin.

It has been generally believed that, because of their hydrophilicity and large molecular size, peptide/protein drugs are unlikely to penetrate through a lipophilic barrier such as the stratum corneum. This is probably the reason why not much work has been done in this area of biomedical research and only a few reports exist in the literature (TREGEAR 1966; MENASCHE et al. 1981).

One possible advantage of using a transdermal route for the systemic delivery of peptide/protein drugs is that the skin reportedly has low levels of proteolytic enzymes (PANNATIER et al. 1978). Most of the other non-parenteral routes outlined above have a significant proteolytic enzyme barrier which could drastically reduce the systemic bioavailability of peptides and proteins. Thus, the skin could be a promising site for the administration of peptide/protein drugs provided that their permeation through the skin can be facilitated.

Iontophoresis, which is known to be capable of delivering ions and charged molecules into the body using a physiologically acceptable level of electric current (Fig. 28), appears to be a potential technique for achieving such a goal. A comprehensive review of the principles and technique of iontophoresis-facilitated drug delivery has been completed very recently (BANGA and CHIEN 1988b). Several studies were initiated to investigate the iontophoretic delivery of insulin (STEPHEN 1984; KARI 1986; SIDDIQUI et al.

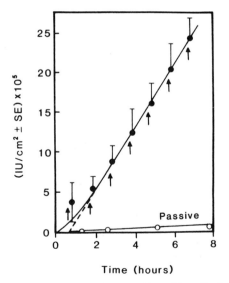

Fig. 29. Comparative in vitro permeation profiles of insulin (pH 7.10) under passive diffusion and iontophoretic transport, across the freshly excised skin of hairless rats. A direct current of 1 mA was applied (↑) periodically every hour for 5 min consecutively for 7 h

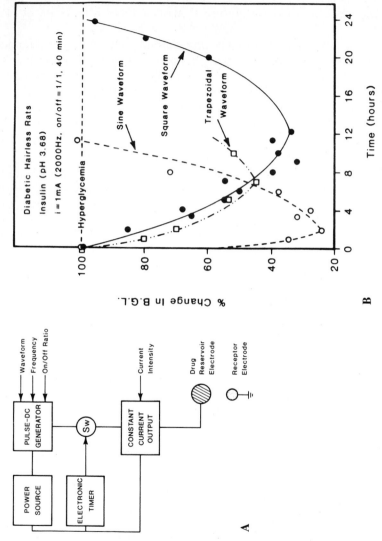

Fig. 30. A Various major electronic components in the transdermal periodic iontotherapeutic system (TPIS) developed at this laboratory. **B** Effect of various wave forms of the pulse current delivered by TPIS on the onset, intensity, and duration of the hypoglycemic effect of insulin, delivered transdermally in streptozotocin-induced diabetic hairless rats

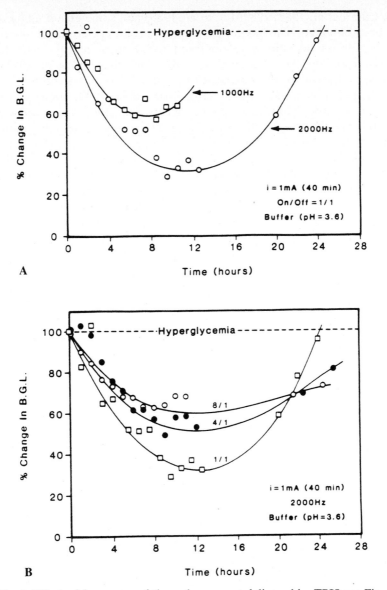

Fig. 31. A Effect of frequency of the pulse current delivered by TPIS see Fig. 30 on the onset, intensity, and duration of the hypoglycemic effect of insulin, delivered transdermally in streptozotocin-induced diabetic hairless rats. **B** Effect of on/off ratio of the pulse current delivered by TPIS on the onset, intensity, and duration of the hypoglycemic effect of insulin, delivered transdermally in streptozotocin-induced diabetic hairless rats. B.G.L., blood glucose level

1987; CHIEN et al. 1987, 1989; LIU et al. 1988) and some encouraging results
have been obtained. The in vitro permeation profiles of insulin across freshly
excised hairless rat skin were observed to be substantially facilitated by
iontophoresis (Fig. 29), (CHIEN et al. 1987, 1989; SIDDIQUI et al. 1987).

Skin is known to be composed of lipids (15%–20%), proteins (40%,
mostly keratin), and water (40%) (ROSENDAL 1942–1943; HARPUDER 1937).
When an electric current is applied across the skin, as in the case of
iontophoresis treatment, the electric potential may alter the molecular
arrangement of the skin components and thus produce some changes in the
skin permeability, especially to charged and hydrophilic penetrants. The
"flip-flop gating mechanism" (JUNG et al. 1983) could be an operating model
for pore formation, which is voltage-dependent, in the keratin-rich stratum
corneum. The flip-flop of keratin (an α-helical polypeptide) may occur to
form a parallel arrangement. Pores are thus opened up as a result of the re-
pulsion between neighboring dipoles, and water molecules and ions will flow
into the pore channels to neutralize the dipole movements. This phenomenon

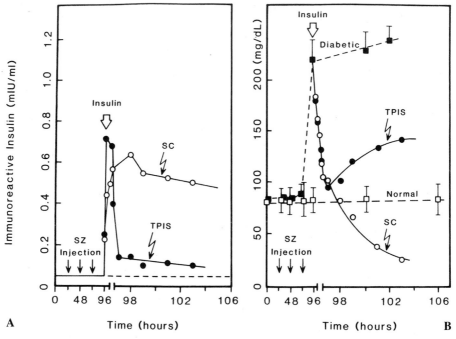

Fig. 32. A Comparative plasma concentration profiles of insulin, determined by
radioimmunoassay, in streptozotocin-induced diabetic rabbits following conventional subcutaneous administration (*SC*) or iontophoretic transdermal delivery by a
transdermal periodic iontotherapeutic system (*TPIS*); SZ, streptozotocin. **B** Comparative blood glucose concentration profiles, determined by glucose analyzer, in
streptozotocin-induced diabetic rabbits following conventional subcutaneous administration (*SC*) of insulin or iontophoretic transdermal delivery of insulin by a TPIS

should lead to an enhancement in skin permeability for peptide and protein molecules (CHIEN et al. 1989).

The upper layers of the skin are also known to have an isoelectric point at pH 3–4; thus the pores in the stratum corneum will have a positive charge when exposed to a solution with pH 3 or lower and a negative charge in a solution with pH 4 or higher (HARRIS 1967; HARPUDER 1937; ROSENDAL 1942–1943). Electro-osmotic flow is also expected to contribute to iontophoretic flux. The direction of electro-osmotic flow will depend on the electrode polarity and skin charge. In addition to ionic conduction and electro-osmosis, other phenomena such as solute-solvent and solute-solute coupling may also account for the observed enhancement in transdermal permeation of drugs, including peptides and proteins, under iontophoresis (CHIEN et al. 1989; WEARLEY et al. 1989; LELAWONGS et al. 1989).

The rate of iontophoretic transdermal delivery of peptide/protein drugs, such as insulin, was found to be dependent upon the physicochemical properties of the formulation, e.g., pH, ionic strength, and electrolyte concentration (CHIEN et al. 1989), and the electronic variables of the iontophoretic delivery systems, e.g., waver form (Fig. 30), frequency, on/off ratio (Fig. 31), current intensity, treatment duration, and mode of current delivery. The iontophoretic transdermal delivery technique provides a noninvasive means for effective systemic delivery of peptide/protein drugs (Fig. 32) and a viable opportunity for pulsatile, modulated, systemic delivery of peptide/protein drugs (Fig. 33).

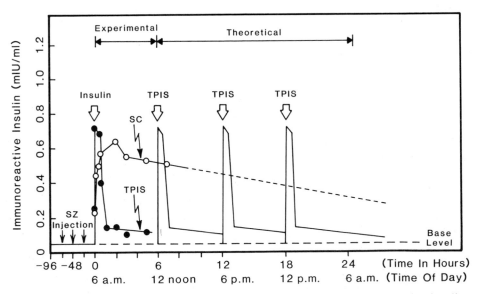

Fig. 33. Comparative daily plasma concentration profiles of immunoreactive insulin in diabetic rabbits following single dose subcutaneous administration (*SC*) and multiple dose chronologic applications by a transdermal periodic iontotherapeutic system (*TPIS*)

An enzyme-responsive transdermal delivery system, which is still in the concept stage, has also been envisioned for insulin delivery (CHECK 1984). An insulin reservoir device which is attached to the skin would generate a minute pulse of electricity to temporarily open the skin pores. While the skin pores are open, the device would take a sample of the blood and process it via a glucose oxidase, by which the device would monitor physiologic indicators and adjust the release of insulin accordingly. A second brief electrical pulse would open the skin pores again to allow the insulin to enter the body. However, no experimental results have been reported yet.

E. Conclusion

As demonstrated by the results outlined in this chapter, transdermal rate-controlled drug delivery can offer one or more of the following potential biomedical benefits:

1. Avoidance of risks and inconveniences of i.v. therapy.
2. Prevention of the variation in absorption and metabolism associated with oral administration.
3. Continuous administration of drugs, especially those with short biological half-lives, without the hazard of i.v. infusion.
4. Increased therapeutic efficacy of drugs that are subject to extensive hepatic "first-pass" elimination.
5. Reduced chance of over- or under-dosing as a result of constant delivery of drug at the required therapeutic rate.
6. Provision of a simplified therapeutic regimen, leading to better patient compliance.
7. Rapid termination of medication, if needed, by simply removing the TDD system from the skin surface.

The intensity of interest in the potential biomedical applications of rate-controlled transdermal drug administration has been demonstrated by a substantial increase in the research and development activities, in many health care institutions, aimed at the development of viable TDD systems for prolonged continuous transdermal infusion of therapeutic agents (RUTGERS 1985; JAEGER et al. 1990). The drug candidates evaluated range from the anti-hypertensive, anti-anginal, antihistamine, anti-inflammatory, analgesic, anti-arthritic, and steroidal contraceptive to peptide/protein drugs. The future of transdermal rate-controlled drug delivery in biomedical applications is undoubtedly bright. The scope of the biomedical applications for this new mode of drug delivery will be expanding for many years to come, especially with the successful development of new approaches to enhance the skin permeability of drugs.

As a result of the progress made in biotechnology, a growing number of therapeutically important peptides/proteins are being produced commercially and their therapeutic applications have become a reality. Due to their biophysical and biochemical characteristics, however, these potent macro-molecules of biological origin are generally not therapeutically active unless given by repeated parenteral administration. There is a growing belief that commercial success of peptide/protein drugs for medication will depend highly upon the successful establishment of nonparenteral routes of admin-istration for effective systemic delivery of a controlled therapeutic regimen; however, the permeation and enzymatic barriers associated with these non-parenteral routes need to be overcome. More research efforts are required to develop viable physical, chemical, and biochemical means to enhance skin permeation and/or to reduce enzymatic metabolism so as to maximize systemic delivery of this new generation of therapeutic agents.

References

Armstrong PW, Armstrong JA, Marks GS (1979) Blood levels after sublingual nitroglycerin. Circulation 59:585

Armstrong PW, Armstrong JA, Marks GS (1980) Pharmacokinetic-hemodynamic studies of nitroglycerin ointment in congestive heart failure. Am J Cardiol 46:670

Arndts D, Arndts K (1984) Pharmacokinetics and pharmacodynamics of transdermally administered clonidine. Eur J Clin Pharmacol 26:79

Aungust BJ, Rojers NJ, Shefter E (1988) Comparison of nasal, rectal, buccal, sublingual and intramuscular insulin efficacy and the effects of a bile salt absorp-tion promotor. J Pharmacol Exp Ther 244:23–27

Banga AK, Chien YW (1988a) Systemic delivery of therapeutic peptides and proteins. Int J Pharm 48:15

Banga AK, Chien YW (1988b) Iontophoretic drug delivery: fundamentals, develop-ment and biomedical application. J Control Kelease 7:1

Check WA (1984) Blundell, TL, Wood SP (1975) Is the evolution of insulin Darwinian or due to selectively neutral mutation? Nature 257:197–203. Am J Hosp Pharm 41:1536–1547 New drugs and drug delivery systems in the year 2000.

Chien YW (1982) Novel drug delivery systems: fundamentals, developmental con-cepts and biomedical assessments. Dekker, New York

Chien YW (1983) Logics of transdermal controlled drug administration. Drug Dece Ind Pharm 9:497

Chien YW (1984a) Long-term controlled navel administration of testosterone. J Pharm Sci 73:1064

Chien YW (1984b) Microsealed drug delivery systems: theoretical aspects and bio-medical Assessments. In: Anderson JM, Kim SW Recent advances in drug delivery systems. (eds), plenum, New York, p 367

Chien YW (1984c) Pharmaceutical considerations of transdermal nitroglycerin delivery: the various approaches. Am Heart J 108:207

Chien YW (1985a) Microsealed drug delivery systems: methods of fabrication. Methods Enzymol 112:461–470

Chien YW (1985b) The use of biocompatible polymers in rate-controlled drug delivery systems. Pharm Tech 9(5):50–66

Chien YW (1987) Transdermal controlled systemic medications. Dekker, New York

Chien YW, Lambert HJ (1976a) Microsealed pharmaceutical delivery devices. US patent #3,946,106

Chien YW, Lambert HJ (1976b) Method for making a microsealed delivery device. US patent #3,992,518

Chien YW, Lambert HJ (1977) Microsealed pharmaceutical delivery device. US patent #4,053,580

Chien YW, Lee CS (1985) Enhancement in transdermal controlled drug delivery. I. Development of a skin-permeation-enhancing transdermal therapeutic system (Abstr). the 39th National Meeting and Exposition of the Academy of Pharmaceutical Sciences, Oct 20–24, Minnesota

Chien YW, Keshary PR, Huang YC, Sarpotdar PP (1983) Comparative controlled skin permeation of nitroglycerin from marketed transdermal delivery systems. J Pharm Sci 72: 968

Chien YW, Valia KH, Doshi UB (1985) Long-term permeation kinetics of estradiol. V. Development and evaluation of transdermal bioactivated hormone delivery system. Drug Dev Ind Pharm 11:1195–1212

Chien YW, Lee CS, Chiang CC (1986) Transdermal drug delivery system with enhanced skin permeability. ACS Symposium on Recent Advances in Controlled Release Technology, April 15–17, New York,

Chien YW, Siddiqui O, Sun Y, Shi WM, Liu J-C (1987) Transdermal iontophoretic delivery of therapeutic peptides/proteins: (I) Insulin. Ann NY Acad Sci 507: 32

Chien YW, Siddiqui O, Shi W-M, Lelawongs P, Liu J-C (1989) Pulse DC-iontophoretic transdermal delivery of peptide and protein drugs. J Pharm Sci 78:376

Cooper ER (1985) Permeability enhancement in skin permeation (Abstr). 1985 International Pharmaceutical R & D Symposium on Advances in Transdermal Controlled Drug Administration for Systemic Medications, June 20–21, College of Pharmacy, Rutgers University,

Dence JB (1980) Steroids and peptides: selected Chemical aspects for biology, biochemistry and medicine. Wiley, New York

Durrheim H, Flynn GL, Higuchi WI, Behl CR (1980) Permeation of hairless mouse skin. I. Experimental methods and comparison with human epidermal permeation by alkanols. J Pharm Sci 69:781

Gerardin A, Hirtz, J, Fankhauser P, Moppert J (1981) Achievement of sustained plasma concentrations of nitroglycerin (TNG) in man by transdermal therapeutic system. AphA/APS 31st National Meeting Abstracts 11(2):84

Goldman P (1984) World Congress of Clinical Pharmacology (1984) Symposium on Transdermal Delivery of Cardiovascular Drugs, Aug 5,1983, Washington. Am Heart J 108(1):195–236

Good WR (1983) Transderm-nitro: controlled delivery of nitroglycerin via the transdermal route. Drug Dev Ind Pharm 9:647

Good WR, Powers MS, Campbell P, Schenkel L (1985) A new transdermal delivery system for estradiol. J Control Release 2:89–97

Harpuder K (1937) Electrophoresis in Physical therapy. Arch Phys Ther X Ray Radium 18:221

Harris R (1967) Jontophoresis In: Licht, S (ed). Therapeutic electricity and ultraviolet radiation. Wiley, Baltimore

Hey DH, John DI (1973) Amino acids, peptides and related compounds. University Park Press, Baltimore (Organic chemistry, ser 1, vol 6)

Jacob SW, Francone CA (1970) Structure and function of Man, 2nd edn. Saunders. Philadelphia, pp 55–60

Jaeger H et al. (eds.) (1990) Proceedings of Neu-Ulm Conference on Transdermal Drug Delivery Systems, Dec 1–3, 1986. ipa, Neu-Ulm

Jung G, Katz E, Schmitt H, Voges KP, Menestrina G, Boheim G (1983) Conformational requirements for the potential-dependent pore formation of the peptide antibiotics alamethicin, suzukacillin and trichotoxin. In: Spach G (ed) Physical chemistry of transmembrane ion motion. Elsevier, New York.

Kari B (1986) Control of blood glucose levels in alloxan-diabetic rabbits by iontophoresis of insulin. Diabetes 35:217

Karim A (1983) Transdermal absorption: unique opportunity for constant delivery of nitroglycerin. Drug Dev Ind Pharm 9:671

Karim A (1986) Comparative pharmacokinetics of different GTN patches. Neu-Ulm Conference on Transdermal Drug Delivery Systems, Dec 1–3, Neu-Ulm

Kastrip EK, Boyd JR (1983) Drug: facts and comparisons. Mosby, St Louis, pp 1634–1708

Keith AD (1983) Polymer matrix considerations for transdermal devices. Drug Dev Ind Pharm 9:605

Keshary, PR, Chien YW (1984) Mechanism of transdermal controlled nitroglycerin administration (I): Development of finite-dosing skin permeation system. Drug Dev Ind Pharm 10:883–913

Keshary, PR, Huang YC, Chien YW (1985) Mechanism of transdermal controlled nitroglycerin administration. III. Control of skin permeation rate and optimization. Drug Dev Ind Pharm 11:1213–1254

Kydonieus AF (1986) Transdermal delivery from solid multilayered polymeric reservoir systems. In: Kydonieus AF, Berner B (eds) Transdermal delivery of drugs, vol 1. CRC, Boca Raton

Laufer LR, de Fazio JL, Lu JKH, Meldrum DR, Eggena P, Sambhi MP, Hershman JM, Judd HL (1983) Estrogen replacement therapy by transdermal estradiol administration. Am J Obstet Gyncol 146:533

Lee VHL Peptide and protein drug delivery systems. (1988) Biopharm Manufact 1:24–31

Lelawongs P, Liu J-C, Siddiqui O, Chien YW (1989) Transdermal iontophoretic delivery of arginine vasopression: (I) Physicochemical considerations. Int J Pharm 56:13–22

Liu J-C, Sun Y, Siddiqui O, Chien YW, Shi WM, Li J (1988) Blood glucose control in diabetic rats by transdermal iontophoretic delivery. Int J Pharm 44:197–204

Mathews DM (1975) Intestinal absorption of peptides. Physiol Rev 55:537

Menasche M, Jacob MP, Godeau G, Robert AM, Robert L (1981) Pharmacological studies on elastin peptides: Blood clearance, percutaneous penetration and tissue distribution. Pathol Biol 29:548–554

Michaels AS, Chandrasekaran SK, Shaw JE (1975) Drug permeation through human skin: theory and in vitro experimental measurement. AIChE J 21:985 National Formulary (NF) (1946) 8th edn

Noonan PK, Gonzalez MA, Ruggirello D, Tomlinson J, Babcock-Atkinson E, Ray M, Golub A, Cohen A (1986) Relative bioavailability of a new transdermal nitroglycerin delivery system. J Pharm Sci 75:688

Oslo A, et al. (1980) Remington's pharmaceutical sciences, 16th edn. Mack, Easton, p 1534

Pannatier A, Jenner P, Testa B, Etter JC (1978) The skin as a drug-metabolizing organ. Drug Metab Rev 8:319–343

Robinson JR (1987) Constraints of nonparenteral routs of administration. Pharm Tech 11:34

Roseman TJ, Bennett RM, Biermacher JJ, Tuttle ME Spilman CH (1984) Design criteria for carbopost methyl controlled release devices. In: Meyers WE, Dunn RL (eds) Proceedings of 11th International Symposium on Controlled Release Bioactive Materials. The Controlled Release Society, Fort Lauderdale, p 50

Rosendal T (1942–1943) Acta Physiol Scand 5:130–151

Rutgers' (1982) Industrial Pharmaceutical R & D Symosium on Transdermal Controlled Release Medication, Jan 14–15, 1983, Rutgers' College of Pharmacy. Piscataway, Drug Dev Ind Pharm 9(4):497–744

Rutgers' (1985) International Pharmaceutical R & D Symposium on Advances in Transdermal Controlled Drug Administration for Systemic Medications, June 20–21, College of Pharmacy, Rutgers University

Sanvordeker DR, Cooney JG, Wester RC (1982) Transdermal nitroglycerin pad. *US patent #4,336,243*

Schenkel L (1986) Experience with estradiol patches. Neu-Ulm 1986 Conference on Transdermal Drug Delivery Systems, Dec 1–3, Neu-Ulm

Schenkel L, Balestra J, Schmitt L, Shaw J (1983) Transdermal oestrogen substitution in the menopause. 2nd International Conference on "Drug Absorption Rate Control in Drug Therapy", Sept 21–23, Edinburgh

Shaw JE (1983) Development of transdermal therapeutic systems. Drug Dev Ind Pharm 9:579–603

Shaw JE (1984) Pharmacokinetics of nitroglycerin and clonidine delivered by the transdermal route. Am Heart J 108:217

Shaw JE, Chandrasekaran SK (1978) Controlled topical delivery of drugs for systemic action. Drug Metab Rev 8:223

Shaw JE, Chandrasekaran SK, Michaels AS, Taskovich L (1975) Controlled transdermal delivery, in vitro and in vivo. In: Maiboch H (ed) Animal models in dermatology. Livingstone, Edinburgh

Shaw JE, Bayne W, Schmidt L (1976a) Clinical pharmacology of scopolamine. Clin Pharmacol Ther 19:115

Shaw JE, Chandrasekaran SK, Campbell P (1976b) Percutaneous absorption: controlled drug delivery for topical or systemic therapy. J Invest Dermatol 67:677

Siddiqui O, Chien YW (1987) Non-parenteral administration of peptide drugs. CRC Crit Rev Ther Drug Carrier Syst 3:195–208

Siddiqui O, Sun Y, Liu JC, Chien YW (1986) Facilitated transdermal transport of insulin. 13th International Symposium of Controlled Release of Bioactive Materials, Aug 3–6, Norfolk

Siddiqui O, Sun Y, Liu JC, Chien YW (1987) J Pharm Sci 76:341

Sitruk-Ware R, deLignieres B, Basdevant A, Mauvais-Jarvis P (1980) Absorption of percutaneous oestradiol in postmenopausal women. Maturitas 2:207

Stephen RL (1984) Biomed Biochim Acta 43:553–558

Sun Y, Siddiqui O, Liu JC, Chien YW, Shi W, Li J (1986) Transdermal modulated delivery of polypeptides – effect of DC pulse waveform on enhancement. 13th International Symposium of Controlled Release of Bioactive Materials, Aug 3–6, Norfolk

Tojo K, Ghannam M, Sun Y, Chien YW (1985a) In vitro apparatus for controlled release studies and intrinsic rate of permeation. J Control Release 1:197–203

Tojo K, Masi JA, Chien YW (1985b) Hydrodynamic characteristics of an in vitro drug permeation cell. Ind Eng Chem Fundam 24: 368–373

Tojo K, Valia KH, Chotani G, Chien YW (1985c) long-term permeation kinetics of estradiol. IV. A theoretical approach to the simultaneous skin permeation and bioconversion of estradiol esters. Drug Dev Ind Pharm 11:1175

Tregear RT (1966) Movement of charged molecules-The electric properties of skin. J Invest Dermatol 46:16

United States Pharmacopeia (USP) (1950) 14th edn

Valia KH, Chien YW (1984a) Long-term skin permeation kinetics of estradiol. I. Effect of drugs solubilizer-polyethylene glycol 400. Drug Dev Ind Pharm 10:951

Valia KH, Chien YW (1984b) Long-term skin permeation kinetics of estradiol. II. Kinetics of skin uptake, binding and metabolism. Drug Dev Ind Pharm 10:991

Valia KH, Tojo K, Chien YW (1985) Long-term permeation kinetics of estradiol. III. Kinetic analyses of the simultaneous skin permeation and bioconversion of estradiol esters. Drug Dev Ind Pharm 11:1133

Wearley L, Liu JC, Chien YW (1989) Iontophoresis-facilitated transdermal delivery of verapamil. II. Factors affecting the reversibility of skin permeability. J Control Release 9:231–242

Weber MA, Drayer JIM (1984) Clinical experience with rate-controlled delivery of antihypertensive therapy by a transdermal system. Am Heart J 108:231

Wolff M, Cordes G, Luckow V (1985) In vitro and in vivo release of nitroglycerin from a new transdermal therapeutic system. Pharm Res 1:23–29

Zanowiak P, Jacobs MR (1982) Topical anti-infective products. In: Laitin Sc(ed) Handbook of nonprescription drugs, 7th edn. American Pharmacentical Association, Washington, pp 525–529

CHAPTER 7

Chemical Delivery Systems

N. Bodor and M.E. Brewster

A. Introduction

One of the most sought after yet elusive goals of the medicinal chemist is the development of site- or organ-targeted drug delivery systems. The realization of Ehrlich's "magic bullet" would be a boon to therapeutic intervention in many disease states. The reason for this, of course, is selectivity. If a systemically or orally administered agent concentrates in its pathophysiologically relevant site, not only would the efficiency of the drug be enhanced but also the toxicity of the material may well be mitigated. This latter point is a consequence of attenuating non-target site drug levels. Lowering the toxicity of a drug is of equal importance to enhancing potency in terms of optimizing the therapeutic index, i.e., the ratio of the median effective and toxic doses.

Numerous techniques have been examined as site-targeting delivery methods including physical, biological, and chemical approaches. This chapter aims to review various chemically mediated delivery systems, including chemical delivery systems (CDSs) for drug targeting to the eye and CNS.

B. Site and Stereospecific Drug Delivery to the Eye

The eye has not traditionally been considered to be an organ for which site-targeted drug delivery is necessary due to its accessibility to topical treatment. This organ is, however, relatively well protected from various foreign substances, including drugs, by the cornea, which allows only a small portion of an applied agent to gain entry to various intraocular sites. The continuous flow of tears causes that part of an applied dose which is not absorbed to pass through the nasal-lacrimal canal and then into the nasal and gastric mucosa. These vascularized sites are excellent areas for drug uptake into the general circulation. Another important limitation to current ophthalmologic therapy is that many of the drugs currently used have not been optimized for the eye, but are simply systemic drugs such as β-adrenergic agonists or antagonists which have found applicability in ocular medicine. Thus, dangerous systemic side effects can be precipitated after topical dosing of drugs in the eye. When, for example, β-blockers such as timolol or betaxolol are used in the treatment of glaucoma, peripheral bron-

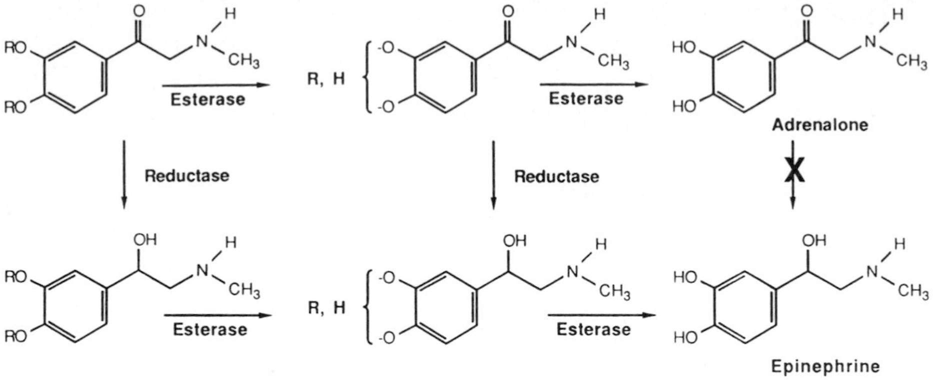

Fig. 1. Ketone reduction of adrenalone esters followed by ester hydrolysis results in release of epinephrine

chial β-adrenoreceptor blockade can occur, resulting in respiratory distress and even death (SCHOENE et al. 1981, 1984; RICHARDS and TATTERSFIELD 1985; FRAUNFELDER and BARKER 1985; AHMAD 1979). Timolol has been shown to significantly alter heart rate after use of 0.5% eye drops (MEKKI et al. 1984). A method which would allow for selective drug delivery to the eye could, therefore, greatly increase the safety of drugs intended for ophthalmologic indications by dramatically reducing the toxicity of the drug. One method appropriate for this purpose is a reduction/hydrolysis-driven CDS.

Adrenalone is the keto-derivative of epinephrine and is itself without sympathomimetic activity when applied as a potential mydriatic agent to the eye. Interestingly, when adrenalone is esterified with lipophilic carboxylic acids, the diesters exert potent mydriatic effects (BODOR et al. 1978). In addition, it has been shown that the adrenalone esters undergo an initial ketone reduction in vivo in the eye followed by ester hydrolysis resulting in the release of epinephrine (Fig. 1) (BODOR and VISOR 1984a,b). The reduction of adrenalone esters appears to occur selectively at the site of action of this drug, namely, the iris-ciliary body, while in other eye compartments only inactive adrenalone is generated (Table 1) (BODOR and VISOR 1984a). As indicated, adrenalone is itself not a reductase substrate, as administration of adrenalone did not lead to elevation of epinephrine levels even though the ketone readily penetrated into most ocular compartments, including the iris-ciliary body.

The potent mydriatic effects of these epinephrine-CDS derivatives could be useful diagnostically and in various surgical procedures, including vitrectomy, lens removal, or lens implantations. In cases where dilatory effects should be of short duration, as in eye examinations, the ester portion of this system can be manipulated since it has been shown that conversion

Table 1. Tissue concentrations of adrenalone and adrenaline at various time intervals following topical administration of diisovaleryl adrenalone[a]

	Concentration of adrenalone[b] (μg/g)			Concentration of adrenaline (μg/g)		
	15 min	30 min	60 min	15 min	30 min	60 min
Cornea	4.47 ± 1.14	7.75 ± 1.92	2.77 ± 0.84	–[c]	–	–
Aqueous humor	0.3 ± 0.09	0.87 ± 0.27	0.52 ± 0.12	–	–	–
Iris-ciliary body	0.42 ± 0.14	2.51 ± 0.72	1.11 ± 0.18	0.09 ± 0.05	0.58 ± 0.35	0.04 ± 0.01

[a] Dose equivalent to 0.05% adrenaline.
[b] HPLC with electrochemical detection (potential 0.7V).
[c] Below detection limit for adrenaline of $0.35 \, \mu g \, g^{-1}$ tissue.

to epinephrine can only occur via the esterified catechol. Thus, alteration of the stability of the catechol esters can directly affect the duration of mydriatic action. By examining plasma and iris-ciliary body homogenate stability for a series of esters, the O,O-di(ethylsuccinate)adrenalone derivative was found to be the most enzymatically labile and therefore most useful epinephrine-CDS when rapid onset and offset of activity is desirable (BODOR and VISOR 1984a). This compound produced significant pupil dilation within 60 min, but the pupil diameter returned to control values within approximately 2 h.

An extension of this approach has been made to various β-blockers (BODOR et al. 1988). β-Blocking agents have been used in the treatment of glaucoma since 1967 but as indicated earlier have profound and undesirable side effects after ophthalmic use. The observation that lipophilic adrenalone derivatives can be converted to epinephrine suggested that various lipophilic ketones can be used as precursors for active drugs in the eye. This concept was embodied in an attempt to generate ketone analogues of β-hydroxyamino β-blockers which would undergo iris-ciliary body-specific reduction to yield the active drug.

Synthetically, it was not possible to easily generate the requisite precursors of propranolol, timolol, carteolol, and other agents due presumably to the chemical instability of the target β-amino ketones. In order to provide more stable intermediates, a hydrolytically labile oxime function was considered (BODOR et al. 1988). This CDS should undergo oxime hydrolysis to yield the intermediate ketone. This species would then undergo reduction in the iris-ciliary body, the site of action of the drug, to yield the active β-blocker. Since drug activation occurs selectively in the eye, material which escapes the ocular site and enters the systemic circulation would be innocuous thus increasing the safety of the drug.

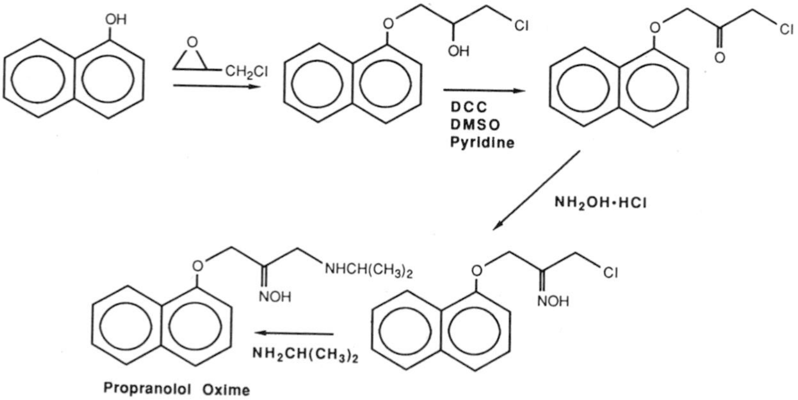

Fig. 2. Preparation of propanolol oxime, DCC, dicyclohexylcarbodiimide

The oxime for propranolol has been prepared as illustrated in Fig. 2. Other β-blockers have been similarly synthesized. Propranolol oxime and timolol oxime were found to exert potent intraocular pressure (IOP) lowering effects in normotensive rabbits and these changes were even greater than those exerted by the parent compounds (EL-KOUSSI and BODOR 1989; BODOR and PROKAI 1990; BODOR et al. 1988). It is interesting to note that, while timolol is more active than propranolol as a mydriatic agent, the oxime derivatives show a reversed order of potency. This may be explained by the relative lipophilicities of the derivatized compounds. As earlier studies have shown, the ketone substrate must be relatively lipophilic to be efficiently reduced by iris-ciliary body enzymes. Thus, adrenalone esters but not adrenalone are converted in vivo to epinephrine, suggesting the greater lipophilic character of the propranolol ketoxime provides for quantitatively better conversion to the parent β-blocker. Pharmacokinetic studies corroborate this suggestion in that relatively high levels of propranolol can be detected in the iris-ciliary body after dosing with the propranolol oxime while the timolol oxime generates relatively little free drug in this and other eye compartments (EL-KOUSSI and BODOR 1989; BODOR 1989).

The generalization that β-blockers with high degrees of lipophilicity should give rise to more active CDSs was tested by synthesis of the oxime derivative of betaxolol (log P = 3.1) which is more lipophilic than propranolol (log P = 2.60). Indeed, betaxolol oxime was highly potent in reducing IOP.

The oxime CDS compounds are isomeric (E/Z) mixtures which are stable in aqueous solutions. Interestingly, separation of the isomeric mixture has indicated that both the Z and E isomers are equipotent. These oximes have also been shown to lack any irritating potential when applied to the eye.

Subsequent work has been completed to carefully examine the conversion of these oxime CDS derivatives to their ultimate drug end product in the eye. This was considered important since the parent β-blockers in many cases exist as enantiomers of differing potency. The S (−) isomer of propranolol, for example, is approximately 100 times more potent than the R (+) enantiomer (HOWE and SHANKS 1966) which is, in turn, metabolically more labile than the S (−) form (KAWASHIMA et al. 1976; WALLE et al. 1984; NELSON and SHETTY 1986). The currently marketed propanolol formulation contains the drug racemate.

When the propranolol or alprenolol ketoxime derivatives are locally applied to the eye, a series of enzymatic events occur as indicated in Fig. 3. Both the intermediate ketone and parent drug are produced. As shown, a mixture of E/Z isomers of the oximes can be detected and studies have confirmed that these geometric isomers are in rapid equilibrium in the eye. The isomerization appears to be enzymatically catalyzed as this process is quite slow in aqueous buffers. Both the E and Z isomers hydrolyze to give a unitary ketone. As shown chromatographically in Fig. 4, the ketone under-

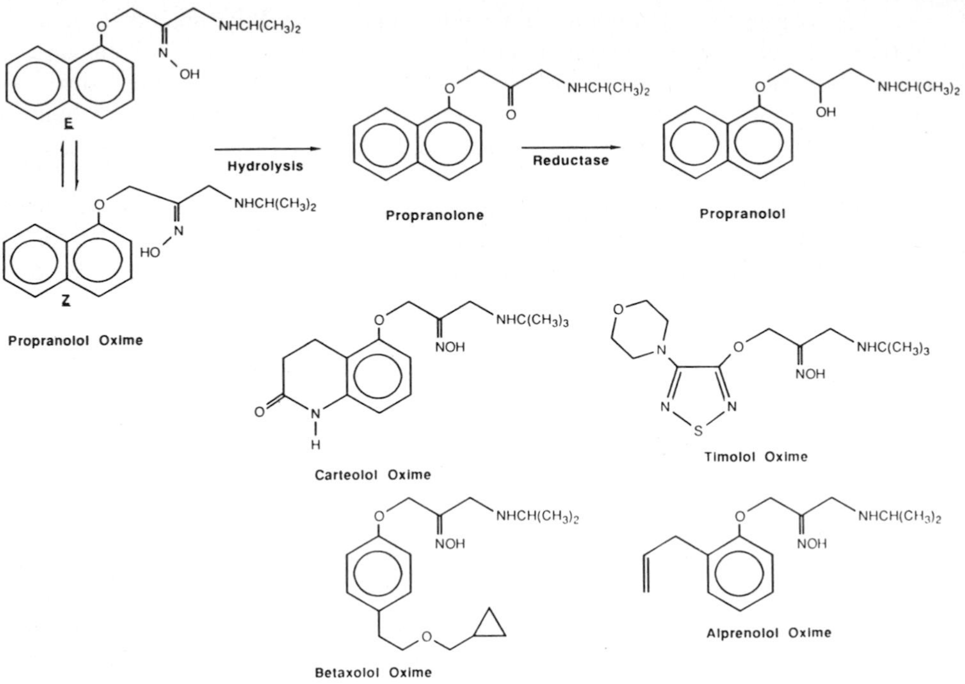

Fig. 3. Enzymatic events that occur following local application of propanolol or alprenolol ketoxime derivatives to the eye

goes reduction to yield stereospecifically the more potent S $(-)$ isomer. Thus, the described CDS provides for a hydrolysis/reduction sequence which is mediated by intraocular enzymes to give an optically active drug. Interestingly, intravenous administration of the propranolol oximes to rats, rabbits, or dogs as either a bolus or 30 min infusion caused *no* cardiovascular effects, the oximes were readily cleared from blood, and no conversion to the active principles could be detected.

Thus by manipulating various enzymatically associated reactions, site- and stereospecific delivery of drugs could be achieved via a sequential hydrolysis/reduction scheme. Agents generated using this approach were more potent and manifested fewer side effects than did the parent β-blockers or catechols. The CDS released drug only at its site of action and systemic administration of the derivatives precipitated no change in resting heart rate or other cardiovascular parameters.

C. Brain-Targeting Drug Delivery

While the eye-based CDS relies on specific enzymatic activation for site selectivity, a CDS useful for enhancing brain levels of various drugs is dependent on organ morphology and physicochemical alterations in the drug structure.

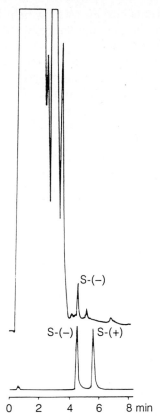

Fig. 4. Chromatographic trace of an extract from the iris-ciliary body of rabbits treated with 1-(isopropylamino)-3-(1-naphthyloxy)-2-propanolone oxime. The homogenate was treated with 2,3,4,6-tetra-*O*-acetyl-β-glucopyrosylisocyanate, a chiral reagent, in acetonitrile. The *S*(-) enantiomer was produced as indicated by authentic *R*(+) and *S*(−) samples (*lower trace*)

I. Background

The inability to effectively deliver agents to and sustain their release in the CNS has caused cerebral disease to be most refractory to therapeutic intervention. The basis of this impermeability is the blood-brain barrier (BBB) (NEUWELT 1989; RAPOPORT 1976; SUCKLING et al. 1986). This functional barricade is derived from evolutionary changes in the cerebral microvasculature. Structurally, the component endothelial cells of the CNS capillaries are joined tightly together precluding intercellular bulk transport (REESE and KARNOVSKY 1967). This architecture forces compounds to diffuse directly through the cell membranes if they are to gain access to the brain parenchyma and, as the cell membranes are phospholipoidal in nature, only lipophilic agents may breach the BBB meaning that many water-soluble substances are excluded. Brain capillaries are also characterized by a high concentration of various enzymes which help to maintain the delicate cerebral milieu by preventing the uptake of blood-borne neurotransmitters and other substances. Enzymes found in high concentration in the cerebral vascular system include monoamine oxidase, catechol-O-methyl transferase, γ-glutamyl transpeptidase, γ-aminobutyric acid transaminase, aromatic amino acid decarboxylase, and others (PARDRIDGE et al. 1975; LEVIN 1977).

These anatomical and enzymatic differences explain the barrier properties of the BBB but incompletely describe the system. Many essential nutrients, such as glucose, and metabolic wastes, including acetate, must be taken up or expelled. These compounds, because of their high polarity, would not be expected to rapidly diffuse through cell membranes and, thus, an apparent problem arises. This paradox is explained by the presence of specialized carrier systems which are located in the BBB (NEUWELT 1989; PARDRIDGE 1981). These protein macromolecular systems are characterized by saturability and high molecular selectivity. Carriers are facilitative in nature and have been identified for hexoses, neutral, acidic, and basic amino acids, monocarboxylic acids, nucleosides and nucleoside bases, choline, and various other biologically important molecules. This avenue, therefore, provides for the bidirectional movement of selective molecules, but, with few exceptions (see GREIG et al. 1987), these systems are not relevant to drug delivery. Thus, the CNS has evolved to exclude polar metabolites and other compounds which may prove harmful. Unfortunately, this barrier system may also exclude many potentially useful therapeutic agents.

General methods for improving drug flux into the brain would, therefore, be useful. Brain uptake of compounds can be improved by derivatization of the drug molecules via prodrug formation (STELLA 1975; BODOR 1981; BODOR and KAMINSKI 1987; BUNDGAARD 1985). A prodrug is a pharmacologically inactive compound which results from transient chemical modification of a biologically active species. The chemical change is designed to improve some deficient physicochemical property of the drug such as membrane permeability or water solubility. After administration, the prodrug, by virtue of its improved characteristics, is brought closer to the receptor site for longer periods of time, where it can convert to the active species. Prodrugs usually require a single activating step. When the BBB is considered, increased drug penetration is usually well correlated with the lipophilicity or the octanol: water partition coefficient of a drug (LEVIN 1980; FENSTERMACHER 1985). In order to improve the entry of a hydroxy-, amino-, or carboxylic acid-containing drug, esterification or amidation may be performed. This greatly enhances the lipid solubility of the drug and, as a result, the drug can better enter the brain parenchyma. Once in the CNS, hydrolysis of the lipophilicity-modifying group will release the active compound. Historically, this is well illustrated in the case of morphine and heroin (RAPOPORT et al. 1980). Heroin is far more potent than morphine even though the two compounds bind comparably to opiate receptors.

Heroin which is the diacetate of morphine is, however, more lipophilic and far more effective in penetrating the BBB.

Unfortunately, simple prodrugs suffer from several important limitations. While increasing the lipophilicity of a molecule may improve its movement through the BBB, the uptake of the compound into other tissues is likewise augmented, leading to a generally greater tissue burden (STELLA and HIMMELSTEIN 1980). This nonselectivity of delivery is especially detrimental when potent drugs such as steroids or cytotoxic agents are considered, in that non-target site toxicities are exacerbated. In addition, while drug uptake into the CNS may be facilitated by increasing the lipophilicity of a drug, its efflux is also enhanced. This results in poor tissue retention of the drug and short biological action. Finally, while the only metabolism associated with prodrugs should be by conversion to the parent drug, other routes can occur and may contribute to the toxicity of the compounds (GORROD 1980). These effects, i.e., poor selectivity, poor retention, and the possibility for reactive catabolism, often conspire to decrease, not increase, the therapeutic index of drugs when masked as a prodrug.

II. Dihydronicotinate CDSs

Some of the limitations associated with the prodrug approach are derived from the fact that only one chemical conversion occurs in the activation of the compound. In many circumstances, multiple facile conversions may not only lead to selectivity in delivery but may also act to decrease the toxicity of a drug as well as sustain its action. A CDS is defined as a biologically inert molecule which requires several steps in its conversion to the active drug and which enhances drug delivery to a particular organ or site (BODOR and BREWSTER 1983; BODOR et al. 1981; BODOR 1987). In designing a CDS for the CNS, the unique architecture of the BBB was exploited. As with a prodrug, a CDS should be sufficiently lipophilic to allow for brain uptake. Subsequent to this step, the molecule should undergo enzymatic, or other, conversions to promote retention within the CNS but, at the same time, to accelerate peripheral elimination of the entity. Finally, the intermediate should degrade, releasing the active compound in a sustained manner. One system which possesses these attributes is summarized in Fig. 5. In this CDS, a carrier molecule is used as a lipophilicity modifier. While many moieties may serve such functions, 1,4-dihydrotrigonellinates have proved to be the most useful. In this approach, a hydroxy-, amino-, or carboxylic acid-containing drug is esterified, amidated, or otherwise covalently linked to nicotinic acid or a nicotinic acid derivative. This compound is then quaternized to generate the 1-methylnicotinate salt or trigonellinate and chemically reduced to give the 1,4-dihydrotrigonellinate or CDS. This dihydro moiety greatly enhances the lipophilicity of the drug to which it is attached. Upon systemic administration, the CDS can partition into several body compartments due to its enhanced lipophilicity, some of which are

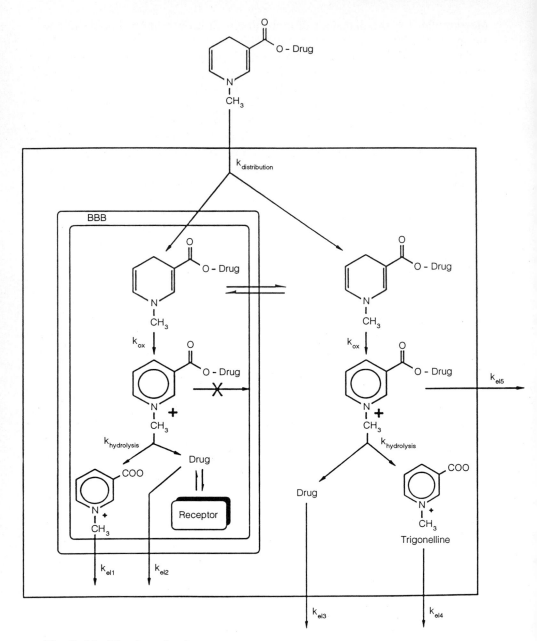

Fig. 5. Modification of a drug to promote retention within the CNS and accelerated elimination is shown. The intermediate is degraded and the active compound is released in a sustained manner

inaccessible to the unmanipulated compound. At this point, the CDS is simply working as a lipoidal prodrug. The carrier molecule is specially designed, however, to undergo an enzymatically mediated oxidation which converts the membrane-permeable dihydrotrigonellinate to a hydrophilic, membrane-impermeable, trigonellinate salt. This conversion occurs ubiquitously. The now polar, oxidized carrier-drug conjugate is trapped behind the lipoidal BBB and is, in essence, deposited in the CNS. Any of this oxidized salt which is present in the periphery will be rapidly lost as it is now polar and an excellent candidate for elimination by the kidney and liver. The conjugate which is trapped behind the BBB can then slowly hydrolyze to give the active species in a slow and sustained manner. By the system design, concentrations of the active drug are very low in the periphery, reducing systemic dose-related toxicities. In addition, the drug in the CNS is present mostly in the form of an inactive conjugate, thus lowering any central toxicities. This approach should allow for a more potent compound in that a larger portion of the administered dose is shunted to its site of action. In addition, this system should allow for an increased dosing interval.

Since it was first proposed in 1978, the brain-targeting CDS has been extensively applied to various pharmacologically active agents. Reviews of work conducted prior to 1983 and 1986 are available (BODOR and BREWSTER 1983; BODOR 1987). It is the purpose of this chapter to concentrate on recent advances of this technology. Specific areas which will be considered include application of this system to neurotransmitters and amino acids, antiviral agents, and estrogenic steroids.

1. Brain-Targeting of Neurotransmitters and Amino Acids

Brain deficiencies of various amino acids or neurotransmitters are thought to figure highly in the etiology of various maladies. Parkinsonism, a disease which affects 100–200 persons per 100 000 of the population, is associated with selective depletion of striatal dopamine (ROLAND 1984). This debilitating malady affects approximately 1% of all individuals over the age of 60 (JANKOVIC 1988). Huntington's disease is associated with diminution of the inhibitory neurotransmitter γ-aminobutyric acid (MARTIN and GUSELLA 1986). Replacement of the deficient neurotransmitter may be of use in treating these diseases and this need suggested the application of the described delivery system. Finally, hypertension is an insidious disease which affects a large percentage of the population and, if untreated, can result in numerous debilitating maladies. One approach to treating hypertension is with tryptophan. Improved delivery of tryptophan to the CNS could, therefore, be useful.

a) Dopamine

Application of the CDS in the case of dopamine was considered particularly apropos since the parent compound does not cross the BBB and, as such, is not useful in replacement therapy (Roos and STEG 1964). L-Dopa, a prodrug of dopamine, has been used clinically for treating parkinsonism but this material exerts peripheral toxicities which can be dose-limiting. A CDS for dopamine was therefore designed and synthesized by first condensing nicotinic acid and dopamine hydrobromide to yield the catechol nicotinamide derivative (Fig. 6) (BODOR and FARAG 1983). Subsequent pivaloylation gave the *bis* ester which was then quaternized and reduced to give rise to the protected dopamine delivery system (DA-CDS). In vitro studies indicated that the necessary transformation required to liberate dopamine occurred, meaning that the DA-CDS was converted to the corresponding quaternary salt (P-DA-Q$^+$) which further underwent sequential ester hydrolysis to give the 1-methylnicotinamide of dopamine (DA-Q$^+$), the ultimate dopamine precursor or prodrug. Systemic administration of the DA-CDS to rats caused high levels of the DA-Q$^+$ to accumulate in the CNS while blood levels were shown to be rapidly cleared. This uncoupling of brain and blood concentration of the administered compounds and its metabolites is a characteristic finding of the CNS approach.

Initial tests used to show dopamine release included such pharmacologic indications as the ability of dopamine to decrease prolactin secretion (BODOR and FARAG 1983; BODOR and SIMPKINS 1983). This action is manifested by the ability of this neurotransmitter to interact with lactophores in the

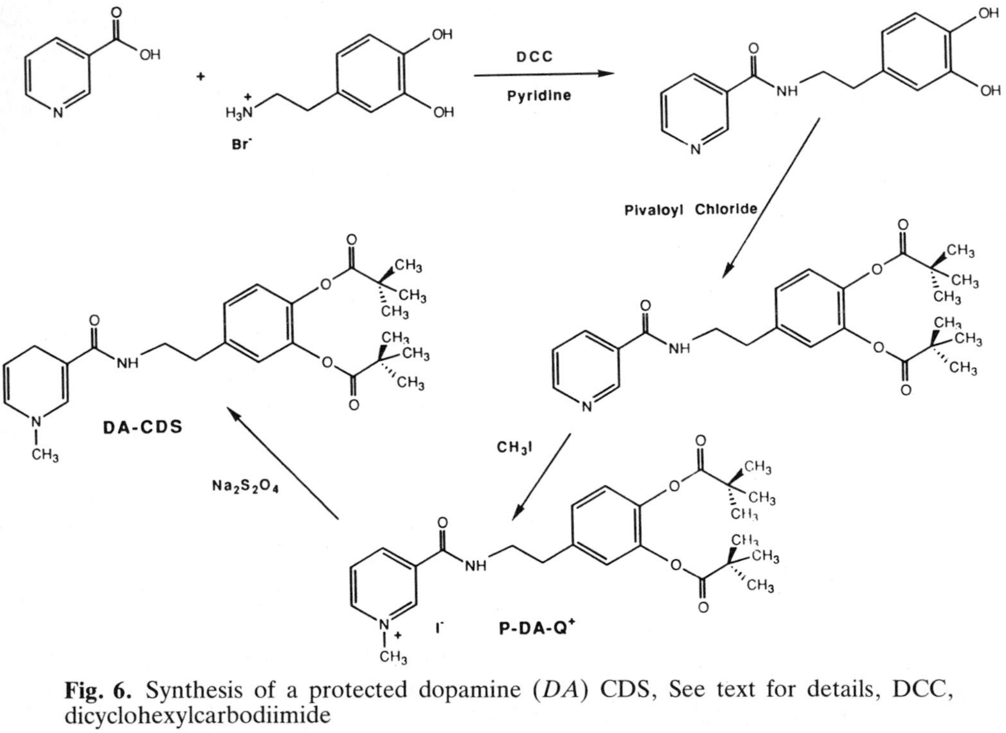

Fig. 6. Synthesis of a protected dopamine (*DA*) CDS, See text for details, DCC, dicyclohexylcarbodiimide

anterior pituitary gland. In testing the DA-CDS, male rats were primed with β-estradiol to elevate serum prolactin. Administration of DA-CDS to these animals resulted in suppression of serum prolactin by approximately 80% for over 12 h. In contrast, the polar dopamine precursor, P-DA-Q$^+$, significantly suppressed prolactin levels only at 30 min, after which serum prolactin returned to control values. These studies, therefore, suggest that dopamine is being slowly released from DA-Q$^+$ after brain sequestration subsequent to DA-CDS administration. The fact that the CDS was, in and of itself, not active, and that hydrolysis was necessary for activity was shown using isolated anterior pituitary glands (BODOR and SIMPKINS 1983). Dopamine at a concentration of 200 nM significantly reduced the rate of prolactin secretion while the DA-CDS had no effect, suggesting it possesses a much lower binding affinity for the pituitary lactophores.

More direct evidence for dopamine release was observed in rats pretreated with the aromatic amino acid decarboxylase inhibitor, m-hydroxybenzylhydrazine (SIMPKINS et al. 1985). Animals administered the DA-CDS demonstrated a dramatic increase of dopamine in the hypothalamus (400%–500%) and significant increases (17%–20%) in the striatum (Fig. 7). In addition, dopamine metabolites, including dihydroxyphenylacetic acid (DOPAC) and homovanillic acid (HVA) were also substantially increased in hypothalamus and striatum after DA-CDS administration.

A second dopamine CDS has also been considered. In this case, an activated carbamate was used as the bridge linking the dihydronicotinamide and the dopamine nitrogen. In the preparation of this material, the dipivaloate of dopamine was treated with chloromethyl chloroformate to give the chloromethyl carbamate derivative. Reaction of this intermediate with the triethylammonium salt of nicotinic acid generated the acyloxyalkyl carbamate which was further methylated and reduced to yield the CDS. In vitro homogenate studies have revealed rapid conversion of this delivery system to the corresponding quaternary salt followed by release of dopamine.

b) γ-Aminobutyric Acid

γ-Aminobutyric acid (GABA) is an inhibitory neurotransmitter and has been implicated in the etiology of epilepsy and Huntington's disease (SAITO 1976; FONNUM 1978). Unfortunately, GABA is, of all neurotransmitters, the one which passes the BBB the least efficiently. Several CDSs were, therefore, devised for GABA. Interestingly, simple nonredox nicotinamides of GABA were shown to have some anticonvulsant activity, albeit in very high concentrations (1 g/kg in mice) (MATSUYAMA et al. 1984). This may indicate that hydrolysis of the amide need not be necessary for GABAminergic activity, unlike in the dopamine case.

Two types of GABA-CDS were considered: derivatives of GABA amides and analogues of GABA (WOODARD et al. 1990). The benzyl (BZ) and cyclohexyl (CH) esters of GABA were condensed with nicotinic acid,

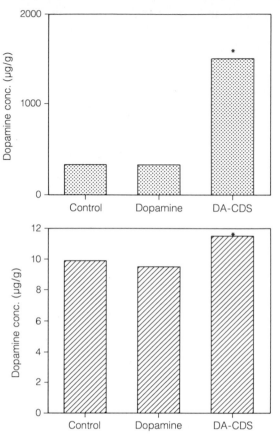

Fig. 7. Effect of DA-CDS on dopamine in hypothalamus (*upper panel*) and striatum (*lower panel*) after *m*-hydroxybenzylhydrazine treatment. Data are represented as mean for 7–13 animals per group. *Asterisks* denote significantly different means ($p < 0.02$)

giving the corresponding GABA ester nicotinamides (Fig. 8). Quaternization of these compounds with methyl iodide provided the nicotinate salts which, upon reduction, afforded Bz-GABA-CDS and CH-GABA-CDS. In providing GABA analogues, the GABA nitrogen was included into the pyridine moiety of the delivery system. Nicotinamide was quaternized with the ethyl ester of 4-bromobutyric acid, giving the nicotinamide salt which was reduced in aqueous basic sodium dithionite to give the GABA-1-CDS. A second analogue was synthesized using an agent useful for converting primary amines to nicotinamide quaternary salts, 1-(2,4-dinitrophenyl)-nicotinamide chloride. The salt was reacted with the diethylacetal of 4-aminobutyraldehyde to give the nicotinate salt which was then reduced to the GABA-2-CDS (Fig. 8). Homogenate studies indicate that facile

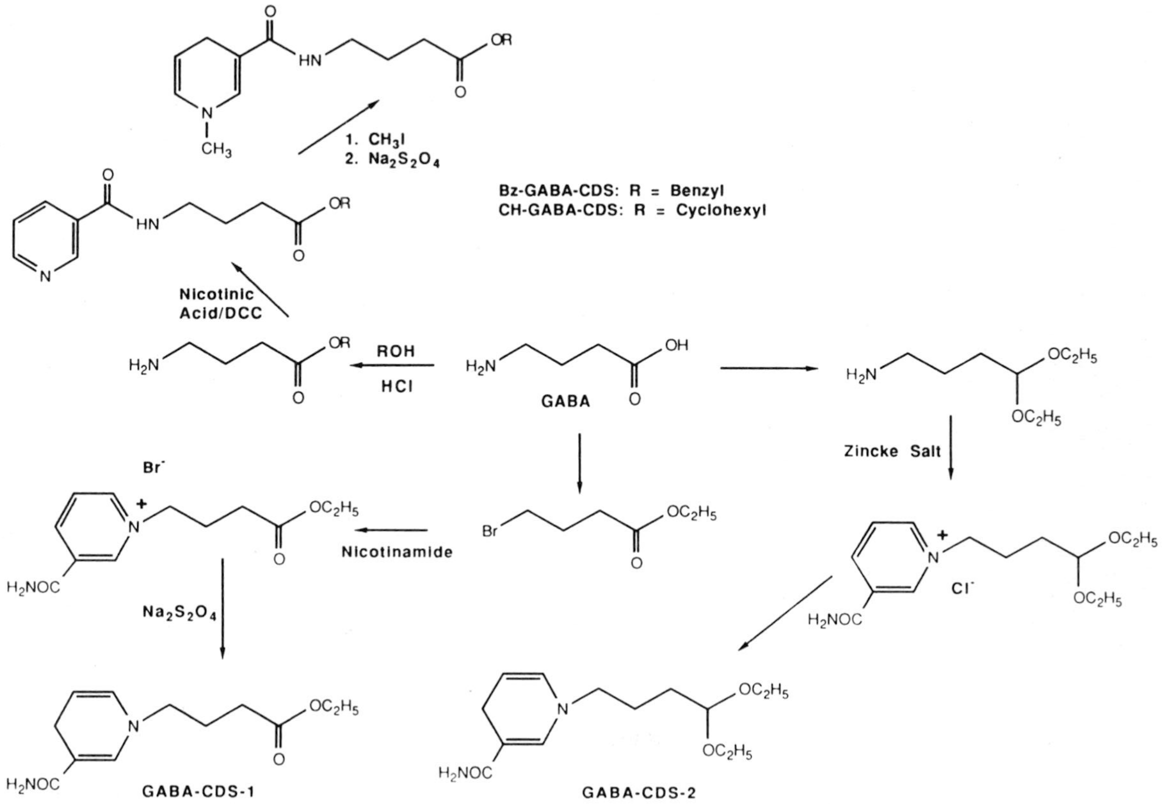

Fig. 8. Synthesis of GABA amide derivatives and GABA analogues. See text for details. DCC, dicyclohexyl-carbodiimide

oxidation and hydrolysis of the synthesized compounds occurred. Oxidation proceeded with varying preferences over hydrolysis. Systemic administration of Bz-GABA-CDS to Sprague-Dawley rats produced sustained concentrations of the corresponding pyridinium salt in the brain. The level of quaternary species was significant up to 12 h, while the salt was undetectable in liver by 4 h, in blood and kidney by 2 h, in heart and lungs by 1 h and in testes at 30 min. The brain penetration index (BPI) for the Bz-GABA-CDS was calculated to be 86% compared to 1% when GABA itself is administered.

The ability of synthesized delivery systems to act as anticonvulsants by antagonizing electroconvulsive shock at 1 min post-dosing was also tested. While CH-GABA-CDS and GABA-2-CDS showed some activity at 40 mg/kg, both Bz-GABA-CDS and GABA-CDS protected animals completely at this dose. The ED_{50} for the benzyl derivatives was found to be 12.1 mg/kg, while the analogue (GABA-1-CDS) generated a value of 17 mg/kg in this model. The anxiolytic properties of Bz-GABA-CDS were also evaluated in male rats by means of drink-foot shock conflict procedure (ANDERSON et al. 1987b). Doses of this compound from 4–25 mg/kg were administered. All doses caused a significant increase in anxiolysis over control levels through 8 h (Fig. 9). A dose-dependent increase occurred up to 10 mg/kg, but no additional increase was seen at 25 mg/kg. No sedation was observed at 2 h with the 10 mg/kg dose as evaluated by open-field behavior.

c) Tryptophan

L-Tryptophan is an essential amino acid which is used pharmacologically as a nutrient and more recently as an antidepressant. A number of reports have indicated that acute administration of tryptophan can lower blood pressure in spontaneously hypertensive, and other, rat models (WOLF and KUHN 1984a,b; SVED et al. 1982; FULLER et al. 1979). In addition, administration of this amino acid to humans has shown a hypotensive effect (FELTKAMP et al. 1984). Many mechanisms have been proposed for the antihypertensive effect of tryptophan, including changes in NaCl ingestion, increased serotonin turnover, and alterations in angiotensin II binding (ITO and SCHANBERG 1972; FULLER et al. 1979; WURTMAN 1981). In any case, the brain figures highly in most of these hypotheses. Tryptophan is transported into the CNS by a stereospecific large neutral amino acid carrier (PARDRIDGE 1985). In addition, tryptophan is the only amino acid which significantly binds to serum albumin. These mechanisms attenuate transport of the amino acid to the CNS and, thus, high systemic doses are required to significantly alter brain levels. Unfortunately, there is evidence that tryptophan can cause bladder cancer and blood dyscrasias, especially eosinophilia, after large oral doses (CATERALL 1988).

Synthesis of a nicotinamide CDS for tryptophan was therefore considered (POP et al. 1990). Tryptophan esters were treated with nicotinoyl

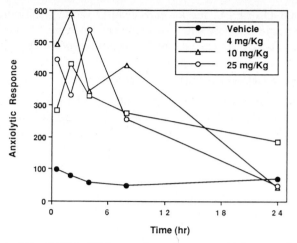

Fig. 9. Effect of Bz-GABA-CDS at various doses or vehicle on anxiolytic response of naive male rats as measured by a drink-foot shock conflict procedure. All Bz-GABA-CDS-treated animals exhibited significant anxiolysis through 8 h. The 4 mg/kg treatment group also demonstrated a significant anxiolytic effect at 24 h

chloride to give the corresponding amide esters (Fig. 10). Quaternization and reduction of these derivatives produced the Try-CDS. The compounds were found to be of sufficient lipophilicity to readily pass the BBB and, also, to convert to the corresponding quaternary salt. The Try-CDS containing an ethyl ester was tested in a deoxycorticosterone acetate (DOCA) model of hypertension (FREGLY and FATER 1986, FREGLY et al. 1987, 1988). While vehicle or tryptophan were ineffective in changing blood pressure, an i.v.

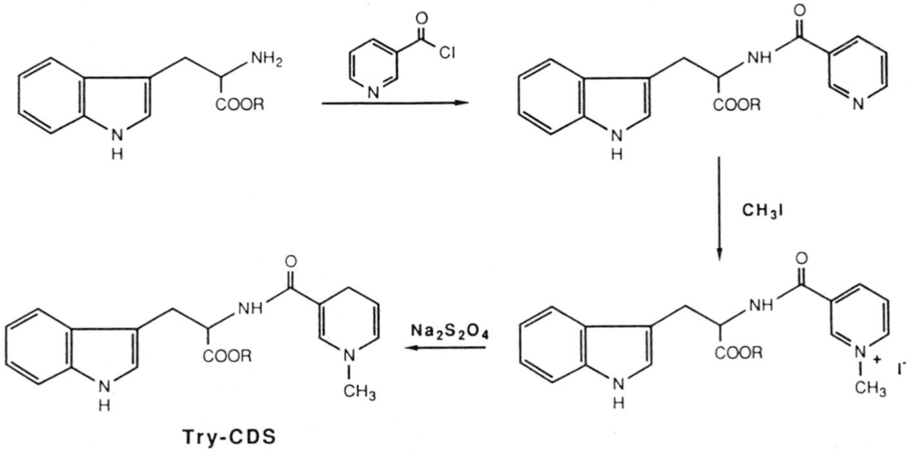

Try-CDS

Fig. 10. Synthesis of a tryptophan CDS. See text for details

dose of the Try-CDS of 14.2 mg/kg significantly reduced blood pressure in rats, 14% by 3 h and 25% by 4 h. Lowering the dose by 63% generated an equivalent hypotensive effect at 3 h which was not as potent at 4 h post-dosing.

2. Brain-Enhanced Delivery of Antiviral Agents

Viral encephalitic diseases are major health problems in the USA and throughout the world. These diseases have the reputation of being extraordinarily pernicious and difficult to treat. The basis of this refractoriness can be traced to several factors, not the least of which is the inability of many potentially useful drugs to penetrate into brain tissue. This section examines the application of the CDS to antiviral agents, specifically drugs useful in the treatment of AIDS, herpes encephalitis, cytomegaloviral encephalitis, and Japanese encephalitis.

a) Antiretroviral Drugs

Zidovudine, or azidothymidine (AZT), is currently the only approved drug for the treatment of AIDS. In a few patients, this modified riboside has been shown to be useful in improving the neuropsychiatric course of AIDS encephalopathy but the doses required to elicit this improvement precipitate severe anemia (YARCHOAN et al. 1987). This usually lends to cessation of therapy. When the drug is withdrawn in response to this neutropenia, all of the abated symptoms promptly return. Interestingly, AZT does enter the cerebrospinal fluid (CSF) after oral or i.v. dosing and achieves significant concentrations (BALIS et al. 1989; KLECKER et al. 1987; BLUM et al. 1988). Unfortunately, these CSF levels appear to greatly overestimate brain parenchymal and neuronal levels as AZT poorly penetrates the BBB (TERASAKI and PARDRIDGE 1988). In an effort to ameliorate the prognosis of AIDS encephalopathy, the CDS approach was applied to AZT (LITTLE et al. 1990; BREWSTER et al. 1988c; GALLO et al. 1989; GOGU et al. 1989; TORRENCE et al. 1988). This antiviral agent has a primary alcohol functionality in the 5'-position which was considered for carrier attachment. As shown in Fig. 11, AZT was treated with nicotinoyl chloride hydrochloride in pyridine to yield the 5'-nicotinate. This ester was subsequently quaternized with methyl iodide to yield the 5'-trigonellinate (1-methylnicotinate) and reduced in basic aqueous sodium dithionite to give the 5'-(1,4-dihydrotrigonellinate) derivative of AZT (AZT-CDS).

The AZT-CDS is a crystalline solid which is stable at room temperature for several months when protected from light and moisture. The lipophilicity of the AZT-CDS and its metabolites, AZT and the AZT-5'-trigonellinate salt (AZT-Q$^+$), is important in determining the efficiency of the CDS. The n-octanol: water partition coefficient (log P) was determined to be 0.06, -2.00, and 1.5 for AZT, AZT-Q$^+$, and AZT-CDS, respectively, as shown in Fig. 11. This indicates that the CDS is 34-fold more lipophilic than the parent riboside and more than 3900-fold more lipophilic than the AZT-Q$^+$.

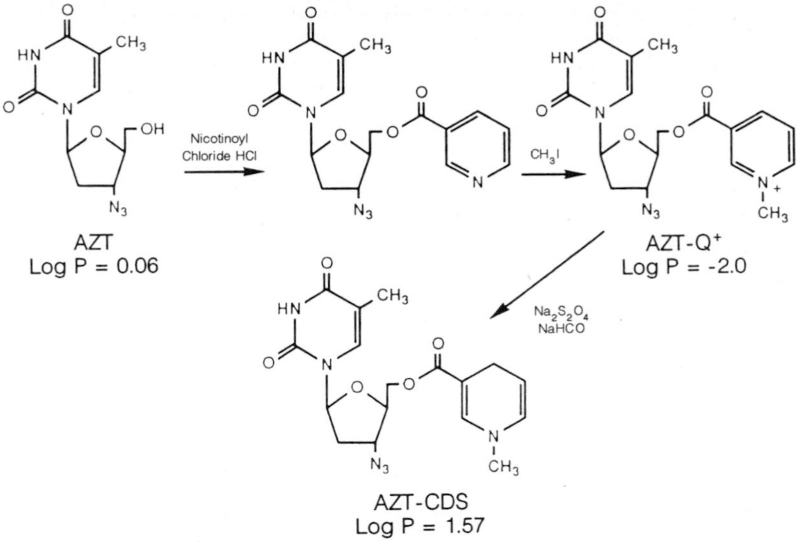

Fig. 11. Synthesis of AZT-CDS. See text for details

These parameters should correlate with rapid brain uptake of the CDS (log P > 1.0) and rapid systemic elimination of the AZT-Q$^+$ (GREIG 1987).

The in vitro stability of the AZT-CDS and its metabolite/precursor, AZT-Q$^+$, was determined in pH 7.4 phosphate buffer, 20% rat brain homogenate, and whole rat blood. The CDS is relatively stable in buffer but rapidly oxidizes in enzymatic media. In addition, the depot form of AZT, i.e., the AZT-Q$^+$, was shown to gradually release the parent compound.

The CDS form of AZT was subsequently examined in a rat model. This study compared the CNS delivery of AZT after dosing animals with either the parent drug itself or the AZT-CDS. Figure 12 gives the brain and blood concentration of AZT after an i.v. dose of 0.136 mmol/kg AZT. As shown, blood levels were initially high, but disappear rapidly with a half-life of approximately 20 min. By 2 h, no AZT was detected. In the brain, AZT levels never surpassed blood concentrations and were at their peak at the first sampling point. AZT was not found in the brain at 60 min. The profile of drug distribution after CDS administration was significantly different. In blood, high levels of the AZT-CDS occurred initially but disappeared rapidly with a half-life of 5 min (Fig. 13). The AZT-Q$^+$ was also present in high levels at early time points, but the concentration of this also fell rapidly ($t_{1/2}$ = 7 min). Finally, low levels of AZT could be detected in blood, but the drug was completely cleared from the body by 2 h. The amount of AZT present in the blood after AZT-CDS administration was much lower than that generated after AZT dosing. In brain (Fig. 14), no CDS was detected,

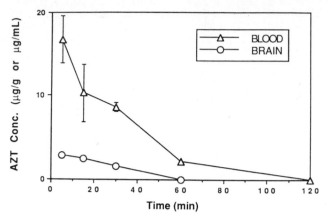

Fig. 12. Brain and blood concentrations of AZT (mean ± SEM) after an i.v. dose of 0.136 mmol/kg AZT using DMSO (0.5 ml/kg) as a vehicle

consistent with its in vitro lability. $AZT-Q^+$ concentrations were characterized by an appearance phase reaching a maximum concentration C_{max} at 15 min and then by a slow decline. The appearance phase is typical for CDS derivatives and is a consequence of the in vivo conversion of the CDS to its corresponding pyridinium salt. $AZT-Q^+$ was detectable in the brain at the last time point examined (4 h). These sustained levels of $AZT-Q^+$ were associated with release of AZT in the CNS which reached peak levels at 30 min post-drug administration and were detectable up to 120 min. When the parent drug was considered, the areas under the brain AZT concentration curve were three-fold higher after AZT-CDS dosing than after AZT

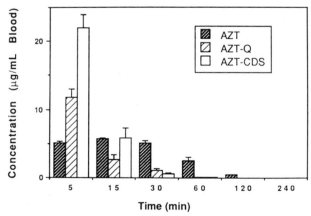

Fig. 13. Blood concentrations of AZT-CDS and its metabolites, $AZT-Q^+$ and AZT, after an i.v. dose of 0.136 mmol/kg of AZT-CDS

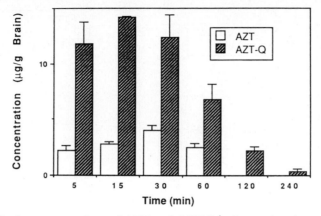

Fig. 14. Brain concentrations of AZT and AZT-Q$^+$ after an i.v. dose of 0.136 mmol/ kg of AZT-CDS

administration (Fig. 15). This was a consequence of not only a higher C_{max} value but also of a longer CNS mean residence time. This is important in that the estimated virustatic concentration of AZT (1.0 μmol/l) is maintained twice as long after AZT-CDS administration as after AZT dosing. This, in combination with the lower blood levels of AZT, results in a favorable increase in the brain/blood ratio for the parent compound when administered as its CDS (Fig. 16).

Subsequent to the investigations in rodents, AZT-CDS was studied in a canine model. In a preliminary study, a mongrel dog (20 kg body weight) was given 11 μmol/kg AZT in a vehicle containing 2.5% DMSO in poly-

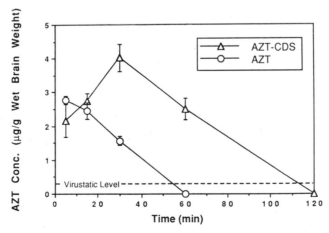

Fig. 15. Brain levels of AZT in rat after a 0.136 mmol/kg dose of either AZT or AZT-CDS

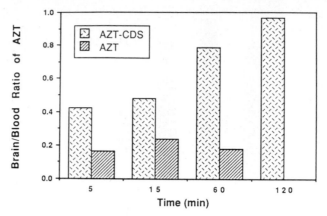

Fig. 16. Brain/blood ratios of AZT in rat after a 0.136 mmol/kg dose of either AZT or AZT-CDS

ethylene glycol (400) followed 1 week later with a dose of 11 µmol/kg AZT-CDS. In both administrations, samples of CSF and blood were obtained. Blood levels of AZT after i.v. administration of either AZT or the AZT-CDS are given in Fig. 17. After administration of the parent compound, blood levels of AZT disappeared in an apparent biphasic manner. Blood levels of AZT after the CDS were much lower initially than those obtained after the parent drug. By 100 min, the blood concentration curves were superimposed after the two treatments. In the CSF (Fig. 18), AZT administration produced significant levels of AZT at early times which were, however, below the 1.0 µmol/l therapeutic threshold for virustatic activity. In addition, these levels fell quickly with an estimated half-life of 30 min. Equimolar AZT-CDS

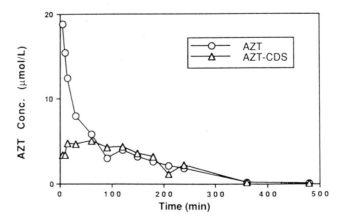

Fig. 17. Blood levels of AZT in dog after an 11 µmol/kg dose of either AZT or AZT-CDS

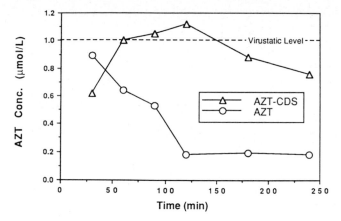

Fig. 18. CSF levels of AZT in dog after an 11 µmol/kg dose of either AZT or AZT-CDS

generated therapeutically significant concentrations of AZT in the CSF for up to 3 h post-dosing. These data indicate that the area under the AZT concentration curve in CSF was doubled after AZT-CDS dosing compared to after AZT administration.

The olefin 2',3'-dideoxy-2',3'-didehydrothymidine (d₄T) has also been derivatized to generate a CDS. This molecule has been found to be equipotent to AZT in vitro in suppressing the cytopathogenicity of HIV-1 but

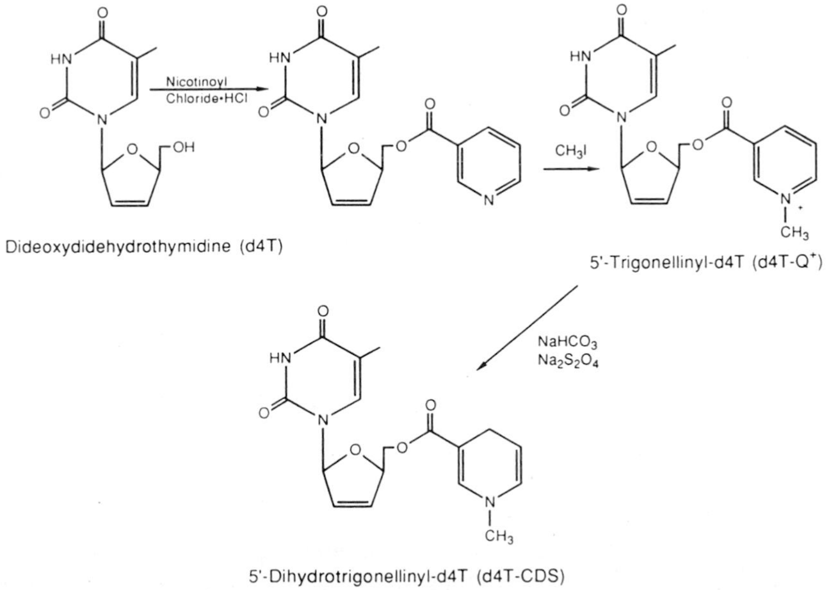

Dideoxydidehydrothymidine (d4T)

5'-Trigonellinyl-d4T (d4T-Q⁺)

5'-Dihydrotrigonellinyl-d4T (d4T-CDS)

Fig. 19. Synthesis of d₄T-CDS. See text for details

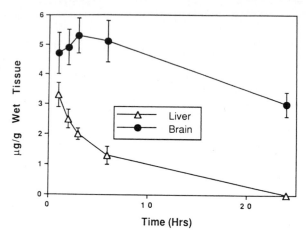

Fig. 20. Brain and liver concentrations of $d_4T\text{-}Q^+$ in mice after an i.v. dose of d_4T-CDS

was also found to be less cytotoxic. The CDS for d_4T was prepared and studied by PALOMINO et al. (1989) at Wayne State University (Detroit, MI, USA). The parent compound was nicotinoylated with the nicotinic acid chloride to give the 5'-nicotinate which was subsequently methylated with methyl iodide to give the d_4T-5'-trigonellinate. Reduction of this species in sodium dithionite generated the 5'-1,4-dihydrotrigonellinate derivative or d_4T-CDS (Fig. 19). The log P for the CDS was 0.85, which was significantly higher than that measured for the parent compound (-0.64).

In the in vivo distribution studies, a dose of 72.5 μmol/kg of d_4T-CDS was administered (i.v.) to a group of BDF/1 mice. At various times post-dosing, animals were killed and brain, blood, and liver were removed, weighed, and subjected to analysis. Brain levels of the d_4T quaternary salt, ($d_4T\text{-}Q^+$) increased from a level of 4.7 μg/g at 60 min to 5.3 μg/g at its C_{max} (3 h). This was followed by a slow efflux ($t_{1/2} = 25$ h). In contrast, the d_4T-Q^+ was readily eliminated from the liver with an estimated half-life of 5 h (Fig. 20). In brain, the deposited salt was associated with a slow but sustained release of the parent compound as shown in Fig. 21. In addition, the oxidized, hydrolyzed, carrier molecule could also be detected and appeared to be more rapidly excreted than the "locked-in" d_4T-Q^+. As shown in Fig. 22, the concentration of trigonelline falls rapidly as a function of d_4T-Q^+ concentrations.

b) Antiherpetic Agents

Acyclovir (ACV) is a synthetic, acyclic analogue of guanine which has a broad spectrum of activity against herpes simplex virus (HSV-1) and varicella zoster virus (VZV). This agent is relatively nontoxic to the host since its

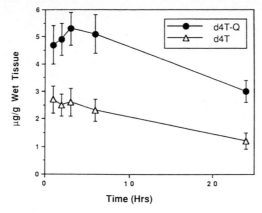

Fig. 21. Brain levels of d_4T-Q^+ and released d_4T in mice after i.v. administration of d_4T-CDS

conversion to the active triphosphate is initiated only in virally infected cells (ELION et al. 1977). While ACV has been used in the treatment of herpes simplex encephalitis, its poor ability to penetrate the BBB has limited its use. The application of the CDS to ACV was, therefore, considered (VENKATRAGHAVAN et al. 1986). The synthesis of the brain-targeting derivative is summarized in Fig. 23. Since ACV is susceptible to alkylation, the trigonellinate unit had to be attached in a single step rather than the conventional acylation/alkylation approach. This was done via the development of a trigonellinating reagent, trigonelline anhydride (BREWSTER et al. 1987b). Reaction of ACV with this activated anhydride produced the

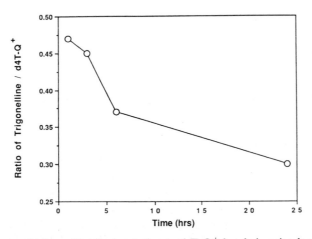

Fig. 22. Rate of trigonelline loss relative to d_4T-Q^+ levels in mice brain after an i.v. dose of d_4T-CDS

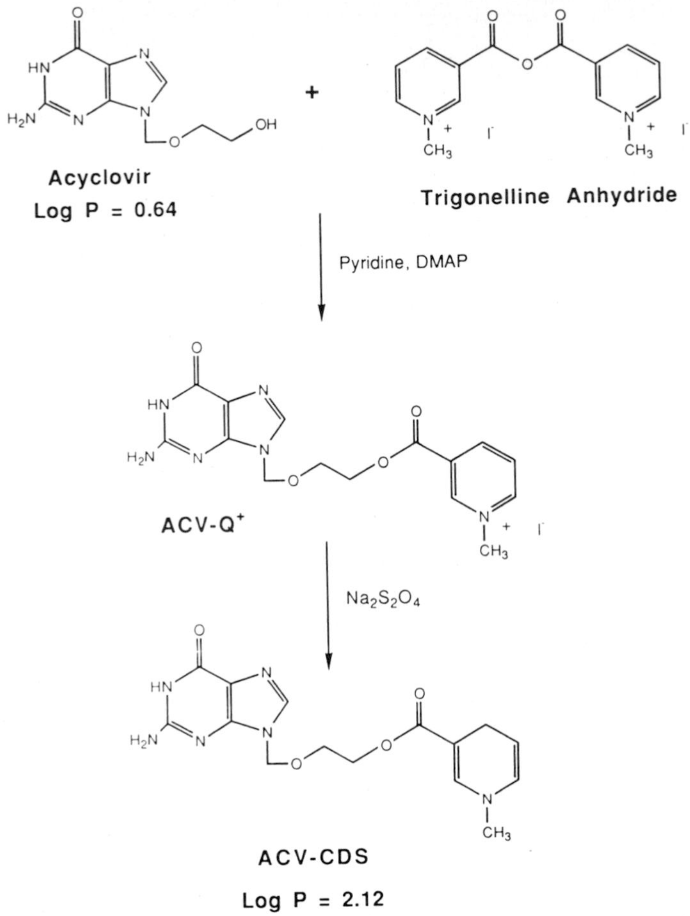

Fig. 23. Synthesis of the brain-targeting ACV-CDS. See text for details. DMAP, dimethylaminopyridine

trigonellinate salt (ACV-Q^+). Subsequent reduction produced the dihydro-trigonellinate CDS (ACV-CDS). This manipulation greatly increased the lipophilicity of ACV as indicated by a log k' system (ACV = 0.64, ACV-CDS = 2.12).

Tissue distribution studies were carried out in Sprague-Dawley rats and the dose of compound used was 58.2 μmol/kg. Both ACV and ACV-CDS were administered i.v. via the tail vein. ACV produced a tissue distribution consistent with its polar structure. Detectable levels could not be measured in brain and high initial levels of drug were found in blood, liver, and kidney but the drug completely disappeared by 6 h from those organs. The ACV-CDS produced a dramatically different pattern. The CDS easily penetrated the BBB and produced sustained levels of the ACV-Q^+. The $t_{1/2}$ for loss of

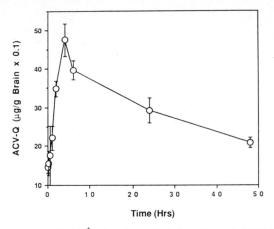

Fig. 24. Brain levels of ACV-Q$^+$ after i.v. administration of ACV-CDS

ACV-Q$^+$ in the brain was almost 2 days (Fig. 24), while the material was rapidly cleared from liver and kidney. Thus, after 4 h, the brain was the only organ with detectable concentrations of ACV-Q$^+$. These prolonged levels of acyclovir were associated with a sustained release of the parent compound in the brain. ACV released after ACV-CDS dosing could not be detected in blood and was not detectable in liver after 1 h, in kidney after 4 h, in lung after 30 min, and in testis after 1 h. Brain levels of ACV persisted through the end of the experiment (48 h) with a $t_{1/2}$ of disappearance of 54 h (Fig. 25). This is one of the best demonstrations of brain-selective delivery using a CDS.

Trifluorothymidine (TFT) is useful in the treatment of herpes infection of the eye but its relatively high systemic toxicity has precluded its use

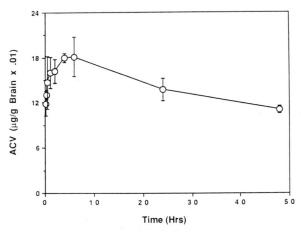

Fig. 25. Brain levels of ACV after i.v. administration of ACV-CDS

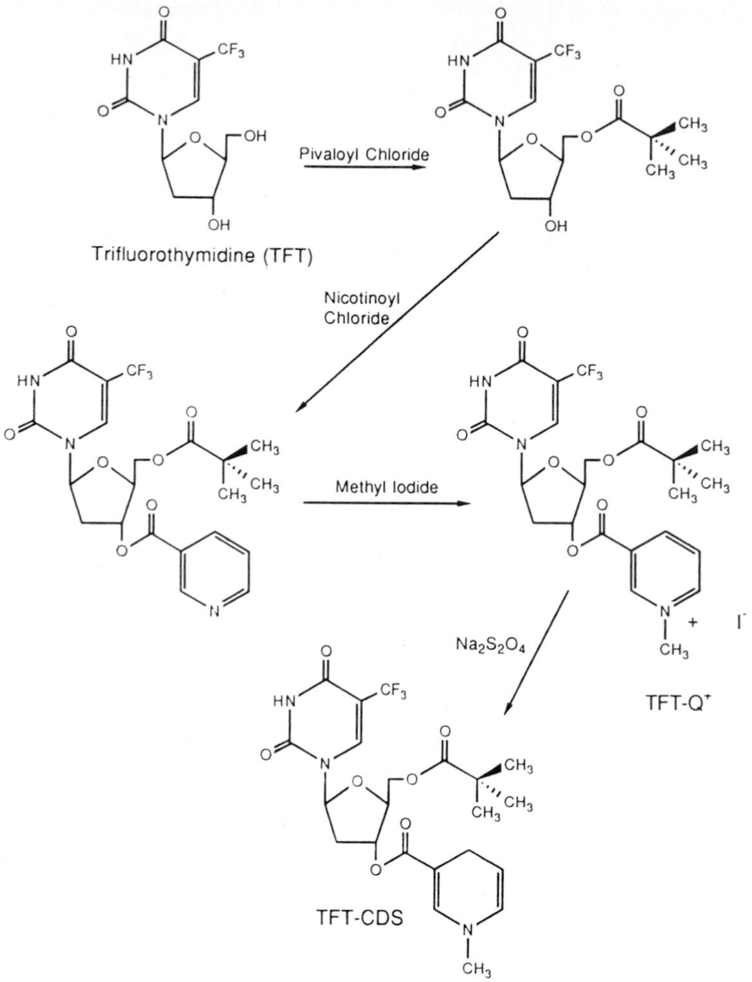

Fig. 26. Synthesis of TFT-CDS. See text for details

intravenously. Application of the CDS to this agent was made to improve the toxicologic profile of this agent as well as to enhance its delivery to the CNS. The TFT-CDS was prepared according to Fig. 26 (EL-KOUSSI and BODOR 1987; RAND et al. 1986). TFT was selectively 5'-pivaloated using pivaloyl chloride. The deoxyriboside was then treated with nicotinoyl chloride to give the 5'-pivaloyl-3'-nicotinoyl compound. Methylation of this *bis* ester gave TFT-Q$^+$ and subsequent reduction produced the transport compound TFT-CDS. This delivery system must undergo a variety of transformations prior to release of TFT. These are summarized in Fig. 27. In vitro homogenate studies indicate that the preferred path is oxidation of

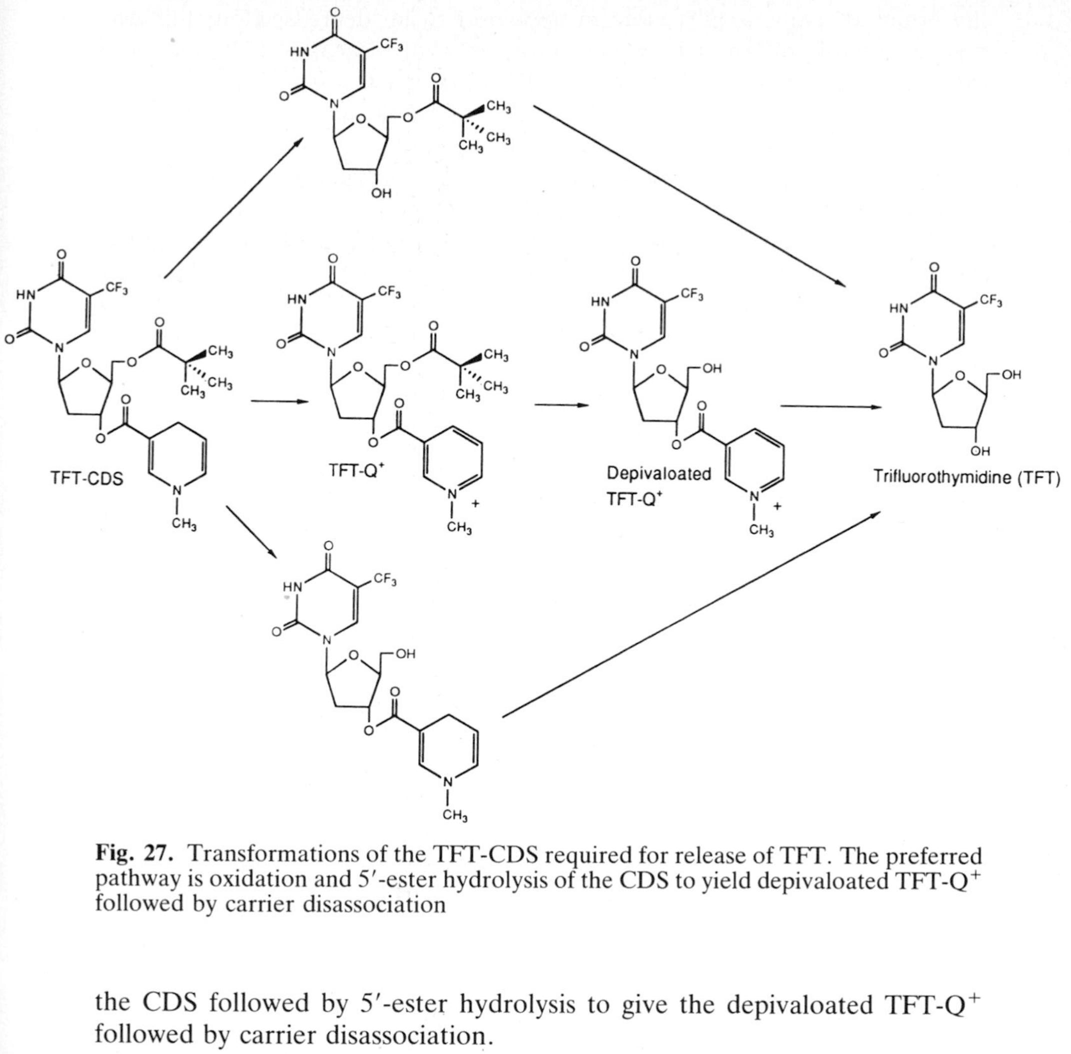

Fig. 27. Transformations of the TFT-CDS required for release of TFT. The preferred pathway is oxidation and 5′-ester hydrolysis of the CDS to yield depivaloated TFT-Q⁺ followed by carrier disassociation

the CDS followed by 5′-ester hydrolysis to give the depivaloated TFT-Q⁺ followed by carrier disassociation.

Administration of a 20 mg/kg dose of the TFT-CDS to rats resulted in accumulation of the depivaloated TFT-Q⁺ in rat brain. Levels measured were 7–8 µg/g at 1 h and 13.5 ± 0.8 µg/mL at 4 h. In addition, low but detectable levels (0.3 ± 0.5 µg/g) of TFT could be detected in the brain of rats 18 h after CDS administration. No TFT could be found in rat brain 1, 4, or 18 h after i.v. administration of equimolar TFT. Two subsequent in vivo experiments were performed using the TFT-CDS to treat rats inoculated intercerebrally with HSV-1 virus (RAND et al. 1986). In the first, 100–150 g Fischer rats were inoculated with 4 × 10⁴ plaque-forming units (pfu) of HSV (>10 000 LD₅₀) in 20 µl of media, intracranially. These animals were then treated with 20 mg/kg TFT-CDS i.v., once daily for 5–7 days. All animals developed signs of CNS infection and died. The titer of HSV-1 isolated from the brains of animals post-mortem appeared to be decreased but this was not significantly different from the untreated control group. This study was repeated using a dose of 40 mg/kg TFT-CDS twice a day for 5–7 days. While there were no cures, viral titers were significantly decreased compared to the untreated control group.

Thus, the CDS of TFT allowed it to cross the BBB and penetrate into the brain parenchyma. The deposited form of the CDS appeared to be the depivaloated TFT-Q$^+$ and low levels of release of TFT could be detected in the brain of rats at later time points after TFT-CDS dosing. Although survival was not prolonged in the rat model used, the inoculum contained extremely high levels of virus. Treatment of animals with the TFT-CDS did significantly reduce viral titers.

c) Agents Useful in the Treatment of "Exotic" Viral Diseases

Ribavirin (RV) was first synthesized in 1972 and since that time has been shown to be a useful broad-spectrum antiviral agent (CONNER 1984; HUGGINS et al. 1984; SIDWELL et al. 1979; CANONICO et al. 1988). This riboside has been demonstrated to inhibit the cytopathicity of various RNA viruses and has been found to be clinically useful in the treatment of respiratory syncytial virus (RODRIGUEZ and PARROTT 1987) and Lassa fever (McCORMICK et al. 1986). RV is, however, highly water-soluble and poorly lipophilic (log P = −2.06) (SIDWELL et al. 1979). This property renders this potentially useful drug useless in the treatment of RNA viral encephalitic diseases such as Japanese B encephalitis, Rift Valley fever, and Dengue fever. Application of the CDS to RV may, therefore, improve its spectrum of activity. RV has three hydroxy groups (2′,3′ and 5′-positions) which are amenable to derivatization. The brain-targeting 1,4-dihydrotrigonellinate moiety can be placed at any or all of these loci. In addition, the underivatized hydroxy groups can be masked with lipophilicity-modifying ester to optimize delivery. The simple 5′-1,4-dihydrotrigonellinate derivative of RV was prepared according to Fig. 28. RV was protected as the 2′,3′-acetonide. This compound was then nicotinoylated with nicotinic anhydride and deprotected using formic acid. The 5′-nicotinate was then methylated to give the 5′-trigonellinate of RV (RV-Q$^+$) and reduced in aqueous dithionite to give the RV-5′-CDS. This compound, independently prepared, was tested in C57BL/6 mice which had been infected i.p. with ten LD$_{50}$s of the Peking strain of Japanese encephalitic virus. The CDS was administered i.p. at doses of 45 mg/kg/day for 9 days. A survival rate of 40%–50% was described even though vehicle or RV itself were totally ineffective (100% mortality) (CANONICO et al. 1988). Other derivatives of RV are presently under development.

3. Application of the Brain-Targeting CDS to Estrogens

Estrogens are lipophilic steroids which are not impeded in their entry to the CNS. These compounds readily penetrate the BBB and achieve high central levels after peripheral administration. Unfortunately, estrogens are poorly

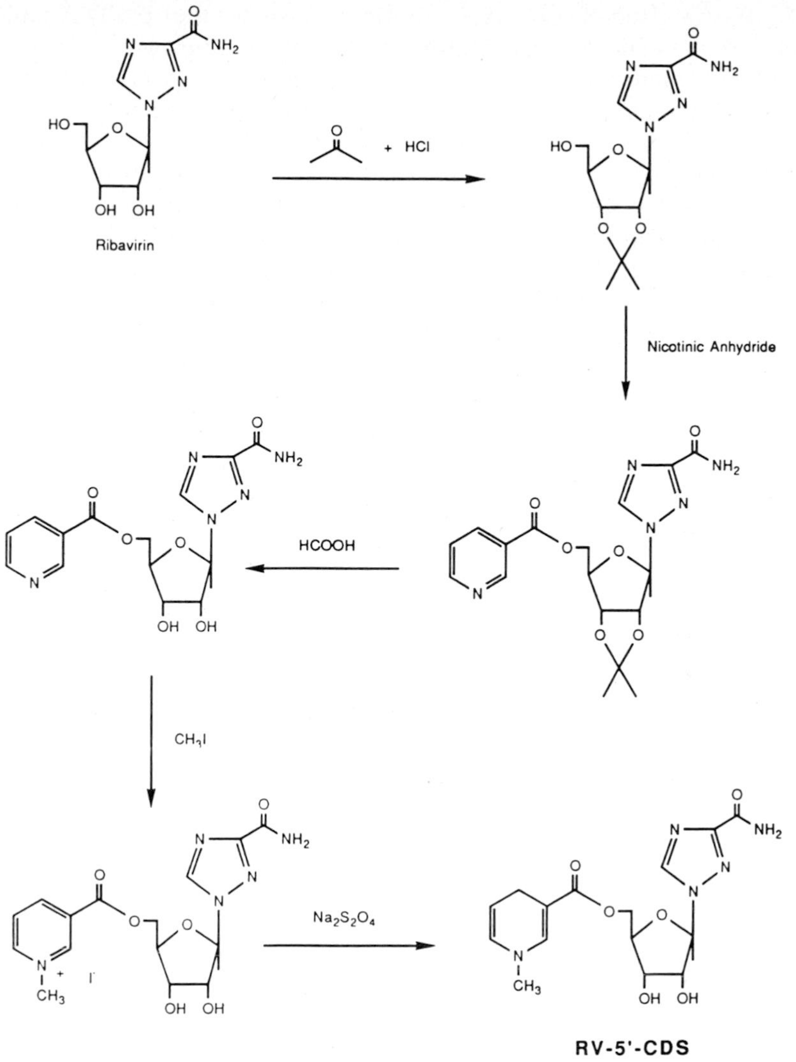

Fig. 28. Synthesis of RV-5'-CDS. See text for details

retained by the brain. This circumstance requires that frequent doses of these steroids be administered to maintain therapeutically significant concentrations. Constant peripheral exposure of estrogen has been related, however, to a number of pathological conditions including cancer, hypertension, and altered metabolism (FOTHERBY 1985; KAPLAN 1978). As the CNS is the target site for many of the actions of estrogens, a brain-targeted delivery form of these compounds may provide for safer and more effective estrogens. Pharmacologically, an estrogen CDS (E-CDS) could be used to reduce the secretion of luteinizing hormone-releasing hormone (LHRH) and hence of luteinizing hormone (LH) and gonadal steroids (BARRACLOUGH and WISE

1982; KALRA AND KALRA 1980, 1983). As such, the E-CDS could be employed to achieve contraception and to reduce growth of peripheral steroid-dependent tumors, such as those of the breast, uterus, and prostate, and to treat endometriosis (HURST and ROCK 1989). Additionally, brain-enhanced delivery of estradiol could be useful in stimulating male and female sexual behavior (CHRISTENSEN and CLEMENS 1974; PFAFF 1970), and in the treatment of menopausal syndrome in which estrogen depletion causes numerous vasomotor symptoms (UPTON 1984; HUPPERT 1987). Other potential uses for the E-CDS, for which estrogens are currently being evaluated, are in the reduction of body weight and in the treatment of depression and various types of dementias, including Alzheimer's disease (MCEWEN 1981; MAGGI and PEREZ 1985).

This broad spectrum of potential clinical applications of E-CDS reflects the wide distribution of estrogen receptors in the brain. Estrogen receptors are found in the hypothalamus and the closely associated preoptic area, where they mediate estradiol effects on LH secretion, sexual behavior in both males and females, appetite, and temperature regulation (SAR and STUMPF 1981; SAR 1984). In addition, estrogen receptors have recently been identified on dopaminergic neurons which innervate the striatum, where estradiol may modulate locomotion and hence may be involved in movement disorders (JOYCE 1983). Also, estrogen receptors have been identified in mesocortical dopamine neurons where they may mediate estradiol effects on mood (LAURITZEN and VANKEEP 1978). Finally, estrogen receptors are found in the region of the nucleus basalis magnocellularis (NBM), a site of cholinergic cell bodies which innervate the cerebral cortex (PFAFF and KEINER 1973). These estrogen receptors may mediate the influence of estrogens on cognitive function.

a) Synthesis and In Vitro and In Vivo Distribution Studies

The most potent natural steroid is estradiol (E_2), which is chemically a diol containing a phenolic 3-moiety and a 17-alcohol group. These synthetic handles provide for three possible CDSs, i.e., the molecule in which the 17-position was manipulated, one in which the 3-position was acylated, and the *bis*-derivatized steroid. Derivatization of either position, but especially the 17-position, should greatly decrease the pharmacologic activity of E_2 as these esters are known not to interact with estrogen receptors (JANOCKO et al. 1984). The preparation of the 17-based CDS and the *bis*-CDS is given in Fig. 29 (BODOR et al. 1987; BREWSTER et al. 1987a). In this summary, E_2 is reacted with nicotinoyl chloride hydrochloride in pyridine to give the 3,17-*bis* nicotinate. This compound is subjected to methanolic potassium bicarbonate which results in selective hydrolysis of the phenolic nicotinate. The resulting secondary ester is quaternized with methyl iodide to give the 17-trigonellinate, or E_2-Q^+, and then reduced using sodium dithionite to give the 17-(1,4-dihydrotrigonellinate), or E_2-CDS. The log Ps for the E_2-CDS and E_2-Q^+

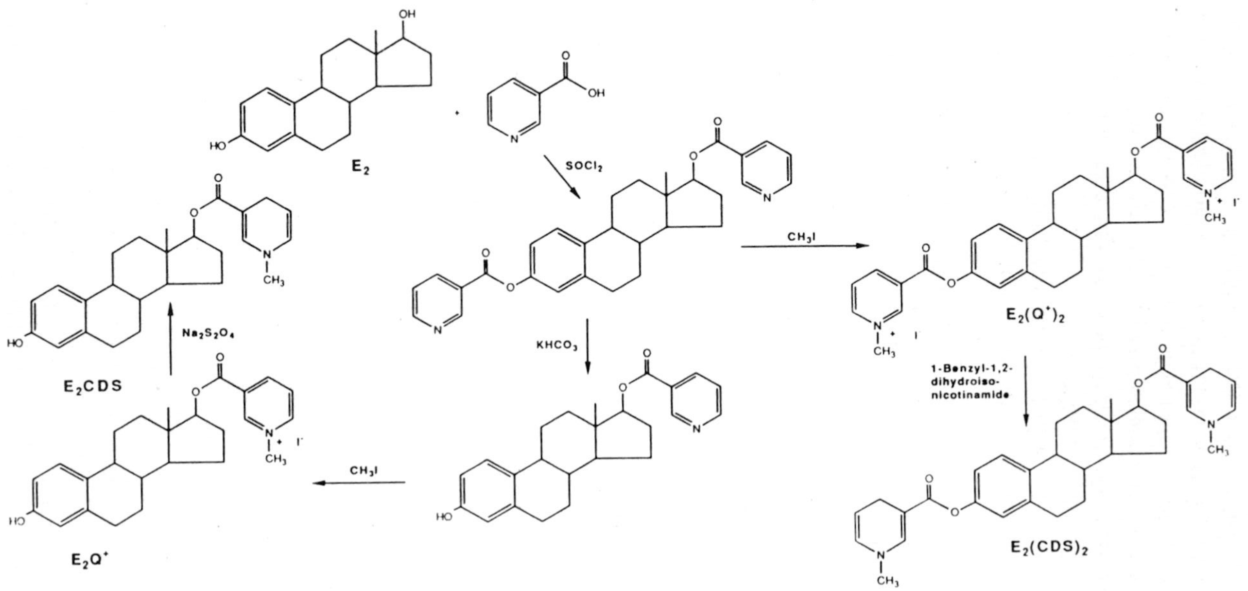

Fig. 29. Synthesis of the 17-based and *bis* forms of estradiol (E_2) CDS. See text for details

were measured using standard procedures and compared to that of E_2. The log of the octanol: water partition coefficient for E_2-CDS was found to be 4.50; for E_2, 3.76; and for the E_2-Q^+ salt, 0.144. This indicates that the quaternary salt form of E_2-CDS is 8000 times more hydrophilic than the parent E_2 and more than 44 000 times more hydrophilic than the E_2-CDS. In addition, the E_2-CDS is approximately five-fold more lipophilic than E_2. These values, which are consistent with other derivatives examined, indicate that the compounds synthesized possess the appropriate physicochemical properties for CDS functioning.

The CDS concept requires that the dihydrotrigonellinate-drug conjugate rapidly converts to the pyridinium salt and that this brain lock-in form slowly hydrolyzes to give the parent drug and the inert carrier molecule (trigonelline). Prior to in vivo study, these assumptions were examined in vitro using rat organ homogenates as the test matrix. The half-life of E_2-CDS in plasma, liver, and brain homogenates was found to be 156.6 min, 29.9 min, and 29.2 min, respectively. Thus, the E_2-CDSs are converted to the corresponding pyridinium salts much faster in the tissue homogenates than in plasma. This is consistent with a membrane-bound enzyme acting as the oxidative catalyst. Candidates for this enzyme include members of the family of NADH transhydrogenase which mediate the redox reactions of NADH, a molecule similar in structure to the active portion of the CDS (Hoek and Rydstrom 1988; Rydstrom 1977). The second metabolic step required is hydrolysis of E_2 from the E_2-Q^+. Initial studies on the disappearance of the E_2-Q^+ from organ homogenates and plasma indicated minimal hydrolysis. To better assay this enzymatic event, the appearance of E_2 was examined. When this was performed, approximately 1.2% of a sample of E_2-Q^+ was found to be converted to free E_2 120 min after incubation of the salt in brain homogenate (Bodor et al. 1987). This conversion factor was 3.1% in whole rat blood and 2.3% in rat liver homogenate given the same incubation period. In plasma, where nonspecific hydrolyses are prominent, approximately 20% of the E_2-Q^+ was converted to the free steroid. This very slow production of E_2 is consistent with a slow and sustained release of E_2 from brain deposits of E_2-Q^+.

Initial studies on the tissue distribution of E_2-CDS involved i.v. administration of high doses (60 mg/kg) of the steroid to conscious restrained rats. The E_2-CDS rapidly disappeared from blood after administration reflecting the enzymatic lability and large volume of distribution of this lipophile. The quaternary metabolite of E_2-CDS was detected in all tissues soon after drug administration. Examinations of the terminal portion of the tissue concentration vs time profiles in these studies indicated the half-life of elimination of the E_2-Q^+ was 46 min in liver, 5.5 h in lung, 8 h in kidney, and almost 1 day in the CNS (Bodor et al. 1987). This first study clearly demonstrated that the E_2-Q^+ was selectively retained in the brain. In addition, the slow decline of E_2-Q^+ formed in situ in the CNS was associated with a small but significant release of E_2 in the brain as measured by radioimmunoassay (RIA) and by spectroscopic means. The dose of drug used in these early studies was extremely high due to the insensitivity of analytical techniques. Clearly a selective and sensitive method for detecting E_2-CDS, E_2-Q^+, and E_2 was necessary if doses of E_2-CDS of physiological significance were to be detected in animals and humans. This problem was solved using a precolumn- enriching HPLC system (MULLERSMAN et al. 1988). In this approach, a large volume (1800 µl) of acetonitrile which had been used to extract various organ homogenates or plasma was injected on a chromatographic precolumn. Under the conditions used, the compound of interest was adsorbed on the precolumn which was washed with an aqueous mobile phase to eliminate proteins and other water-soluble contaminants. The direction of solvent flow was then reversed and an organic mobile phase was used to wash the contents of the precolumn onto the analytical column where separation, detection, and quantitation could be performed. Using this methodology, the limits of accurate detection for plasma samples and organ homogenates were 10 ng/ml or g, E_2-Q^+; 20 ng/ml or g, E_2-CDS; and 50 ng/ml or g, E_2. The improved sensitivity of this system allowed the pharmacokinetics of the E_2-CDS to be examined after much lower parenteral doses. To this end, rats were given 5 mg/kg E_2-CDS and blood and various tissues were monitored up to 48 h post-dosing. As illustrated in Fig. 30, at this dose a significant selectivity was observed for the CNS as the tissue half-life was approximately five-fold greater than that observed in the kidney, heart, lung, testis, eye, or peritoneal fat (MULLERSMAN et al. 1988).

In order to follow E_2 released over time from deposited E_2-Q^+, an RIA technique was developed (SARKAR et al. 1989). In this method, tissue or plasma samples were extracted with hexane: ethyl acetate and purified on a

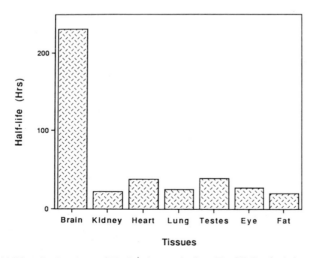

Fig. 30. Half-life elimination of E_2Q^+ formed after E_2-CDS administration in brain, kidney, heart, lung, testis, eye, and fat

Celite column. The column fractions were then assayed using a specific E_2 antiserum which was raised against E_2 conjugated at the 6-position. The profiles of E_2 concentration in the brain region and in plasma are given in Fig. 31. The levels of E_2 in brain tissue after E_2-CDS administration are elevated four to five times longer than after simple E_2 treatment. In addition, the ratio of the concentration of E_2 in brain and plasma after E_2-CDS treatment was approximately 12. This profile confirms that E_2 is generated within the CNS and is not sequestered from peripheral sources. In addition, pharmacokinetic analysis of the brain and plasma assay data indicates that the E_2 present in the periphery at later times after drug administration can be accounted for by leakage of E_2 from the CNS.

b) Pharmacology Studies

The response of LH secretion to E_2-CDS was evaluated in several rat studies as an indication of the pharmacologic potency of this compound. In the first set of experiments, E_2-CDS was administered as a single i.v. injection (3 mg/kg) to male rats which had been orchidectomized 2 weeks previously (SIMPKINS et al. 1986). E_2 was administered to another group of rats at an equimolar dose and dimethylsulfoxide (DMSO) treated rats served as the vehicle controls. Both E_2 and E_2-CDS reduced serum LH equivalently from 4 to 48 h post-drug administration. From 4 to 12 days, LH levels in the E_2 treated rats increased progressively to levels equivalent to those in DMSO treated rats (Fig. 32). By contrast, LH concentrations in animals treated with E_2-CDS remained low and were suppressed by 82%, 88%, and 90% when compared to DMSO treated animals at 4, 8, and 12 days after treatment, respectively. In these animals, serum E_2 levels remained elevated through 2

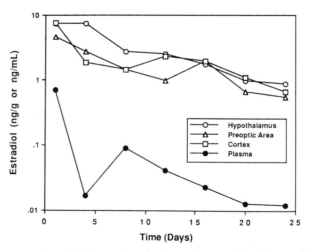

Fig. 31. Concentration of E_2 in various brain regions and in plasma after a 3.0 mg/kg dose of E_2-CDS

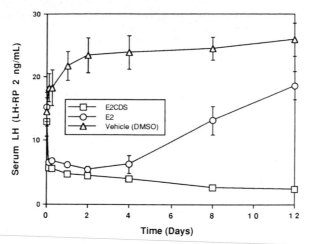

Fig. 32. Serum LH (as measured using LH reference preparation 2, LH RP-2) concentrations following an i.v. dose of either E_2-CDS (3.0 mg/kg), equimolar E_2, or vehicle (DMSO). Each point represents the mean ± SEM for 4–8 rats

days in both rats treated with E_2 and E_2-CDS. By 4 days after drug treatment, E_2 levels in both drug treated groups returned to that observed in vehicle treated orchidectomized male rats. These data indicated that, despite the clearance of E_2 from the plasma, the delivery system achieved chronic suppression of LH secretion for at least 12 days following a single i.v. administration. These data are consistent with the hypothesis that the E_2-CDS causes enhanced brain delivery, lock-in of the E_2-Q^+, and slow release of E_2 to achieve LH suppression.

This study was extended to determine the duration of LH suppression following a single injection of the E_2-CDS. In this second evaluation, orchidectomized rats were treated with E_2-CDS (3 mg/kg, i.v.) or the DMSO vehicle and were examined at 12, 18, and 24 days post-treatment (ESTES et al. 1987). E_2-CDS suppressed LH secretion by 88%, 86%, and 66% relative to DMSO controls at 12, 18, and 24 days, respectively (Table 2) and, as predicted from the first study, E_2 was not elevated relative to the DMSO controls at any sampling time.

To define the dose dependency of the LH suppression caused by E_2-CDS, ovariectomized female rats were injected with various doses of E_2-CDS or equimolar doses of E_2 and evaluated at 12 days for LH suppression (ESTES et al. 1987). While a dose of 10.38 mg/kg of E_2 was required to significantly suppress LH secretion after 12 days, doses of E_2-CDS as low as 2.0 mg/kg reduced LH levels by 76% in this experiment. In subsequent studies, it was found that doses of E_2-CDS as low as 0.5 mg/kg could suppress serum LH by as much as 81% at 18 days post-drug administration.

To ensure that LH suppression observed was, in fact, due to the brain-targeting features of the CDS and not due to a simple peripheral estrogen

Table 2. Response of serum LH and serum estradiol concentrations 12–14 days posttreatment with E_2-CDS (3 mg/kg) or equimolar estradiol in orchidectomized rats

Treatment Group (n)	Days Posttreatment	Serum LH (ng/ml)	Serum E_2 (pg/ml)
DMSO (7)		$6.83 \pm 0.79^{a*}$	$25.5 \pm 3.8 \ (4/7)^{*a}$
E_2-CDS (7)	12	0.76 ± 38^b	$25.9 \pm 3.9 \ (5/7)^a$
Estradiol (6)		12.9 ± 1.65^c	$29.3 \pm 5.9 \ (4/6)^a$
DMSO (7)		14.42 ± 2.50^a	$.20 \ (7/7)^a$
E_2-CDS	18	1.74 ± 0.70^b	$.20 \ (7/7)^a$
Estradiol (6)		12.08 ± 0.91^a	$.20 \ (6/6)^a$
DMSO (7)		8.58 ± 1.73^a	24.4 ± 3^a
E_2-CDS (7)	24	2.94 ± 1.10^b	24.1 ± 3.2^a
Estradiol (7)		11.60 ± 1.35^a	31.2 ± 8.6^a

[a–c] Values within a posttreatment time with different superscripts are significantly different $^*p < 0.05$. Mean values of serum LH and estradiol (E_2) ± standard errors of the mean are provided. The parentheses following E_2 values give the number of samples below E_2 assay detection limits (20 pg/ml) per number of samples per group.

deposit, the biological potency of the E_2-CDS was compared to that of a commonly used, lipophilic, deposited estrogen derivative, estradiol 17-valerate (E_2V) (ESTES et al. 1987). In this experiment both drugs were administered to female rats which had been ovariectomized 2 weeks earlier. The dose of each steroid was 0.5 mg/kg (equimolar to the E_2-CDS). At 12 days post-administration, LH was suppressed 80% in E_2CDS treated animals while E_2V treated animals demonstrated LH values which did not differ from controls.

The dose dependency of LH suppression on the E_2-CDS is highly dependent upon the time of post-drug administration, at which animals are evaluated due to the long duration of action of the CDS. Thus, ovariec-tomized rats were used to examine the dose of E_2-CDS at low concentrations (10 µg/kg–333 µg/kg) administered as a single i.v. injection (ANDERSON et al. 1988a). At 2 days post-drug treatment, serum LH levels were reduced by 5%, 39%, 42%, and 52% relative to DMSO controls at doses of 10, 33, 100, and 333 µg/kg, respectively. Interestingly, serum E_2 concentrations were not significantly greater than controls at the 10 and 33 µg/kg levels and were increased in a dose-dependent manner at the 100 and 333 µg/kg doses. Thus, very low doses of E_2-CDS can suppress LH secretion while not significantly elevating serum E_2. An additional observation was that serum prolactin was increased at higher doses of E_2-CDS, as expected (ANDERSON et al. 1988a).

An alternative approach to document the brain-enhanced delivery of E_2 following E_2-CDS is to administer low doses of CDS repeatedly and evaluate the cumulative LH suppressing effect. To this end, ovariectomized rats were treated every second day for seven administrations (2 weeks) with E_2-CDS at doses of 10–333 µg/kg, i.v. (ANDERSON et al. 1988a). These doses are equivalent to those used in the aforementioned single dose study and thus facilitate comparisons between these two dosing regimens. At 2 days after the last injection, rats were killed and serum LH and E_2 levels determined. Repeated treatment with E_2-CDS reduced serum LH by 32%, 57%, 72%, and 76% at doses of 10, 33, 100, and 33 µg/kg i.v., respectively. This LH suppression occurred without a concomitant significant increase in serum E_2 at doses of 10 and 33 µg/kg. At the higher doses, serum E_2 levels were equivalent to those observed after a single injection of the same dose of E_2-CDS. These data indicated that repeated administration of low doses of E_2-CDS E_2 accumulate in the brain but not in the periphery. What remains to be determined is the duration of LH response following the "loading" of the brain with low doses of the E_2-CDS.

The secretion of LH in rats can be controlled or attenuated by numerous factors, including the action of E_2 both in a positive and negative feedback mode at the pituitary gland. In addition, hypothalamic release of LHRH stimulates LH secretion. Again, LHRH release can be augmented by the interaction of E_2 in the preoptic area (SARKAR et al. 1976). The effect of the E_2-CDS on LHRH release was, therefore, studied (SARKAR et al. 1989). Animals which had been ovariectomized for at least 2 weeks were given a single i.v. dose of E_2-CDS, E_2, or vehicle. At either 1 or 16 days post-drug administration, animals were anesthetized and their pituitary stalks exposed for collection of portal blood samples to be used for LHRH RIA. Subsequent to sample collections, hypothalamic tissue was removed for LHRH assay. Finally, plasma LH was determined in the animals. Portal blood concentrations of LHRH were significantly reduced on day 1 for both E_2 and E_2-CDS. By day 16, however, only the E_2-CDS continued to decrease LHRH secretion, while the E_2 treated animals were not different from vehicle controls. The decreased LHRH secretion was mirrored by an increase in hypothalamic LHRH levels, suggesting that the inhibition of hormone release resulted in a tissue accumulation of the peptide. Again, hypothalamic LHRH concentrations were significantly elevated at day 1 for both E_2-CDS and E_2, but by 16 days only the E_2-CDS produced a significant accumulation. The LH data indicated secretion of LH was closely correlated with LHRH release. Since previous studies have indicated that long-term exposure of E_2 decreases pituitary responsiveness to LHRH (VERJANS and EIK-NES 1976; HENDERSON et al. 1977; LIBERTUN et al. 1974), the results generated strongly suggest that the prolonged inhibitory action of E_2-CDS on LH release is due primarily to sustained suppression of LHRH secretion from the hypothalamus.

Collectively, the data presented demonstrate that the chemical delivery system for E_2 can cause dose-dependent chronic suppression of LH and LHRH secretion following a single intravenous administration. The remarkably long time-course of suppression (at least 24 days) in the face of clearance of E_2 from the periphery provides strong evidence for the *delivery* to the brain of the E_2-CDS, its *conversion* to the E_2-Q^+, which has a slow egress from the brain and the *slow hydrolysis* of the carrier, resulting in the local *release* of estradiol. A more direct confirmation of this proposed

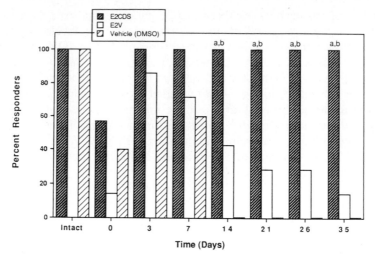

Fig. 33. Effect of 3 mg/kg E_2-CDS, equimolar E_2V, and DMSO on the mounting percentage (percent responders) in castrate male rats from 0–35 days after a single i.v. injection. Groups were analyzed by the Fisher exact test and differences ($p < 0.05$) from control are depicted by *a* and from E_2V by *b*

sequence of brain-enhanced chemical delivery of E_2 includes the previously cited observations of prolonged elevations of E_2-Q^+ in the brain and its rapid clearance from peripheral tissues. Thus, the CDS principle appears to be accurately portrayed in the case of the E_2-CDS.

The E_2-CDS was also used to stimulate male sexual activity. In sexually experienced male rats, orchidectomy results in an expected decline in male sexual behavior (ANDERSON et al. 1987a). As shown in Fig. 33, orchidectomy reduced, but E_2-CDS restored, mounting behavior for 35 days in 100% of rats treated with this system. E_2V was only transiently effective in this regard. Similarly, mount latency, which is an estimate of the rapidity with which the male pursues and mounts the receptive female and, therefore, an estimate of the sexual motivation of the male, was dramatically increased following orchidectomy (Fig. 34). E_2-CDS reduced the mount latency significantly through 28 days post-injection, while E_2V only transiently reduced this parameter. The number of intromissions occurring during the test of sexual behavior was reduced by orchidectomy. E_2-CDS restored intromission behavior to control values for 28 days. Again, E_2V was only transiently effective in this regard. Intromission latency paralleled mount latency, both in response to orchidectomy and to E_2 replacement in that orchidectomy increased, and E_2-CDS decreased the intromission latency for 28 days. E_2V was effective in reducing intromission latency for only 3 days. In contrast to the effect of E_2-CDS on mount and intromission behavior, E_2-CDS had little effect on ejaculatory behavior, a response which requires the stimulation of peripheral tissues by dihydrotestosterone.

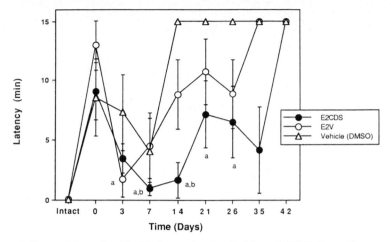

Fig. 34. Effect of 3 mg/kg E_2-CDS, equimolar E_2V, and DMSO on the mounting latency in castrate male rats from 0–42 days after a single i.v. injection. Each point represents the mean ± SEM; *a* denotes significant differences ($p < 0.05$) from DMSO controls and *b* from E_2V treated rats

The observation of the chronic stimulation of male sexual behavior in rats, at a dose and for a time during which peripheral E_2 concentrations are not elevated, indicates that mounting and intromission behavior are dependent upon a local action of E_2 in the brain. Although doubt exists as to the exact site of action of E_2-CDS on copulatory behavior, the localization of aromatase enzymes, which convert testosterone to E_2 in the preoptic area and the amygdala (BEYER et al. 1976; MacLUSKY et al. 1984), suggests that these areas are involved. Additionally, since evidence suggests that E_2 may similarly stimulate libido in human subjects (BANCROFT et al. 1974), this novel chemical delivery system for E_2 may be useful in the treatment of sexual dysfunction in individuals with psychological impotence not complicated by deficits in peripheral androgen-responsive tissue.

Estrogens are known to affect body weight and the E_2-CDS was therefore examined as a potential anorexigenic (WADE 1972; LANDAU and ZUCKER 1976; CZAJA 1983). The effects of E_2-CDS on food intake and body weight have been evaluated in male rats which were sexually mature, in 9-month-old male rats whose obesity was age-related, and in female rats (SIMPKINS et al. 1988, 1989; ANDERSON et al. 1988b; ESTES et al. 1988; SARKAR et al. 1989). In each study involving males, animals were treated with one of three doses of E_2-CDS or with the DMSO vehicle by a single i.v. injection. Body weights and 24 h food intakes were determined prior to the day of treatment and daily for the next 12–14 days and at 3–7 day intervals thereafter. For adult ovariectomized rats, E_2-CDS caused a dose-dependent reduction in the rate of body weight increase (Fig. 35). The dose-dependent reduction in body weight was maintained at each sampling

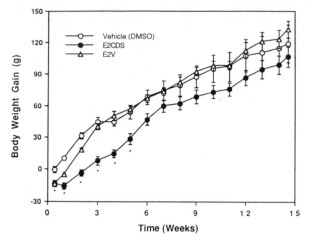

Fig. 35. Effect of E_2-CDS, E_2V, and vehicle on body weight in ovariectomized rats. Each point represents the mean $\pm$ SEM for 6–10 animals. *Asterisks* denote significant differences ($p < 0.05$) from vehicle controls

time and by the last observation day (day 100). Body weights of animals treated with 1 mg/kg dose remained lower than the DMSO control animals. These data indicate that E_2-CDS can chronically suppress body weight following a single administration, despite the clearance of E_2 from the periphery. The local release of E_2 from the E_2-CDS in the brain would appear to be responsible for the chronic reduction in body weight.

c) Toxicity Studies and Human Clinical Trials

Prior to clinical evaluation, extensive safety studies were performed on E_2-CDS to ensure, as much as possible, that the drug would not provoke untoward reactions in humans. The E_2-CDS formulated in 2-hydroxypropyl-β-cyclodextrin (E_2-CDS-CD) was shown to lack mutagenic potential in bacteria as measured in a standard Ames test. This excipient was chosen as it is not parenterally toxic and gives adequate aqueous solubility for the E_2-CDS (BREWSTER et al. 1988a, 1990a). The E_2-CDS-CD system was then tested in Sprague-Dawley rats and cynomolgus monkeys over a period of either 14 (subacute) or 90 (subchronic) days. In the subacute studies, groups of 10 rats (5 males and 5 females) or 2 monkeys (1 male and 1 female) were injected i.v. with either normal saline, 2-hydroxypropyl-β-cyclodextrin in sterile water, or E_2-CDS in the cyclodextrin vehicle at doses of 0.025, 0.25, 1.5, and 5.0 mg/kg. The treatments were administered every second day resulting in cumulative doses of 0.2, 2, 12, and 40 mg/kg; 24 h after the eighth dose, animals were sacrificed and necropsied. During the period of drug administration, animals were monitored for toxic manifestations and macroscopic observation of the animals was made at necropsy. Histo-pathological samples were prepared from various organs and blood was drawn for hematologic and clinical chemistry evaluation. No effects of the vehicle were apparent. The estrogen caused expected changes in hematology (increased neutrophils) in both species. In rats, various expected estrogenic reactions were observed, including weight loss and pituitary hypertrophy. In the subchronic paradigm, 20 rats (10 males and 10 females) and 8 monkeys (4 males and 4 females) were used. Again, one group received normal saline and, another, the cyclodextrin vehicle at a dose of 200 mg/kg. E_2-CDS was administered to monkeys at doses of 1.0 and 5.0 mg/kg and to rats at a dose of 2.5 mg/kg. Drug treatment was performed every other day, resulting in cumulative doses of 46 and 230 mg/kg in monkeys and 115 mg/kg in rats; 24 h after the 46th dose, animals were necropsied and biological samples obtained for evaluation. There were no mortalities in this study as in the subacute trials and no abnormal cageside behaviors were observed. Again, various estrogen-sensitive parameters were significantly altered as a result of E_2-CDS dosing, including decreased body weight and white blood cell count and increased pituitary weight in rats and decreased protein and glucose concentrations with increased triglycerides in monkeys. The toxicologic evaluation of the data obtained from the subchronic studies indicated that the no observable adverse effect dose was the maximum dose used in the protocol, i.e., 5 mg/kg in monkeys and 2.5 mg/kg in rats.

As the CDS, by its design, targets drugs to the CNS, the neurotoxicologic potency of these compounds should be examined. This was done for E_2-CDS by evaluating the effect of the CDS on central neurochemical function (BREWSTER et al. 1988b). In the experiment, E_2-CDS, saline, or the cyclodextrin vehicle was administered to conscious, restrained cynomolgus monkeys i.v. every other day for 2 weeks. The cumulative dose of E_2-CDS ranged from 0.2 to 40 mg/kg and two monkeys (one male and one female) were included in each group; 24 h after the eighth dose, animals were euthanized and samples of striatum removed and frozen. During the study, animals were observed twice a day for locomotor impairment such as rigidity, akinesia, and hypoactivity. No altered motor activity was observed. Neuro-chemical analysis of brain samples was performed by HPLC with electro-chemical detection as earlier described. The results of these assays are given in Table 3 and show that there was no effect of E_2-CDS on striatal dopaminergic concentration. The unaffected dopamine levels and the lack of behavioral changes suggest neurotoxicologic safety of these materials.

The first human examination of E_2-CDS was designed as a rising dose safety study (HOWES et al. 1988; BREWSTER 1990). In this evaluation, meno-pausal women served as the test population in that plasma LH and FSH could be readily assayed as indicators of pharmacologic action. The initial report evaluated ten subjects. In the protocol, all subjects were healthy, post-menopausal females as defined by age and time of last menstrual period (LMP), as confirmed by plasma FSH and LH levels. Each subject received a

Table 3. Effect of repeated dosing (eight injections administered every second day) of E_2-CDS on striatal dopamine and dihydroxyphenylacetic acid and brain levels of E_2-Q^+ in cynomolgus monkeys

Cumulative dose (mg/kg)	Striatum concentration		E_2Q^+ concentration	
	DA (µg/g)	DOPAC (ng/g)	Cortex (ng/g)	Amygdala (ng/g)
0 (saline, vehicle)	12.2, 16.2	594 833	NA	NA
	15.1, 13.5	484 814	NA	NA
0.2	12.3	800	102	200
	11.7	606	230	140
2.0	13.7	714	480	100
	10.0	242	540	450
12.0	14.0	903	2 310	1 445
	13.8	433	3 255	5 940
40.0	11.1	876	4 890	5 700
	12.1	720	8 560	7 900

DA, dopamine; DOPAC, dihydroxyphenylacetic acid. NA, not applicable.

single dose of E_2-CDS as an intravenous injection of the drug dissolved in 20% (w/v) 2-hydroxypropyl-β-cyclodextrin (2-HPCD) as described in Table 4. Subjects remained for 48 h in the clinic and subjective side effects and vital signs were recorded. Blood samples were obtained for analysis of LH, FSH, and 17-β-estradiol at 15 min, 30 min, 1, 2, 4, 8, 24, and 48 h after drug administration. Subjects were then released from the clinic but were asked to return on the morning of day 4 and day 7 for additional blood sampling. In addition, pre- and post-study blood samples were taken for clinical evaluation.

In the study, all subjects met the entry criteria for inclusion. There were no dropouts and all subjects completed the protocol. No adverse effects were

Table 4. Dosing protocol for E_2-CDS complexed in 2-hydroxypropyl-β-cyclodextrin to postmenopausal human volunteers as defined by weight, age, and time of last menstrual period

Subject number	Subject weight (kg)	Dose of E_2-CDS	Dose (µg/kg)	Age (years)	LMP
1	63.8	10 µg	0.16	48	1986
2	63.2	20 µg	0.32	50	1985
3	56.0	40 µg	0.71	61	1978
4	67.0	80 µg	1.19	46	1985
5	57.1	160 µg	2.80	63	1979
6	54.5	320 µg	5.87	50	1986
7	84.5	640 µg	7.57	54	1985
8	63.5	640 µg	10.0	57	many years ago
9	64.5	1.28 mg	19.8	50	1985
10	65.1	1.28 mg	19.7	49	1986

LMP, last menstrual period.

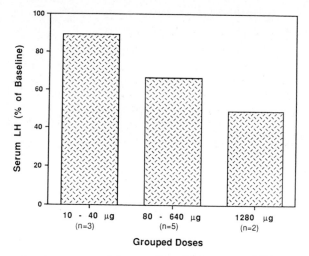

Fig. 36. Effect of various grouped doses of E$_2$-CDS on mean LH suppression relative to baseline values in post-menopausal women

reported which could be attributed to the E$_2$ and all hematologic and clinical chemistry values were unaffected by drug administration. The results of the hormonal assay are summarized in Figs. 36–38 and in Table 4. In examining the data, the results appeared to cluster into three groups: 10–40 µg ($n = 3$), which showed minimal changes; 80–640 µg, which showed threshold effects ($n = 5$); and 1280 µg ($n = 2$), which showed substantial and sustained

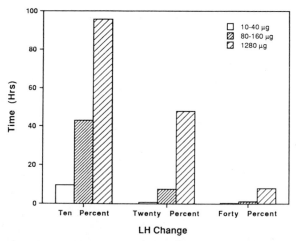

Fig. 37. Effect of various grouped doses of E$_2$-CDS on the duration of action of LH suppression. Duration is measured by return to baseline values in at least two consecutive measurements. Suppression of 10%, 20%, and 40% of LH values are presented

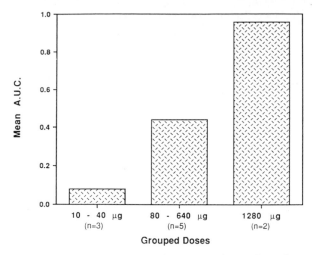

Fig. 38. Mean area under the LH suppression curves for various dose groups of E_2-CDS

decreases in plasma LH levels. Grouping the data for interpretation also has the benefit of reducing the effects of inter-individual variation as only one subject was given a particular dose of drug in most cases.

Figure 36 illustrates the relationship between these three dose groups and the percent maximum fall in LH value. Mean peak decreases of 11%, 34%, and 50% for the three groups were noted. This fall in LH favorably compares to mean peak decreases of 28%–36% seen after 1 month of dosing with E_2 transdermal patches (JUDD 1987; STEINGOLD et al. 1985). Figures 37 and 38 illustrate the duration of LH changes as a function of the magnitude of the LH decrease, i.e., at least 10%, 20%, or 40% decreases from baseline values. The duration of the effect also shows a substantial dose-dependent relationship, e.g., a >20% decrease lasted for up to 48 h after 1280 µg, 18 h at 80–640 µg, and 0 h at 10–40 µg. The area under the curve (AUC) shows comparable dose-related changes in plasma LH. In these studies, it was difficult to quantitate the magnitude of improved action obtained using the CDS relative to the natural hormone E_2 in that no studies have been published which specifically examine the effect of moderate i.v. dose of E_2 on serum LH and E_2. This lack of experimental data was not totally unexpected in that E_2 is poorly water-soluble. This makes parenteral dosing especially difficult when moderate to high E_2 doses are considered. The recent development of non-toxic, highly water-soluble, modified β-cyclodextrins has allowed for the i.v. administration of highly water-insoluble compounds such as sex steroids. The paucity of historic controls and the timely development of safe, useful, and water-soluble inclusion complexes of E_2 led us to conduct an i.v. study using this technology to examine E_2 and LH levels with time after moderate doses of E_2.

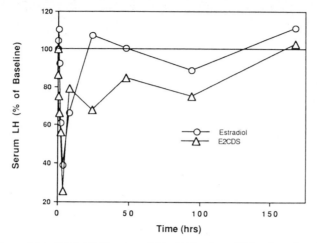

Fig. 39. Effect of E_2-CDS (1280 µg) and E_2 (900 µg) on LH values in a human post-menopausal volunteer. Data are reported as percent of control

Figure 39 illustrates the effect of E_2 and E_2-CDS, both administered in an aqueous-modified β-cyclodextrin vehicle, on LH levels at various times post-treatment in post-menopausal human volunteers. In this study, the dose of E_2 was 900 µg and the equimolar dose of E_2-CDS was 1280 µg. The data were reported as percent of control where control values were obtained by averaging the LH levels obtained at time 0 and on the day prior to treatment. As illustrated in Fig. 39, LH is dampened in a clinically meaningful way through 96 h after E_2-CDS treatment, while LH values have already returned to control by 24 h after E_2 dosing. The LH suppression induced by E_2-CDS returns to control values by 168 h. As would be expected for a long-acting drug such as E_2-CDS, the ratio of the areas under the LH suppression curves, obtained after either E_2-CDS or E_2 dosing, increases as a function of time. In addition, if the initial LH drop which is common to both treatments is discounted, the apparent E_2-CDS/E_2 enhancement is even greater. In this circumstance, the ratio of E_2-CDS to E_2, examining the AUC from 24 h to 168 h, is greater than ten-fold.

The effect of E_2 or E_2-CDS on serum E_2 is given in Fig. 40. Administration of E_2 in an HPCD vehicle rapidly generates high serum E_2 levels as expected and these levels rapidly fall. In contrast, E_2-CDS produces relatively low initial levels of E_2. These concentrations are also rapidly cleared. Past 8 h, the profiles of E_2 elimination are superimposed after either E_2 or E_2-CDS administration. The relative E_2-CDS areas under the E_2 concentration curve increase with time starting at 0.2 at 4 h and approach 1.0 at 168 h.

Two important pieces of information are derived from this study: (1) The initial levels of plasma E_2 generated by E_2-CDS are five- to ten-fold less than those generated after E_2. This dampened surge should improve the

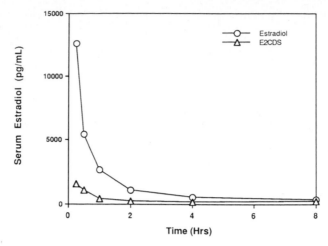

Fig. 40. Effect of E_2-CDS or E_2 on E_2 levels in a human post-menopausal volunteer. The data point at 15 min, obtained after E_2 treatment, represented E_2 levels which were too high to be calculated with the standard curve used in the assay (>6000 pg/ml). This point was estimated using a curve-fitting procedure. The model used was $y = a + b/x + c/x^2$ which gave an $r^2 > 0.999$

therapeutic index of E_2-CDS relative to E_2, especially in circumstances where estrogens are contraindicated such as in breast cancer. The levels of E_2 following E_2-CDS treatment do, however, seem to be sufficient to support bone development in post-menopausal women. (2) LH is clearly suppressed at 24 h, 48 h, and 96 h in a clinically relevant manner after E_2-CDS treatment, while *no* LH suppression is evident at 24 h and beyond after E_2 treatment. This occurs in spite of the fact that the serum levels of immunoreactive E_2 are similar for the two groups. This strongly suggests that E_2-CDS is indeed working via a brain-mediated mechanism in that serum differences in E_2 cannot account for the LH suppression.

4. Conclusion

The ability to deliver pharmacologically active agents to their site of action can be actualized via a number of techniques. This chapter has suggested two: a reduction/hydrolysis-driven chemical delivery system for targeting drugs to the eye and a dihydropyridine-pyridinium salt approach for selectively enhancing drug concentrations in the CNS. Both of these techniques have been fruitful, as indicated by the entry of both eye- and CNS-based delivery systems into human clinical trials. The basic approach taken here can be extended to other organ systems. Importantly, while sequential enzymatic or other conversions are the cornerstone of these delivery approaches, each tissue is associated with distinct biochemical processes which must be understood prior to developing efficient delivery methods.

References

Ahmad S (1979) Cardiopulmonary effects of timolol eye drops. Lancet 2:1028

Anderson WR, Simpkins JW, Brewster ME, Bodor N (1987a) Evidence for the reestablishment of copulatory behavior in castrated male rats with a brain-enhanced estradiol-chemical delivery system. Pharmacol Biochem Behav 27: 265–271

Anderson WR, Simpkins JW, Woodard PA, Winwood D, Stern WC, Bodor N (1987b) Anxiolytic activity of a brain delivery system for GABA. Psychopharmacology (Berlin) 92:157–163

Anderson WR, Simpkins JW, Brewster ME, Bodor N (1988a) Evidence for suppression of serum LH without elevation of serum estradiol or prolactin with a brain-enhanced redox delivery system for estradiol. Life Sci 42:1493–1502

Anderson WR, Simpkins JW, Brewster ME, Bodor N (1988b) Effects of a brain-enhanced chemical delivery system for estradiol on body weight and serum hormones in middle-aged rats. Endocrinol Res 14:131–148

Balis F, Pizzo P, Murphy R, Eddy J, Jarosinski P, Fallon J, Broder S, Poplock D (1989) The pharmacokinetics of zidovudine administered by continuous infusion in children. Ann Intern Med 110:279–285

Bancroft J, Tennent G, Loucas K, Cuss J (1974) The control of deviant sexual behaviour by drugs: behavioral changes with oestrogens and antiandrogens. Br J Psychiatry 125:310–315

Barraclough CA, Wise PM (1982) The role of catecholamines in the regulation of pituitary luteinizing hormone and follicle-stimulating hormone secretion. Endocr Rev 3:91–119

Beyer C, Morali G, Naftolin F, Larsson K, Perez-Palacio G (1976) Effect of some antiestrogens and aromatase inhibitors on androgen induced sexual behavior in castrate male rats. Horm Behav 7:353–362

Blum R, Liao S, Good S, deMiranda P (1988) Pharmacokinetics and bioavailability of zidovudine in humans. Am J Med [Suppl 2A] 85:189–194

Bodor N (1981) Novel approaches to prodrug design. Drugs Future 6:165–182

Bodor N (1987) Redox drug delivery for targeting drugs to the brain. Ann NY Acad Sci 507:289–306

Bodor N (1989) Designing safer ophthalmic drugs. In: vander Goot H, Domany G, Pallos L, Timmerman H (eds) Trends in medicinal chemistry '88. Elsevier, Amsterdam, pp 145–164

Bodor N, Brewster M (1983) Problems of delivery of drugs to the brain. Pharmacol Ther 19:337–386

Bodor N, Farag H (1983) Improved delivery through biological membranes. XIII. Brain-specific delivery of dopamine with a dihydropyridine-pyridinium salt type redox delivery system. J Med Chem 26:528–534

Bodor N, Kaminski J (1987) Prodrugs and site-specific chemical delivery systems. Annu Rep Med Chem 22:303–313

Bodor N, Prokai L (1990) Site and stereospecific drug-delivery by sequential enzymatic bioactivation. Pharm Res 7:723–725

Bodor N, Simpkins J (1983) Redox delivery system for brain-specific, sustained release of dopamine. Science 221:65–67

Bodor N, Visor G (1984a) Formation and adrenaline in the iris-ciliary body from adrenalone diesters. Exp Eye Res 38:621–626

Bodor N, Visor G (1984b) A site-specific chemical delivery system as a short-acting mydriatic agent. Pharm Res 1:168–173

Bodor N, Kaminski JJ, Roller R (1978) Improved delivery through biological membranes. VI. Potent sympathomimetic adrenalone derivatives. Int J Pharm 1: 189–196

Bodor N, Farag H, Brewster M (1981) Site-specific, sustained release of drugs to the brain. Science 214:1370–1372

Bodor N, McCornack J, Brewster, ME (1987) Improved delivery through biological membranes. XXII. Synthesis and distribution of brain-selective estrogen delivery systems. Int J Pharm 35:47–59

Bodor N, El-Koussi A, Kano M, Nakamura T (1988) Improved delivery through biological membranes. Design, synthesis and pharmacological activity of a novel chemical delivery system for β-adrenergic blocking agents. J Med Chem 31: 100–106

Brewster ME (1990) Brain-targeted delivery of estrogens. Rev Neurosci 12:9

Brewster ME, Estes KS, Bodor N (1987a) Improved delivery through biological membranes. XXXII. Synthesis and biological activity of brain-targeted delivery systems for various estradiol derivatives. J Med Chem 31:244–249

Brewster ME, Venkatraghavan V, Shek E, Bodor N (1987b) Facile, one-step preparation of trigonellinate esters. Synthetic Commun 17:451–455

Brewster ME, Estes K, Loftsson T, Perchalski R, Derendorf H, Mullersman G, Bodor N (1988a) Improved delivery through biological membranes. XXXI. Solubilization and stabilization of an estradiol chemical delivery system by modified β-cyclodextrins. J Pharm Sci 77:981–985

Brewster ME, Estes KS, Perchalski R, Bodor N (1988b) A dihydropyridine conjugate which generates high and sustained levels of the corresponding pyridinium salt in the brain does not exhibit neurotoxicity in cynomolgus monkeys. Neurosci Lett 87:277–282

Brewster M, Little R, Venkatraghavan V, Bodor N (1988c) Brain-enhanced delivery of antiviral agents (Abstr). Antiviral Res 9:127

Brewster ME, Estes KS, Bodor N (1990a) An intravenous toxicity study of 2-hydroxypropyl-β-cyclodextrin, a useful drug solubilizer, in rats and monkeys. Int J Pharm 59:231–243

Brewster ME, Simpkins JW, Bodor N (1990b) Brain-targeted delivery of estrogens. Rev Neurosci 2:241–285

Bundgaard H (ed) (1985) Design of prodrugs. Elsevier, Amsterdam

Canonico P, Kende M, Gabrielsen B (1988) Carrier-mediated delivery of antiviral agents. Adv Virus Res 35:271–312

Caterall WC (1988) Tryptophan and bladder cancer. Biol Psychiatry 24:733–734

Christensen LW, Clemens LG (1974) Intrahypothalamic implants of testosterone or estradiol and resumption of masculine sexual behavior in long-term castrated male rats. Endocrinology 95:984–990

Conner CS (1984) Ribavirin. Drug Intell Clin Pharm 18:137–138

Czaja JA (1983) Body weight and growth rates throughout the guinea pig pregnancy: evidence for modulation by endogenous estrogens. Physiol Behav 30:197–201

Elion G, Furman P, Fyfe J, deMiranda P, Beauchamp L, Schaeffer H (1977) Selectivity of action of an antiherpetic agent, 9-(2-hydroxyethoxymethyl) guanine. Proc Natl Acad Sci USA 74:5716–5720

El-Koussi A, Bodor N (1987) Improved delivery through biological membranes. XXV. Enhanced and sustained delivery of trifluorothymidine to the brain using a dihydropyridine-pyridinium salt type redox delivery system. Drug Design Delivery 1:275–283

El-Koussi A, Bodor N (1989) Formation of propranolol in the iris-ciliary body from its propranolol-ketoxime precursor–a potential antiglaucoma drug. Int J Pharm 53:189–194

Estes KS, Brewster ME, Simpkins JW, Bodor N (1987) A novel redox system for CNS-directed delivery of estradiol causes sustained LH suppression in the castrate rat. Life Sci 40:1327–1334

Estes KS, Brewster ME, Bodor N (1988) A redox system for brain targeted estrogen delivery causes chronic body weight decrease in rats. Life Sci 42:1077–1084

Feltakamp H, Meurer KH, Godchardt F (1984) Tryptophan-induced lowering of blood pressure and changes of serotonin uptake by platelets in patients with essential hypertension. Klin Wochenschr 62:1115–1119

Fenstermacher JD (1985) Current models of blood-brain transfer. Trends Neurol Sci 8:449–452

Fonnum F (1978) Comment on localization of neurotransmitters in the basal ganglia. In: Fonnum F (ed) Amino acids as chemical transmitters. Plenum, New York, pp 143–153

Fotherby K (1985) Oral contraceptives, lipids and cardiovascular disease contraception 31:367–394

Fraunfelder FT, Barker AF (1985) Respiratory effects of timolol. N Engl J Med 311:1441

Fregly MJ, Fater DC (1986) Prevention of DOCA-induced hypertension in rats by chronic treatment with tryptophan. Clin Exp Pharmacol Physiol 13:767–776

Fregly MJ, Lockley, OE, vanderVoort J, Sumner C, Henley W (1987) Chronic dietary administration of tryptophan prevents the development of deoxycorticosterone acetate salt induced hypertension in rats. Can J Physiol Pharmacol 65:753–764

Fregly MJ, Lockley OE, Cade JR (1988) Effect of chronic dietary treatment with L-tryptophan on the development of renal hypertension in rats. Pharmacology 36:91–100

Fuller RW, Holland DR, Yen TT, Bemis KG, Stamm N (1979) Antihypertensive effects of fluoxetine and L-5-hydroxytryptophan in rats. Life Sci 25:1237–1242

Gallo J, Boubinot F, Doshi D, Etse J, Bhandti V, Schinazi R, Chu CK (1989) Evaluation of brain targeting of anti-HIV nucleosides delivered via dihydropyridine prodrugs (Abstr). Pharm Res 6:S161

Gogu SR, Aggarwal SK, Rangan SR, Agrawal KC (1989) A prodrug of zidovudine with enhanced efficacy against human immunodeficiency virus. Biochem Biophys Res Commun 160:656–661

Gorrod J (1980) Potential hazards of the prodrug approach. Chem Ind 11:458–462

Greig NH (1987) Optimizing drug delivery to brain tumors. Cancer Treat Rev 14:1–28

Greig NH, Momma S, Sweeney DJ, Smith QR, Rapoport SI (1987) Facilitated transport of melphalan at the rat blood-brain barrier by the large neutral amino acid carrier system. Cancer Res 47:1571–1576

Henderson SR, Baker G, Fink G (1977) Oestradiol-17β and pituitary responsiveness to luteinizing hormone releasing factor in the rat. J Endocrinol 73:441–453

Hoek JB, Rydstrom J (1988) Physiological roles of nicotinamide nucleotide transhydrogenases. Biochem J 254:1–10

Howe R, Shanks RG (1966) Optical isomers of propranolol. Nature 210:1336–1338

Howes J, Bodor N, Brewster ME, Estes K, Eve M (1988) A pilot study with PR-63 in post-menopausal volunteers (Abstr). J Clin Pharmacol 28:951

Huggins J, Robins R, Canonico P (1984) Synergistic antiviral effects of ribavirin and the C-nucleoside analogs of tiazofurin and selenazofurin against togaviruses, bunyaviruses and arenaviruses. Antimicrob Agents Chemother 26:476–480

Huppert LC (1987) Hormone replacement therapy: benefits, risks, doses. Med Clin North Am 71:23–29

Hurst BS, Rock JA (1989) Endometriosis: pathophysiology, diagnosis and treatment. Obstet Gynecol Surv 44:297–304

Ito A, Schanberg SM (1972) Central nervous system mechanism responsible for blood pressure elevation induced by p-chlorophenylalanine. J Pharmacol Exp Ther 181:65–74

Jankovic J (1988) Parkinson's disease: recent advances in therapy. South Med J 81:1021–1027

Janocko L, Larner J, Hochberg RH (1984) The interaction of C-17 esters of estradiol with the estrogen receptor. Endocrinology 114:1180–1186

Joyce JN (1983) Multiple dopamine receptors and behavior. Neurosci Biobehav Rev 7:227–256

Judd H (1987) Efficacy of transdermal estradiol. Am J Obstet Gynecol 156:1326–1331

Kalra SP, Kalra PS (1980) Modulation of hypothalamic luteinizing hormone-releasing hormone levels by intracranial and subcutaneous implants of gonadal steroids in castrated rats: effects of androgen and estrogen antagonists. Endocrinology 106:390–397

Kalra SP, Kalra PS (1983) Neural regulation of luteinizing hormone secretion in the rat. Endocr Rev 4:311–351

Kaplan NM (1978) Cardiovascular complications of oral contraceptives. Annu Rev Med 29:31–40

Kawashima D, Levy A, Spector S (1976) Stereospecific radioimmunoassay for propranolol isomers. J Pharmacol Exp Ther 196:517–523

Klecker R, Collins J, Yarchoan R, Thomas R, Jenkins J, Broder S, Myer C (1987) Plasma and cerebrospinal fluid pharmacokinetics of 3'-azido-3'-deoxythymidine: a novel pyrimidine analog with potential application for the treatment of patients with AIDS and related diseases. Clin Pharmacol Ther 41:407–412

Landau T, Zucker I (1976) Estrogenic regulation of body weight in female rats. Horm Behav 7:29–39

Lauritzen C, vanKeep PA (1978) Potential beneficial effects of estrogen substitution in the post-menopause – a review. Front Horm Res 5:1–25

Levin E (1977) Are the terms blood-brain barrier and brain capillary permeability synonymous. Exp Eye Res 25:191–199

Levin VA (1980) Relationship of octanol/water partition coefficients and molecular weight to rat brain capillary permeability. J Med Chem 23:682–684

Libertun C, Orias R, McCann SM (1974) Biphasic effect of estrogen on the sensitivity of the pituitary to luteinizing hormone-releasing factor (LRF). Endocrinology 94:1094–1100

Little R, Bailey D, Brewster M, Estes K, Clemmons R, Saab A, Bodor N (1990) Improved delivery through biological membranes. XXXIII. Brain-enhanced delivery of azidothymidine. J Biopharm Sci 1:1–16

MacLusky NJ, Phillip A, Hurlburt C, Naftolin F (1984) Estrogen metabolism in neuroendocrine structures. In: Celotti F, Naftolin F, Martini L (eds) Metabolism of hormonal steroids in the neuroendocrine structures. Raven, New York, pp 103–116

Maggi A, Perez J (1985) Role of female gonadal hormones in the CNS: clinical and experimental aspects. Life Sci 37:893–906

Martin JB, Gusella JF (1986) Huntington's disease: pathogenesis and management. N Engl J Med 315:1267–1276

Matsuyama K, Yamashita C, Noda A, Goto S, Nodo H, Ichimaru Y, Gomita Y (1984) Evaluation of isonicotinoyl-γ-aminobutyric acid (GABA) and nicotinoyl-GABA as prodrugs of GABA. Chem Pharm Bull (Tokyo) 32:4089–4095

McCormick J, King I, Webb P, Scribner C, Craven R, Johnson K, Elliott L, Belmont-Williams R (1986) Lassa fever: effective therapy with ribavirin. N Engl J Med 314:20–26

McEwen BS (1981) Neural gonadal steroid action. Science 211:1303–1311

Mekki QA, Warrington SJ, Turner P (1984) Ocular and cardiovascular effects of timolol and pindolol eyedrops in normal volunteers. Br J Clin Pharmacol 17: 632–633

Mullersman G, Derendorf H, Brewster ME, Estes KS, Bodor N (1988) High performance liquid chromatographic assay of a central nervous system (CNS)-directed estradiol chemical delivery system and its application after intravenous administration in rats. Pharm Res 5:172–177

Nelson W, Shetty H (1986) Stereoselective oxidative metabolism of propranolol in the microsomal fraction from rat and human liver. Use of deuterium labeling and pseudoracemic mixtures. Drug Metab Dispos 14:506–508

Neuwelt EA (ed) (1989) Implications of the blood-brain barrier and its manipulations. Plenum, New York

Palomino E, Kessel D, Horwitz J (1989) A dihydropyridine carrier system for sustained delivery of 2',3'-dideoxynucleosides to the brain. J Med Chem 32: 622–625

Pardridge WM (1981) Transport of nutrients and hormones through the blood-brain barrier. Diabetologia 20:246–254

Pardridge WM (1985) Strategies for drug delivery through the blood-brain barrier. In: Borchardt R, Repta A; Stella VJ (eds) Directed drug delivery. Humana, Clifton, pp 83–96

Pardridge WM, Connor JD, Crawford IL (1975) Permeability changes in the blood-brain barrier: causes and consequences. CRC Crit Rev Toxicol 3:159–199

Pfaff DW (1970) Nature of sex hormone effects on rat sex behavior: specificity of effect and individual patterns of response. J Comp Physiol Psychol 73:349–358

Pfaff DW, Keiner M (1973) Atlas of estradiol-concentrating cells in the central nervous system of the female rat. J Comp Neurol 151:121–158

Pop E, Anderson W, Prokai-Tatrai K, Brewster M, Fregly M, Bodor N (1990) Antihypertensive activity of redox derivatives of tryptophan. J Med Chem 33:2063–2065

Rand K, Bodor N, El-Koussi A, Raad J, Miyake A, Houck H, Gildersleeve N (1986) Potential treatment of herpes simplex virus encephalitis by brain-specific delivery of trifluorothymidine using a dihydropyridine-pyridinium salt type redox delivery system. J Med Virol 20:1–8

Rapoport SI (1976) The blood-brain barrier in physiology and medicine. Raven, New York

Rapoport SI, Klee WA, Pattigrew KD, Ohno K (1980) Entry of opioid peptides into the central nervous system. Science 207:84–86

Reese B, Karnovsky MJ (1967) Fine structural localization of a blood-brain barrier to exogenous peroxides. J Cell Biol 34:207–217

Richards R, Tattersfield E (1985) Brochial β-adrenoreceptor blockade following eye drops of timolol and its isomer L-714, 465 in normal subjects. Br J Clin Pharmacol 20:459–462

Rodriguez W, Parrott R (1987) Ribavirin aerosol treatment of serious respiratory syncytial virus infection in infants. Infect Dis Clin North Am 1:425–439

Roland L (ed) (1984) Marritt's textbook of neurology. Lea and Febiger, Philadelphia, p 526

Roos BE, Steg G (1964) The effect of 3,4-dihydroxyphenylalanine and 5-hydroxytryptophan on rigidity and tremor induced by reserpine, chlorpromazine and phenoxybenzamine. Life Sci 3:351–360

Rydstrom J (1977) Energy-linked nicotinamide nucleotide transhydrogenases. Biochim Biophys Acta 463:155–184

Saito K (1976) Immunochemical studies of GAD and GABA-T. In: Roberts E, Chase TN, Tower DB (eds) GABA in nervous system function. Raven, New York, pp 103–111

Sar M (1984) Estradiol is concentrated in tyrosine hydroxylase containing neurons of the hypothalamus. Science 223:938–940

Sar M, Stumpf WE (1981) Central noradrenergic neurons concentrate ^{3}H-oestradiol. Nature 289:500–502

Sarkar DK, Chippa SA, Fink G, Friedman HM (1976) Gonadotropin-releasing hormone surge in proestrus rats. Nature 264:461–463

Sarkar DK, Friedman SJ, Yen SSC, Frautschy SA (1989) Chronic inhibition of hypothalamic-pituitary-ovarian axis and body weight gain by brain-directed delivery of estradiol-17β in female rats. Neuroendocrinology 50:204–210

Schoene RB, Martin TR, Chavan NB, French DL (1981) Timolol induced bronchospasm in asthmatic bronchitis. JAMA 245:1460–1461

Schoene RB, Ward R, Abuan T, Beasley CH (1984) Effect of topical betaxolol, timolol and placebo on pulmonary function in asthmatic bronchitis. Am J Ophthalmol 97:86–92

Sidwell R, Robins R, Hillyard I (1979) Ribavirin: an antiviral agent. Pharmacol Ther 6:123–146

Simpkins JW, Bodor N, Enz A (1985) Direct evidence for brain-specific release of dopamine from a redox delivery system. J Pharm Sci 74:1033–1036

Simpkins J, McCornack J, Estes KS, Brewster ME, Shek E, Bodor N (1986) Sustained brain specific delivery of estradiol causes long-term suppression of luteinizing hormone secretion. J Med Chem 29:1809–1812

Simpkins JW, Anderson WR, Dawson R, Seth A, Brewster M, Estes K, Bodor N (1988) Chronic weight loss in lean and obese rats with a brain-enhanced chemical delivery system for estradiol. Physiol Behav 44:573–580

Simpkins JW, Anderson WR, Dawson R, Bodor N (1989) Effect of a brain-enhanced chemical delivery system for estradiol on body weight and food intake in intact and ovariectomized rats. Pharm Res 6:592–600

Steingold KA, Lauter L, Chetkowski RJ, Defazio J, Matt DW, Meldrum DR, et al. (1985) Treatment of hot flashes with transdermal estradiol administration. J Clin Endocrinol Metab 61:627–632

Stella VJ (1975) Prodrugs: an overview and definition. In: Higuchi T, Stella VJ (eds) Prodrugs as novel drug delivery systems. American Chemical Society, Washington, pp 1–115

Stella VJ, Himmelstein KJ (1980) Prodrugs and site-specific drug delivery. J Med Chem 23:1275–1282

Suckling AJ, Rumsby MG, Bradbury MW (eds) (1986) The blood-brain barrier in health and disease. VCH, Chichester

Sved A, van Itallie CM, Fernstrom JD (1982) Studies on the antihypertensive action of L-tryptophan. J Pharmacol Exp Ther 221:329–333

Terasaki T, Pardridge W (1988) Restricted transport of 3'-azido-3'-deoxythymidine and dideoxynucleosides through the blood-brain barrier. J Infect Dis 158: 630–632

Torrence P, Kinjo J, Lesiak K, Balzarini J, DeClercq E (1988) AIDS dementia: synthesis and properties of a derivative of 3'-azido-3'-deoxythymidine (AZT) that may become "locked" in the central nervous system. FFBS Lett 234:134–140

Upton V (1984) Therapeutic considerations in the management of the climacteric. J Reprod Med 29:71–79

Venkatraghavan V, Shek E, Perchalski R, Bodor N (1986) Brain-specific chemical delivery systems for acyclovir (Abstr). Pharmacologist 28:145

Verjans HL, Eik-Nes KB (1976) Serum LH and FSH levels following intravenous injection of a gonadotropin releasing principle in normal and gonadectomized adult male rats with estradiol-17β or 5α-dihydrotestosterone. Acta Endocrinol (Copenh) 83:493–505

Wade GN (1972) Gonadal hormones and behavior regulation of body weight. Physiol Behav 8:523–534

Walle T, Walle U, Wilson MJ, Fagan TC, Gaffney T (1984) Stereoselective ring oxidation of propranolol in man. Br J Clin Pharmacol 18:741–748

Wolf WA, Kuhn DM (1984a) Antihypertensive effects of L-tryptophan are not mediated by brain serotonin. Brain Res 295:356–359

Wolf WA, Kuhn DM (1984b) Effect of L-tryptophan on blood pressure in normotensive and hypertensive rats. J Pharmacol Exp Ther 230:324–329

Woodard P, Winwood D, Brewster ME, Estes K, Bodor N (1990) Improved delivery through biological membranes. XXI. Brain-targeted anti-convulsive agents. Drug Design Delivery 6:15–28

Wurtman RJ (1981) Process and composition for reducing blood pressure in animals. US Patent 4,296,119

Yarchoan R, Berg G, Brouwers R, Fischl M, Spitzer A, et al. (1987) Response of human immunodeficiency-virus-associated neurological disease to 3'-azido-3'-deoxythymidine. Lancet 1:132–135

CHAPTER 8

In Vivo Behavior of Liposomes:
Interactions with the Mononuclear Phagocyte
System and Implications for Drug Targeting*

G.L. SCHERPHOF

A. Introduction

Several years before BANGHAM et al. (1965a,b) formulated the concept of the liposome as a closed compartment separated from its aqueous environment by one or more lipid bilayers, and even longer before GREGORIADIS and RYMAN (1972a) first suggested the use of such liposomes as a potential drug carrier system, intravenous administration of aqueous dispersions of phospholipids was proposed as an anti-atherogenic treatment, facilitating the elimination of cholesterol from the body (FRIEDMAN et al. 1957). Even before that, a patent was obtained for the creation of a local depot of steroids, created by applying phospholipid/steroid mixtures, which clearly must have had the structural features of what we now call liposomes (JOHNSON 1934, cited according to PAGANO and WEINSTEIN 1978). However, the enormous boost in liposome literature that we have seen in more recent years did not start before the early 1970s, when GREGORIADIS and RYMAN (1972b) proposed the enzyme-loaded liposome as an approach to the treatment of (lysosomal) storage diseases. Ever since then, we have seen an exponential growth of literature on the potentials of the liposome as a drug carrier system, culminating over the past 3 or 4 years in a large number of reports on clinical trials concerning a limited number of applications. Much of the work published on liposomes deals with their in vivo behavior, both from a fundamental point of view and with respect to direct applications. Although a considerable share of this latter work serves to moderate the over-enthusiastic conclusions frequently drawn from in vitro experiments with liposomes and cells, it cannot be denied that sometimes spectacular results are reported, mostly on the therapeutic utility of liposomes in animal models of disease. Such observations maintain the interest in the liposome as a drug carrier system at a high level. At the same time, however, they serve to make us aware that we still do not fully understand the ways in which liposomes interact with the various

*The work from this laboratory referred to was financially supported by grants from the Netherlands Organization for Scientific Research, the Dutch Cancer Foundation and Ciba Geigy AG, Basel.

components of the animal body with which they come in contact upon in vivo administration. In this review I will discuss current knowledge of the in vivo behavior of liposomes, with an emphasis on the fate of intravenous administration, and attempt to correlate this with the possibility of successfully using the liposome as a drug targeting system.

B. Interactions with Body Fluids

For the liposome to act as a useful drug carrier it should be able to retain an encapsulated drug for a sufficiently long time after its administration in order to appropriately alter the pharmacokinetics of the drug. If the action of the drug is to involve an interaction of the drug-carrier complex with any type of cell, this means that the drug should be retained long enough to accomplish this interaction. It was observed more than 10 years ago that blood plasma contained factors that were able to drastically enhance the rate at which encapsulated solutes were released from liposomes (ZBOROWSKI et al. 1977) and that mainly high density lipoproteins were responsible for these liposome destabilizing effects (SCHERPHOF et al. 1978). Further studies, mainly by the groups of Allen (ALLEN and CLELAND 1980; ALLEN 1981; ALLEN and EVEREST 1983), Gregoriadis (KIRBY et al. 1980a,b; KIRBY and GREGORIADIS 1980, 1981; SENIOR and GREGORIADIS 1982a,b; SENIOR et al. 1983) and Scherphof (SCHERPHOF et al. 1979, 1983b; DAMEN et al. 1979, 1980, 1981, 1982; SCHERPHOF and MORSELT 1983), revealed details of the detrimental effects of plasma components on liposomal integrity and also showed that there are relatively simple means to render liposomes quite resistant to such effects. Incorporation of high proportions of cholesterol, for example, was shown to reduce the plasma-induced leakage of encapsulated solutes quite substantially (KIRBY et al. 1980a,b; KIRBY and GREGORIADIS, 1980, 1981), as was the use of phospholipids with relatively high gel to liquid crystalline phase transition temperatures (SENIOR and GREGORIADIS 1982a; SCHERPHOF et al. 1979). Also, the exploitation of phospholipid analogues, such as ether phospholipids, was shown to have a beneficial effect on plasma stability of liposomes (GUPTA et al. 1981; BALI et al. 1983; HERMETTER and PALTAUF 1983; AGARWAL et al. 1986a,b).

The interactions of liposomes with plasma constituents leading to enhanced solute release are elaborately described and discussed in an excellent review on factors controlling the in vivo fate of liposomes, recently published by SENIOR (1987). From all evidence available it becomes clear that by properly manipulating the lipid composition of liposomes and by choosing the appropriate preparation technique liposomes can be prepared with any required degree of stability towards plasma proteins. Thus, one could achieve, for instance, a pre-meditated controlled rate of drug release from a dose of long-circulating liposomes (see below) as easily as a nearly perfect liposomal retention of the drug for the more than 24 h that such liposomes may circulate. The choice will only be determined by the particular goal one is aiming for, i.e., either sustained intravascular release to make drug gradually available to target sites or maximal retention to accomplish direct and maximal interaction of the intact drug-carrier complex with target cells.

Upon administration along other routes, such as intraperitoneally, intratracheally, or orally, fluids of other composition may jeopardize the integrity of the liposomes. Upon intraperitoneal injection liposomes appear in the bloodstream with a delay of several minutes to a few hours, depending on the animal species (ELLENS et al. 1981, 1983). The route they take is very likely to be via the lymphatics (PARKER et al. 1981); thus, the proteins of the lymph may contribute to the destabilization of the liposomal permeability barrier before they enter the bloodstream. Since (high density) lipoproteins are present in the lymph in appreciable concentrations (RUDRA et al. 1984), the mechanism of destabilization is probably similar to that in plasma. Hence, the factors influencing the liposomal instability will also be the same, i.e., cholesterol content and phospholipid composition. Also intratracheal administration will lead to contact with protein-containing fluids before interaction with cells can take place. No studies have been published from which conclusions to that effect can be drawn, probably because of obvious difficulties in obtaining these fluids in undiluted form. Besides, it should be realized that the composition of such fluids may greatly vary with physiological or pathological conditions. Ophthalmological application of liposomes involves exposure to tear fluid, which can relatively easily be collected. In this case, for maximal stability similar requirements of liposomal composition have been reported as for plasma (BARBER and SHEK 1986). A quite different situation is met when liposomes are administered orally. Several attempts have been made to improve intestinal absorption of orally given drugs by encapsulation in liposomes (see WOODLEY 1986 for a review). The strongly acidic environment of the stomach is generally rather well taken by the liposomes; however, the combination of high bile salt concentrations and pancreatic phospholipase A activity in the upper intestine demands very special properties of a liposome for it to survive. Resistance against a variety of bile salts has been reported for liposomes consisting of phospholipids containing saturated long-chain acyl residues and a high cholesterol content (ROWLAND and WOODLEY 1980, 1981). Resistance against phospholipase activity can be achieved by using, for example, ether analogues of glycerophospholipids (DESMUKH et al. 1978, 1981; STEIN et al. 1984a,b). Thus, theoretically an almost perfectly stable liposome might be constructed with the ability to survive even the very hostile environment of the gut. It is likely, however, that such a liposome would also provide a nearly perfect permeability barrier to any encapsulated water-soluble drug. Since it is unlikely that intact liposomes can be transferred from the lumen of the intestine to the blood circulation (DESMUKH et al. 1981; PATEL et al. 1985), such a liposome would seem to be of little avail in enhancing blood concentrations of an encapsulated drug as it would also be expected to be resistant to intracellular degradation within the intestinal epithelial cells. Only if massive liposome uptake by such cells from the intestinal lumen could be achieved could this lead to the formation of substantial intracellular depots of an encapsulated drug from which appreciable concentrations of drug could gradually diffuse into the circulation.

C. Interactions with Cells

The general objective of using liposomes as drug carriers is to achieve specific interaction of the carrier with a particular type of cell or tissue followed by internalization of the drug or the drug/carrier complex by the cells. Whether or not the drug, after this has been achieved, will reach its intended intracellular target site will greatly depend on the mechanism of internalization and on the specific characteristics of the drug as well as of the carrier. For liposomes, it has been postulated that there are a number of ways in which they can interact with a cell (PAGANO and WEINSTEIN 1978), i.e., stable or transient adsorption, fusion with the plasma membrane, or endocytosis. In case the liposome remains adsorbed, internalization of the drug will depend on its release from the liposome followed by cellular uptake along the regular route, e.g., diffusion through the plasma membrane. The liposome then would serve merely to concentrate the drug at the surface of the target cell. The feasibility of such an approach has been questioned because drug released from the liposomes at the cell surface was believed to diffuse too rapidly into the medium, viz. the circulation, to result in any increased uptake by the target cells (BLUMENTHAL et al. 1982). On the other hand, a direct transfer of liposome-associated drug from the liposome to the cell has been postulated (WEINSTEIN and LESERMAN 1984). The likelihood of such a mechanism might increase with increasing hydrophobicity of the drug. For example, enhanced specific transfer of liposomal phosphatidylcholine from liposomes to hepatocytes has been reported to take place during receptor-mediated interaction of galactose-bearing liposomes and the galactose receptor of these cells (HOEKSTRA et al. 1980).

Evidence for fusion of liposomes with cells has been presented in the past by several research groups (PAPAHADJOPOULOS et al. 1974; PAGANO and HUANG 1975; MARTIN and MacDONALD 1974; WEINSTEIN et al. 1978; KIMELBERG and MAYHEW 1978). Later it became clear that in these studies probably phenomena other than liposome fusion with the plasma membrane of the cell were to be held responsible for the reported cytoplasmic transfer of liposomal contents (MAYHEW et al. 1980; SZOKA et al. 1980; ALLEN et al. 1981; STRAUBINGER et al. 1983). SZOKA et al. (1981) demonstrated that under more rigorous conditions it is possible to let liposomes fuse with the plasma membrane of cells. After achieving specific interaction of glycolipid-containing liposomes with cell-surface lectins in vitro, the liposomes could be made to fuse in the presence of high concentrations of polyethylene glycol. In more recent years a number investigators have claimed to have succeeded in designing various fusogenic liposomes of very specific composition. Virtually all of these concerned liposomes specifically designed to trigger fusion upon acidification of the medium (CONNOR et al. 1984; STRAUBINGER et al. 1985; ELLENS et al. 1985; NAYAR and SCHROIT 1985). This implies that, for in vivo application, internalization of the liposome-encapsulated drug would still have to depend on an endocytic mechanism involving acidified endocytic vacuoles (VAN RENSWOUDE et al. 1982) from which the drug might be transfused into the cytoplasm. Extracellular conditions of sufficiently low pH are very unlikely to be met in the in vivo situation and will probably be restricted to in vitro conditions where liposomes may be made to fuse directly with the plasma membrane. In spite of the considerable number of papers devoted to "fusogenic liposomes" which have been published lately, it is by no means firmly established that in all these cases it is really fusion of membranes that is responsible for the observed transfer of liposome-encapsulated solutes to the cytoplasmic compartment of the cell. For example, recently it was demonstrated that the delivery of nucleotides to the cytoplasm by means of pH-sensitive liposomes was likely to be accomplished by a nucleotide translocase present in the membranes of the endocytic vacuole, upon disintegration of the liposome in the acidic environment of the endosome, rather than by direct transfer through a fusion process (BROWN and SILVIUS 1989). With or without involving fusion processes, endocytosis appears to be the most common mechanism by which liposomes are internalized by cells. This has been most thoroughly established for phagocytic cells such as macrophages (MUNN and PARCE 1982; MEHTA et al. 1982; RAZ et al. 1981; HAFEMAN et al. 1980; HOWARD et al. 1982; DIJKSTRA et al. 1984a,b, 1985a-c), but also for several non-phagocytic cells endocytosis has been described as the major if not only mechanism of liposome uptake (POSTE and PAPAHADJOPOULOS 1976; FRALEY et al. 1980, 1981). This implies that the internalized liposome, via the endosome compartment where destabilization or perhaps even fusion may occur (see above), will end up in the lysosomal system. There, degradation of the constituent (phospho) lipids by lysosomal acidic hydrolases will take place and the released drug, if resistant to this rather hostile environment and if of sufficiently small molecular size, may escape from the lysosomal compartment and find its way to the intended intracellular target site. It has been argued that also non-fusogenic liposomes may release some of their encapsulated solute into the cytoplasm before hydrolytic enzymes access them, for instance, during the fusion of the endosome with the primary lysosome which may involve a transiently leaky stage (STRAUBINGER et al. 1983). Such imperfections may cause a fraction of the encapsulated material to escape from enzymatic degradation; this would seem to be especially relevant for substances which are particularly sensitive to such hydrolytic actions and, in addition, display intracellular activities at (very) low concentrations, such as DNA or enzymes.

D. Anatomical Barriers

Once brought into the body by means of any administration route, the liposome, be it targeted or not, will face the physical limitations of the site of application. Subcutaneous or intramuscular administration has been shown to lead to long or even very long retention times at the site of injection (TUMER et al. 1983). The physicochemical characteristics of the liposome will mainly determine to what extent an encapsulated solute will be retained as well. It is basically the narrowness of the interstitial spaces that sets diffusion restraints on the injected vesicles; it is not surprising therefore that large liposomes are generally retained longer than small vesicles such as small unilamellar vesicles (SUV) (TUMER et al. 1983). This route of administration will, as a rule, be resticted to the purpose of eliciting an immune response (ALVING 1987) or to applications involving the establishment of a local sustained-release depot from which the drug is supposed to be gradually released. Also, accumulation in regional lymph nodes will be achieved by subcutaneous injection (MANGAT and PATEL 1985; PATEL et al. 1984). Eventually, subcutaneously injected liposomes may reach the blood circulation (STEVENSON et al. 1982), although for large liposomes this may take a virtually infinite period of time.

Intratracheal administration of liposomes has mostly been aimed at alveolar macrophages, which are in direct contact with the air-water interface in the lung. This means that for this application there are basically no major morphological obstacles, provided that the dose can be applied sufficiently deep in the respiratory tract. Other cells lining the airways will be equally accessible; thus, specific interaction will probably have to be designed, e.g., by means of proper receptor-ligand interaction, in order to overcome the competition of the strongly phagocytic macrophages, as discussed below for the liver.

Intraperitoneal administration of liposomes has been shown repeatedly to lead to more or less delayed appearance of intact, solute-retaining liposomes in the main circulation (PARKER et al. 1981, 1982a,b; ELLENS et al. 1981). The length of the time period required for the liposomes to enter the blood compartment is probably related to the size of the animal involved (WEISSMANN et al. 1978; KIMELBERG and MAYHEW, 1978; ELLENS et al. 1983). For human application the i.p. route is less relevant and probably of little use except perhaps in cases where tumors accessible from the peritoneal cavity are under consideration, such as ovarian cancers. Senior has extensively discussed the fate of i.p. administered substances (SENIOR 1987).

In recent years the percutaneous route of administration of liposome-associated agents has received a great deal of attention, mainly because of the application in cosmetic preparations. Formidable physical barriers in the skin await such dermally applied liposome-based formulations, if penetration deeper than into the stratum corneum would be required. It cannot be expected that intact liposomes will succeed in reaching the deeper layers of the skin beyond the more superficially located keratinocytes. Claims that "normal" liposomes can fuse with the lamellar lipid structures in the skin (ABRAHAM et al. 1988) will have to await confirmation before they can be considered seriously. Recently, however, it was reported that liposomes composed of lipids extracted from these multilamellar structures do fuse with (skin) cells (ABRAHAM and DOWNING 1990). In this way the penetration of, in particular, hydrophobic substances, associated with the liposomal lipid bilayers, may be facilitated (LASCH and WOHLRAB 1986). Similar to what was discussed concerning the processing of liposomes in the digestive tract, such applications of liposomes would also not involve the intracellular uptake of intact liposomes.

By far the most extensively investigated route of liposome administration is the intravenous route. The very first reports on the use of liposomes as a carrier of biologically active substances dealt with the i.v. administration of liposome-encapsulated enzymes intended for the alleviation of lysosomal storage diseases (GREGORIADIS and RYMAN 1972a). Very soon it was established that, as a rule, intravenously injected liposomes localize mainly in spleen and liver (GREGORIADIS and RYMAN 1972b; McDOUGALL et al. 1974; Juliano and STAMP 1975)). The initial assumption was that the macrophages in those tissues, as major representatives of the reticuloendothelial system (RES) or, as it is called nowadays, mononuclear phagocyte system (MPS), were to be held responsible for this preferential localization. This was firmly established for the liver, where the Kupffer cells were confirmed to account for the bulk of the total hepatic contribution to liposome clearance from the blood (FREISE et al. 1980; SCHERPHOF et al. 1980; ROERDINK et al. 1981; RAHMAN et al. 1982; POSTE et al. 1982). For spleen as well as for the other organs which were shown to contribute to some extent to liposome elimination, namely bone marrow and lung (ABRA and HUNT 1981; ABRA et al. 1983; POSTE et al. 1984), solid evidence for a major role of macrophages is less abundant, but it is generally assumed to be true. The reason for this important role of macrophages is not only that these cells, professional phagocytes as they are, have a "natural" affinity for particulate substances like liposomes. Although this high affinity is an established fact, as can be concluded from comparison of in vitro experiments with isolated macrophages (MEHTA et al. 1982; DIJKSTRA et al. 1984a; ALVING 1988) and other non-phagocytic cells (HOEKSTRA et al. 1978; VAN RENSWOUDE et al. 1979), other factors play a role as well. A very important one is the initially overlooked or at least ignored circumstance that only relatively few cell types in the body are directly accessible from the blood stream because of the tightness of the vascular system. In most tissues the vascular system is lined with a continuous layer of endothelial cells, often even supported by a complex basement membrane, which virtually excludes extravasation of particles such as liposomes. Exceptions to this rule have been observed; for example, the massive accumulation of (SUV) of long circulation time in certain types of solid tumors (PROFFITT et al. 1983) and the demonstration of substantial amounts of liposomes inside the tumor cells provide indirect evidence that such small liposomes may under certain conditions be able to escape from the vascular system (HWANG et al. 1982). This may be favored by the condition that the endothelium in tumor tissue has been found to be less tight than that in normal tissue. Also, under conditions of fever, which might be deliberately elicited, the endothelial lining of the vessel wall may be more permeable even to small particulate matter such as liposomes.

A number of organs, such as liver and bone marrow, do have a naturally fenestrated endothelium which allows an intravenously administered dose of liposomes to interact with tissue cells other than macrophages and endothelial cells. The best described example is the liver where the fenestrated endothelium has been thoroughly investigated. The hepatic endothelial fenestrae are arranged in clusters, have a diameter of between 100 and 200 nm, and vary in number and size in the periportal and perivenous areas of the liver sinusoid (WISSE et al. 1983). The fraction of the surface area of the hepatic endothelium covered with fenestrae, i.e. its porosity, amounts to approximately 7% on average. For liposomes it has been clearly shown that, when they are sufficiently small, they can directly interact with the parenchymal tissue, the hepatocytes, underneath the endothelial lining. SUV of various compositions have been demonstrated to be endocytosed by hepatocytes upon intravenous administration (ROERDINK et al. 1984; KUIPERS et al. 1986). Also for the spleen, uptake of liposomes by cells other than macrophages has been reported, in particular lymphocytes (GROSSE et al. 1984). To what extent non-phagocytic cells in the bone marrow may participate in liposome uptake from the blood is not known. It should be emphasized that isolation and identification of cell types of most tissues is far more complicated than for liver, which has a relatively simple makeup with respect to the number of cell types present. In addition to the macrophages or Kupffer cells, the hepatocytes, and the endothelial cells, only two other cell types have been identified in liver tissue: the fat-storing cells and the pit cells or large granular lymphocytes (WISSE et al. 1982). We do not know whether the latter two cell types participate to any extent in liposome uptake. Well established is the lack of participation by endothelial cells, which in our hands consistently failed to show any trace of liposome uptake (ROERDINK et al. 1981; SPANJER et al. 1986). Lack of affinity of a particular cell type for liposomes may be relieved by attaching cell-specific ligands to the liposomal surface (see also Sect. F). The possibility of raising antibodies specific to the surface of vascular endothelial cells in a specific organ (HUGHES et al. 1989) would provide a means to target liposomes carrying such antibodies attached to the surface to these cells. Numerous methods have been reported over the past 10 years for the (covalent) attachment of proteins and other possible cell-specific ligands to the liposomal surface (TORCHILIN et al. 1978, 1984; HEATH et al. 1980; LESERMAN et al. 1980; HUANG et al. 1980; MARTIN et al. 1981; DERKSEN and SCHERPHOF 1985; see TORCHILIN (1987); WRIGHT and HUANG (1989) for recent reviews). Many of the proposed applications, however, suffer from the lack of a concept concerning the limited access liposomes are likely to have to nearly all cells in the normal or diseased body with but a few exceptions.

In addition to the limited number of tissue cell types that may come within reach of intravenously administered particulate matter, such as liposomes, circulating blood cells form another obvious target. Not only have white cells such as monocytes (MEHTA et al. 1982; FOGLER and FIDLER 1986) served as potential targets for liposome-associated drugs, also the numerically overwhelming erythrocyte population has attracted attention in this respect. For example, red cells infected with the malaria parasite could be selectively removed from the circulation upon specific interaction with liposomes carrying an infected erythrocyte-specific antibody (PEETERS et al. 1989).

E. Factors Influencing Liposome Uptake by Cells

Once direct contact between a liposome and a target cell, be it a tissue macrophage, an anatomically accessible extravascular cell, or a circulating blood cell, has been established, the question arises whether the cell will proceed to internalize the liposome or otherwise accommodate it together with its associated drug. It should be kept in mind that it will depend on the particular goal one is aiming for whether uptake is really required. For example, for imaging purposes it would obviously suffice for the liposome to establish a firm, but specific, interaction with the surface of the cells involved, e.g., tumor cells or even only the cells of the tumor vasculature. For therapeutic purposes, on the other hand, it will in most cases be required that the surface-associated liposome is internalized by the cells in order for the associated drug to become available to the intracellular target sites.

The two major mechanisms by which a liposome could conceivably be accommodated by a cell following its interaction with the cell surface are endocytosis and fusion (WEINSTEIN and LESERMAN 1984). There is overwhelming evidence that, generally, fusion of the liposomal membrane with the cell membrane is a rare event and that endocytosis is the major if not only route by which a liposome delivers its contents to the cell interior (STRAUBINGER et al. 1983). In recent years, however, several investigators have made successful attempts to design liposomes containing fusogenic constituents. In nearly all cases the design of the liposome was geared to low pH instability. By incorporation of a lipid with a weakly acidic head group, a moderate drop in pH, e.g., to a value of 5–6, will lead to protonation of the head group. Examples of such lipids that have been reported on are succinylated cholesterol (ELLENS et al. 1985), oleic acid (DUZGUNES 1985), succinylated phosphatidylethanolamine (NAYAR and SCHROIT 1985), and acylated amino acids (YATVIN et al. 1980). Because of the additional presence in the liposomal bilayer of phospholipids such as unsaturated phosphatidylethanolamines, which are unfavorable for stable bilayer formation, the resulting change in configuration of the head group leads to a destabilization of the bilayer structure; this, in turn, is presumed to lead to fusion of the two membranes and subsequent delivery of liposomal contents directly to the cytosol. The required drop in pH could be achieved by temporary acidification of the extracellular medium, but this approach would, obviously, limit the applicability of this method to in vitro conditions. Alternatively, the physiological drop in pH in the endosomal compartment arising during the first steps of the endocytic process (VAN RENSWOUDE et al. 1982) may be exploited for this purpose. The acidic environment of the endosome will allow the acid-sensitive membrane of the liposome to fuse with the endosomal membrane from within the endosome. As long as this occurs before the hydrolytic enzymes of the primary lysosomes access the endosomal compartment, the liposome-encapsulated substance will escape from the lysosomal hydrolases and be delivered into the cytoplasm of the cell, similar to the conditions attained upon extracellular acidification. However, by making use of the endocytic route, in vivo application becomes feasible. Obviously, we will still have to deal with the anatomical restrictions and the competition with the MPS discussed above; in addition, this route of delivery will still be limited to cells with an endocytic capacity. In the past few years a number of investigators have reported significant delivery of liposome-encapsulated substances to the cytoplasm of various cell types in vitro by making use of pH-sensitive liposomes (STRAUBINGER et al. 1985; CONNOR and HUANG 1985, 1986).

A word of caution is appropriate here: Recent observations have shown that cytoplasmic delivery of liposomal contents by means of acid-labile liposomes may be achieved without the involvement of low pH-induced fusion of the liposomal bilayer and the endosomal membrane. Mere acid-induced destabilization of the liposomal bilayer in the endosomal compartment followed by uptake of the released solute through carrier-mediated transport was demonstrated to suffice as an explanation for cytoplasmic delivery of nucleotides by means of pH-sensitive liposomes (BROWN and SILVIUS 1989). Nonetheless, WANG and HUANG (1987) recently reported convincing evidence for the functional delivery of DNA into cells in vivo by means of pH-sensitive liposomes. In addition to the use of fusogenic lipids, attempts have been made to construct fusogenic liposomes by inserting naturally fusogenic components such as the fusion proteins of membrane viruses into the liposomal membrane. Successful delivery of solutes encapsulated in such liposomes to the cytoplasm has thus been claimed. Because of the presence of potentially highly antigenic peptides on the surface of such liposomes, in vivo application would seem rather remote in this case. Nonetheless, such virosomal systems might be very powerful for in vitro use, e.g., for transfection purposes. A lipid system with reportedly very high transfection efficiency involves the use of synthetic cationic amphiphiles, which, when incorporated into liposomes, result in highly increased binding of DNA (FELGNER et al. 1987). Certainly for this system, irrespective of its extremely high efficiency, it remains to be established to what extent fusion plays a role. In any case, the potential advantages of systems capable of delivering biologically active substances directly to the cytoplasm, without involvement of the lysosomal compartment, are straightforward. In this way compounds which are susceptible to enzymatic hydrolysis can circumvent the lysosomal compartment and, in addition, we no longer have to deal with restrictions with respect to molecular size, limiting the diffusion of substances from the lysosomal compartment into the cytosol.

The efficiency of cytoplasmic delivery by means of pH-sensitive liposomes, in addition to being dependent on the fusogenic potential of the liposomes, still remains, of course, a function of the endocytic capacity of the cell. This, in turn, has been shown to vary greatly with the physical and chemical features of the liposomes applied. Numerous reports have demonstrated that the rate of (endocytic) uptake of liposomes by cells is strongly dependent on both size and composition of the liposomes.

I. Liposome Size

Liposomes may vary in size from approximately 20 nm to as large as several μm. As discussed previously, all of these sizes are too large to allow free access to extravascular spaces. Only for small liposomes, i.e., smaller than about 100 nm, has extravascular localization been reported for tissues with a fenestrated vascular endothelial lining, such as the liver (ROERDINK et al. 1981; SCHERPHOF et al. 1983a; RAHMAN et al. 1982). Besides this microanatomical consideration, liposome size will determine whether or not a liposome, once having established contact with a cell surface, will be endocytosed. Nonphagocytic cells will, in general, not be capable of endocytosing particles with a size exceeding that of the diameter of the coated pit, i.e., about 120 nm. STRAUBINGER et al. (1983), for example, demonstrated clearly that endocytic uptake of liposomes by monkey kidney cells proceeds through coated pit-mediated endocytosis. (Endocytic uptake of large (multilamellar) liposomes by non-phagocytic cells, such as hepatocytes (GHOSH et al. 1982), are likely to suffer from contaminating small vesicles in such liposomal preparations. The often provided morphological evidence of internalization of large multilamellar liposomes by non-phagocytic cells, by demonstrating the presence of intracellular myelin-like structures, should be considered of little value. Such structures have been repeatedly observed by us in cells which were never exposed to liposomes (ROERDINK et al. 1977). Professionally phagocytic cells, i.e., macrophages, are capable of endocytosing (phagocytosing) particles up to very large sizes; as far as liposomes are concerned, they appear even to prefer large over small vesicles. This property has been observed under in vitro conditions (ROERDINK et al. 1986), but is even more clearly reflected in the in vivo situation, where the rate of liposome clearance from the blood is found to increase steeply with liposome size (JULIANO and STAMP 1975; ABRA and HUNT 1981; ALLEN and EVEREST 1983; SENIOR et al. 1985). It is generally agreed that the rate of elimination of liposomes from the bloodstream is dictated mainly by the phagocytic activity of the cells of the MPS. Only when these cells have a low affinity for the type of liposome administered and the plasma elimination rate therefore is low, do other cells have a chance to participate in liposome uptake from the blood. This has been shown repeatedly: (a) for SUV, particularly when uncharged (Beaumier and Hwang 1983; Senior et al. 1985; Spanjer et al. 1986); (b) for larger liposomes under conditions of MPS blockade, causing a slowdown of blood elimination (Abra et al. 1980, 1981; Kao and Juliano 1981; Souhami et al. 1981; Ellens et al. 1982); and (c) in the use of "stealth" liposomes which are designed to be largely ignored by the MPS (Allen et al. 1989, 1989; Gabizon and Papahadjopoulos 1988; Gabizon et al. 1989a).

II. Liposome Composition

For liposomes of similar size but of different lipid composition both the rate of elimination from the blood and the organ or, within one organ, the cellular distribution can vary greatly. One of the first factors which were shown to be of importance in this respect is liposomal surface charge. Negative surface charge, which can be conferred by incorporation into the liposomal bilayer of anionic lipids such as phosphatidylserine, phosphatidylglycerol, cardiolipin, phosphatidic acid, or nonphospholipid structures such as dicetylphosphate, appears to have an accelerating effect on blood elimination (see Senior 1987). Also in vitro, such effects of negative surface charge on the uptake of liposomes by cells have been reported repeatedly (Fraley et al. 1980; Allen et al. 1981; Heath et al. 1985b; Spanjer et al. 1986). Work from the group of Fidler has provided evidence that there may be more to this than just surface charge: Phosphatidylserine has been claimed to interact in a specific manner with macrophages and thus to be far superior to other negatively charged lipids in this respect (Schroit and Fidler 1982). As was pointed out by Senior (1987), the incorporation of negatively charged lipids in the liposomal bilayer may cause alterations in the permeability properties of the liposomal membrane; this may, in turn, influence the observations on blood clearance, particularly when labeled encapsulated solutes are being used as a marker of the fate of the liposome. In view of that consideration the use of (nondegradable and non-exchangeable) lipid markers, such as long-chain cholesteryl ethers, for monitoring the intravenous fate of liposomes is preferred (Derksen et al. 1987; New et al. 1990).

Observations on positively charged liposomes are far less abundant. There are several reasons for this. First of all, the choice of positively charged amphiphiles has been limited for many years. Stearylamine has been applied most widely in spite of reports of toxicity. A general disadvantage of the use of single-chain amphiphiles such as stearylamine may be that they may easily exchange with other membranes as was observed in our laboratory by Wilschut (unpublished observations). Another single-chain cationic lipid that has been used for conferring positive charge to the liposomal surface is the more natural compound sphingosine. It may suffer from the same drawback as stearylamine. In vitro, positively charged liposomes tend to stick to the culture dishes and thus may cause erroneous results (Dijkstra et al.

1985b). Positive charge was also introduced by incorporating cholesterol derivatives of aminosugars, particularly 6-aminomannose, as was reported some years ago by Baldeschwieler and his colleagues (MAUK et al. 1980; WU et al. 1981; BALDESCHWIELER 1985). Incorporation of the aminomannosyl cholesterol derivative was found to increase the interaction of liposomes with macrophages in vitro by more than an order of magnitude. It was not clearly established whether this effect could be fully ascribed to the presence of the positive charge or that receptor-mediated interaction was to some extent involved. Others have claimed that there is little difference between stearylamine and 6-aminomannosyl cholesterol in augmenting the uptake of liposomes by peritoneal macrophages, implying that the aminomannose effect is merely a matter of positive charge (SCHWENDENER et al. 1984). In vivo use of these liposomes showed extreme stability following subcutaneous application (MAUK et al. 1980). Upon systemic administration aminomannosyl liposomes were found to be very rapidly eliminated from the circulation, probably due to strong aggregation upon exposure to plasma (ROERDINK et al. unpublished observations).

III. Cholesterol and Opsonization

The presence of cholesterol in the liposomal membrane is another factor of potential influence on the rate of blood elimination. The general observation is that inclusion of cholesterol causes a decrease in the elimination rate. The group of Patel (PATEL et al. 1983a; DAVE and PATEL 1986; MOGHIMI and PATEL 1988, 1989a,b) has investigated the cholesterol effect in more detail. Also, Gregoriadis and his associates addressed this item in their studies on the stability of SUV in plasma (SENIOR and Gregoriadis 1982a,b, 1984). Both groups tend to explain the differences in rates of elimination from plasma in terms of different degrees or mechanisms of opsonization. It has been proposed that cholesterol, because of its rigidifying effect on phospholipid bilayers, would impede the adsorption or penetration of opsonic proteins at the liposomal surface, thus diminishing their affinity for macrophages (SENIOR and GREGORIADIS 1982a). This effect was further enhanced by replacing egg phosphatidylcholine as the major liposomal phospholipid by phospholipids containing saturated long-chain acyl groups such as distearoyl phosphatidylcholine. A general correlation was observed between the ability of liposomes to retain an encapsulated solute in the presence of serum or plasma and the rate at which they were eliminated from blood, both decreasing with increasing "rigidity" of the liposomal bilayer. As discussed extensively by SENIOR (1987), the degree of hydrophobicity of the liposomal surface may be a more meaningful parameter in this respect than rigidity of the bilayer, although the two are likely to be related. For bacteria, hydrophobic surfaces were shown to present conditions unfavorable for phagocytosis and different degree of hydrophobicity may be imposed by adsorption of different opsonic factors, e.g., alpha-1 glycoprotein vs alpha-2 glycoprotein (VAN OSS et al. 1974a,b). By contrast, the adsorption of certain synthetic amphiphilic polymers to the surface of very hydrophobic polystyrene microspheres was reported to cause a dramatic decrease in the rate of elimination of these spheres from the blood (ILLUM and Davis 1984; ILLUM et al. 1986, 1987).

These observations, although apparently conflicting, indicate that hydrophobicity of particle surfaces probably plays a role in the elimination of such particles from the vascular system. This may be achieved either directly or indirectly, by determining the nature and the degree of opsonization by plasma opsonic factors. In spite of the uncertainty concerning the involvement of opsonic factors in the uptake of liposomes from the circulation, it is generally agreed that liposomes do adsorb proteins when incubated with plasma (BLACK and Gregoriadis 1976; JULIANO and LIN 1980; HOEKSTRA et al. 1981; DAMEN et al. 1982). Large variation exists, however, in the proteins reported to adsorb to liposomes this way. Few of those reports have unequivocally identified any of these proteins as being responsible for possible opsonic effects; fibronectin and alpha-2 macroglobulin are among these. Recently, apolipoprotein E was identified as a protein which, after being bound to the liposomal surface, enhanced the uptake of liposomes by liver cells, presumably through specific interaction with the apoE receptor (BISGAIER et al. 1989). Interestingly, this stimulating effect of apoE was counteracted by apolipoproteins A-IV and A-I, which were shown to displace apoE from phosphatidylcholine liposomes. Thus, it was proposed that apoA-I and apoA-IV might have a modulating influence on in vivo uptake of liposomes by cells through the apoE receptor. In this connection, it is interesting to note that, although in rat plasma apoA-IV is normally found as a constituent of the HDL fraction, in fasting human plasma virtually none of the plasma apoA-IV is associated with lipoproteins (GREEN et al. 1980). Experiments by DAMEN (1982) in our laboratory revealed a 45 kDa protein, tentatively identified as apoA-IV, as the main protein associating with phosphatidylcholine/cholesterol liposomes upon incubation with lipoprotein-free human plasma.

The work done in this area by MOGHIMI and PATEL (1988, 1989a) is of particular interest since it also points to not only the involvement of opsonic factors in liposome uptake processes in vivo, but additionally reveals the existence of different opsonic activities, one delivering preferentially to liver macrophages and the other mainly to spleen macrophages. The observed differentiation is brought about by differences in liposome composition. Cholesterol-poor or cholesterol-free liposomes were shown to bind opsonic factors that caused an increase in uptake by liver macrophages in vitro, whereas cholesterol-rich liposomes bound proteins which resulted in a strong increase in uptake by spleen cells. It was shown that cholesterol-poor liposomes, during an incubation with rat serum, adsorbed substantially higher quantities of serum proteins than cholesterol-rich liposomes. No obvious differences in the pattern of adsorbed proteins could be shown, however, when the liposomes were washed after the incubation with serum. The "liver-specific" and "spleen-specific" opsonins were further characterized and found to differ in heat stability and cofactor requirement (MOGHIMI and PATEL 1989a). Furthermore, additional experiments by this group showed that the phospholipid composition of the liposomes also had an extensive influence (MOGHIMI and PATEL 1989b). When the egg yolk phosphatidylcholine used in the earlier studies was replaced by sphingomyelin or disaturated phosphatidylcholines, incubation in the presence of serum led to a decrease in uptake by liver macrophages, irrespective of the amount of cholesterol present in the bilayers. This was put forward as an explanation for the frequently observed long circulation times of liposomes with this lipid composition. Unfortunately, the presence of the negatively charged lipid dicetylphosphate in the liposomes used by MOGHIMI and Patel (1988, 1889a,b) complicates this interpretation, as negative charge by itself has a strong influence on liposome-cell interaction and thus on their in vivo behavior.

The very long half-lives of liposomes in circulation that were observed by many investigators referred to neutral liposomes, in particular those of small size (HWANG et al. 1980; SENIOR et al. 1985; SPANJER et al. 1986). Thus, any effect of anti-opsonization or dysopsonization factors would be expected to show up much more readily with these types of liposomes than with the negatively charged large vesicles used by PATEL et al.. In this connection it is worthwhile mentioning that in absence of any serum proteins, the uptake of sphingomyelin/cholesterol SUV by liver macrophages in vitro is extremely low (SPANJER et al. 1986), making it unlikely that under in vivo conditions dysopsonization of such vesicles plays a major role in their slow elimination from the circulation. This consideration presents a general problem in these studies; also, the incorporation of cholesterol in the liposomal bilayer by itself causes a reduction in the affinity of such liposomes for the macrophage; any additional effect of (dys)opsonic proteins can easily be obscured by this phenomenon. With respect to the identity of these proteins no data are available to date. It is tempting, however, to refer in this connection to the work of BISGAIER et al. (1989) on the apolipoproteins A-I, A-IV, and E, discussed above.

Irrespective of any role of opsonic factors in the in vivo behavior of liposomes, we have stressed the point that in the absence of any (plasma) proteins there are very substantial differences in the affinity for (phagocytic) cells between liposomes of different lipid composition. We have tentatively explained this phenomenon at the level of the interaction of the liposomal surface with cell-surface proteins, since protease treatment of liver macrophages was shown to abolish liposome-cell interaction completely (DIJKSTRA et al. 1985b). Plasma proteins were described as having more or less easy access to the lipid-water interface of liposomes, depending on the liposomal lipid composition. This leads to decreased stability and increased rates of elimination from the circulation (SENIOR et al. 1985). Similarly, cell-surface proteins may penetrate liposomal bilayers of different composition more or less readily and in this way give rise to different affinities towards cells.

An interesting observation relating to liposome/plasma protein interactions, if not to opsonization, was described recently by LIU et al. (1989) and
LIU and HUANG (1989b). They reported the stabilization of cholesterol-free
(!) dioleoyl phosphatidylethalonamine (DOPE)/oleic acid liposomes as a
result of incubation with human plasma. This type of vesicle was designed as a
pH-sensitive liposome but was expected to be destabilized upon contact with
plasma as the oleic acid moiety would be readily extracted from the bilayer.
This would leave the non-bilayer-forming DOPE as the only constituent of
the remaining liposomes which would consequently collapse. Surprisingly,
however, these vesicles displayed a dramatically increased stability after
incubation with plasma, which was ascribed to the insertion into the vesicle
bilayer of amphipathic plasma peptides. Although it was claimed that such
stabilized vesicles revealed a relatively low affinity for both liver and spleen
upon intravenous administration to mice, the results as presented (LIU et al.
1989) leave room for some doubts concerning the validity of that conclusion.

IV. Prolonged Circulation Time

The desire for prolonged circulation times of liposomes so as to increase
chances of interaction with cells other than macrophages has led a number of
investigators to try and mimic the cell surface of blood cells such as erythrocytes, which normally have very long circulation times before being removed
from the vascular compartment. Out of a large number of glycosphingolipids
and gangliosides, Allen and co-workers found ganglioside GM1 to be superior in delaying the elimination of large liposomes, both large unilamellar
vesicles (LUV) and multilamellar vesicles (MLV), from the circulation, with
a concomitant decrease in the extent of accumulation in liver and spleen
(ALLEN and CHONN 1987; ALLEN et al. 1989; ALLEN and MEHRA 1989; ALLEN
1989). A molar fraction of 10%–15% in a variety of differently composed
liposomes was shown to be optimal to obtain several-fold increases in circulation time. A mixture of sphingomyelin, egg phosphatidylcholine (PC) and
cholesterol served best as a carrier of the ganglioside (ALLEN et al. 1989).
Other relatively rigid carrier lipids, such as distearoyl PC, in combination
with cholesterol produced substantial avoidance of the MPS when incorporating 10%–15% GM1. Similar observations were made by GABIZON
et al. (1989a) and GABIZON and PAPAHADJOPOULOS (1988). These authors
also obtained remarkable prolongation of liposome circulation times with a
combination of cholesterol and fully hydrogenated phospholipids, including phosphatidylinositol, without the incorporation of any glycolipid. The
ganglioside effect observed by ALLEN et al. (1985, 1989) parallels the inhibiting effect this lipid was shown to have on both solute release from liposomes
and the release or exchange of liposomal lipids under the influence of plasma
proteins. Therefore, the retarding effect of GM1 on blood elimination could,
by analogy (see above), be attributed to the involvement of opsonization, the
ganglioside either inhibiting adsorption of opsonins or stimulating the binding
of dysopsonins. Alternatively, a direct inhibitory effect of the ganglioside on

liposome-cell interaction might be involved. No in vitro data proving or disproving this possibility appear to be available as yet.

Another approach that has been taken to achieve prolonged circulation times of liposomes involves blockade of the phagocytic capacity of the cells of the MPS. Two basically different approaches seem to be at hand for that purpose: (1) saturation of the MPS with one or more predoses of ("empty") liposomes or another substance that can be phagocytosed by these cells, such as carbon particles, dextran sulfate, latex particles, red cells, etc. and (2) inhibition of the phagocytic potency of the cells of the MPS. Reversible depression of the phagocytic capacity of liver and spleen by predosing with liposomes has been observed by numerous investigators (e.g., ABRA et al. 1980; KAO and JULIANO 1981; ELLENS et al. 1982). The effectiveness of the depression seems to depend on liposome dose and number of consecutive doses as well as on liposomal parameters such as composition and size. A generally observed phenomenon is that initially (low dose, single dose) the phagocytic capacity of the liver is blocked, the spleen showing increased uptake of the test dose under these conditions, whereas at higher or multiple doses the phagocytic capacity of the spleen also is impaired. The effects of chronic administration of liposomes have been described by ALLEN (1984) and RICHARDSON et al. (1988/1989). The severity of the impairment depends on the liposomal composition; mice receiving repeated daily injections of relatively rigid liposomes showed more rapid hepatic granuloma formation than animals injected with fluid-type liposomes (ALLEN 1984). RICHARDSON et al. (1988/1989) claim only moderate histological alterations in liver, spleen, and bone marrow after up to 17 injections of dipalmitoyl phosphatidyl choline (DPPC)/cholesterol liposomes into mice over a period of more than 2 years. Effects on liposome elimination by particulate substances other than liposomes have also been observed repeatedly (SOUHAMI et al. 1980; FREISE et al. 1981; PATEL et al. 1983b). The effects of different blockading agents on the MPS has been reviewed recently by ALLEN (1988).

Temporary inhibition of spleen and/or liver phagocytic activity was also observed following i.v. injection of gadolinium chloride (ROERDINK et al. 1981; LAZAR et al. 1989) or dichloromethylene diphosphonate (DMPD) (VAN ROOIJEN and VAN NIEUWMEGEN 1984; VAN ROOIJEN et al. 1985). Gadolinium chloride administration caused a shift in intrahepatic distribution of egg PC/ cholesterol/phosphatidylserine SUV from the Kupffer cells to the hepatocytes, whereas identically composed MLV, which because of their large size cannot reach the hepatocytes, showed a shift in uptake from the large Kupffer cells to the smaller ones (LAZAR et al. 1989). It appears as though the larger cells are irreversibly poisoned by the Gd salt and are forced out of the liver (HARDONK and KOUDSTAAL, unpublished observations). This would explain why it takes almost a day for the inhibitory effect on phagocytic activity to develop following Gd administration. Recovery of hepatic phagocytic activity takes approximately 1 week and is apparently achieved by repopulation of the liver with new (large) macrophages. Also the effect of liposome-encapsulated DMPD on liver and spleen macrophages appears to involve elimination of

macrophages from these organs (VAN ROOIJEN et al. 1985). Restoration of
phagocytic potency of these organs will also require a repopulation process.

F. Surface Modification

Several approaches have been proposed over the past few years to achieve
specific interaction of liposomes with selected target cells following in vivo
administration. Obviously, such attempts are often frustrated by unfavorable
conditions created by anatomical constraints preventing the liposomes from
escaping from the vascular bed, as pointed out above. In addition, as far as
the target cells are not macrophages, the strong competition on the part of the
latter cells in liver and spleen will also contribute to limited success. The two
major targeting strategies applied involve the addressing of carbohydrate-
specific receptors by means of carbo-hydrate-bearing liposomes and of cell-
specific antigenic sites by means of antibody-linked liposomes. Numerous
methods have been published in recent years to achieve covalent or non-
covalent coupling of proteins (see WRIGHT and HUANG 1989 for a recent
review) or carbohydrates (GREGORIADIS and NEERUNJUN 1975; MAUK et al.
1980; HOEKSTRA et al. 1980; GHOSH et al. 1982; SPANJER and SCHERPHOF 1983;
SZOKA and MAYHEW 1983; GREGORIADIS and SENIOR 1984; SPANJER et al. 1984,
1985; TAKADA et al. 1984; DAS et al. 1985; DRAGSTEN et al. 1987; HAENSLER
and SCHUBER 1988; MULLER and SCHUBER 1989) to the liposome surface.
Most of these studies involved the insertion of glycolipids in the liposomal
membrane. Exceptions are the use of asialoglycoproteins (e.g., GREGORIADIS
and NEERUNJUN 1975) and coating of the liposomes with polysaccharides
(e.g., TAKADA et al. 1984). Also, ligands for other cell-surface specific
structures, such as specific ecto-enzymes, have been explored as homing
devices for liposomes (SALORD et al. 1986; SALORD and SCHUBER 1988).
Increased interaction of specific antibody-bearing liposomes with antigen-
specific target cells in vivo has been reported by a number of investigators.

Of the more recent findings, mention is made of the work by
PAPAHADJOPOULOS and GABIZON (1987) on the combination of antibody-
specific targeting with long-circulating liposomes. The incorporation of GM1
ganglioside in the liposomal lipid formulation conferred a long circulation
half-life on the liposomes as discussed above. This allowed more time for
the surface-coupled anti-Thy 1.1 antibody to find its antigen on the target,
AKR/J lymphoma cells, in the mouse. As was pointed out by the authors,
the use of whole antibody, including the Fc portion, probably influenced the
results unfavorably; nonetheless a small but significant concentration of
immunoliposomes in the tumor areas was observed. Accessibility is one of the
obvious prerequisites that have to be fulfilled in order to allow a liposome to
interact with its target cell. Thus, target cells preferably should be either
circulating white or red blood cells or cells of the endothelial lining of the
vascular system. An example of successful targeting of immunoliposomes to
red blood cells was recently reported by PEETERS et al. (1989). Liposomes

bearing covalently coupled anti-mouse red blood cell Fab' fragments on their surface were far more effective than free chloroquine or chloroquine in control liposomes in preventing malaria infection in rats that were infected with malaria parasite-containing mouse red blood cells. Remarkably high liposome accumulation in the lung was recently reported by HUGHES et al. (1989) using liposomes bearing a monoclonal antibody against lung capillary endothelial cells. Up to 5 h after liposome administration, the absolute amounts of liposome label associated with lung exceeded that of liver several-fold; per gram of organ, lung showed a more than 20-fold excess of liposome uptake over liver and spleen. In this way the liposome may serve as a local organ-specific depot for antineoplastic drugs, accumulating in the vicinity of the tumor cells to be attacked without the need for the drug carrier to interact with or to be taken up by these cells. Obviously, application of this approach is restricted to "liposome-independent" drugs, i.e., drugs that by themselves are able to enter the target cells after having been released from the cell surface-attached liposomes (HEATH et al. 1985a). In this connection it is interesting to note that Huang and co-workers designed what they called "target-sensitive immunoliposomes," i.e., antibody-targeted liposomes that are destabilized upon interaction with their target cell surface antigen (Ho et al. 1987) leading to rapid release of their contents. The authors pointed out that this approach to organ-specific targeting, in addition to circumventing problems relating to inadequate anatomical accessibility of target tumor cells, also avoids the problem of antigenic heterogeneity among tumor cells (HUGHES et al. 1989). For effective immunotargeting of drugs directly to tumor cells, the construction of a range of different monoclonal antibodies may be required.

Another important factor to be considered is that the use of liposome-dependent drugs requires not only direct interaction between target cell and liposome but also internalization of the liposome by the cell. Recent work by MATTHAY et al. (1989) emphasized the important role of the liposome-associated ligand in determining the rate and/or extent of endocytic liposome uptake by cells. Thus, liposomes liganded with an antibody against the transferrin receptor were more efficiently internalized by a number of human T cell leukemic cell lines than liposomes carrying antibodies against the surface antigens CD2, CD3, or CD5 of these cells.

Another interesting in vivo application of antibody-targeted liposomes was described recently by PATEL and WILD (1988), who observed Fc receptor-mediated transport of high molecular weight solutes encapsulated in immunoglobulin-coated liposomes across epithelial barriers in vivo. Liposome-encapsulated polyvinylpyrrolidone (PVP) was shown to be transported across yolk sac endoderm of pregnant rabbits; encapsulated inulin was demonstrated to pass across the small intestine of newborn rats after intragastric administration. The data concerning the yolk sac experiments are particularly impressive, as the concentration of PVP in fetal blood was shown to increase several hundred-fold by encapsulation of the solute in (human)

IgG-coated liposomes. By using a liposomal lipid marker, cholesteryl-[^{14}C]oleate, the authors provided evidence that not only the transport of liposomal contents but also that of the lipid across the epithelial barrier was enhanced by coating the liposomes with IgG. Based upon this observation, the authors suggested that intact liposomes were crossing the barrier; this conclusion should be considered premature, however, since the lipid label they used is readily metabolizable. The resulting labeled oleate will, at least in part, be released by the cells either in free form or as the triglyceride constituent of lipoproteins (DERKSEN et al. 1987). The results presented on the appearance of lipid label in the fetal blood serve to indicate that the IgG coating caused enhanced liposome internalization and intracellular processing.

In suckling rats it was shown that the intragastric administration of [^{3}H]inulin encapsulated in IgG-coated liposomes gave rise to several-fold higher blood inulin levels as compared to the administration of free inulin. Of particular relevance in this connection is the observation that administration of insulin encapsulated in IgG-coated liposomes caused a more than 30% lowering of blood glucose in 12-day-old sucklings, whereas in 22-day-old rats a significant reduction in glucose concentration could not be detected. These results indicate that under favorable conditions systemic delivery of liposome-associated substances by means of oral administration may be achieved or even enhanced. Earlier conflicting reports on sytemic delivery of liposome-encapsulated insulin after oral admiistration eventually led to serious doubts about the feasibility of this approach, while a single report on the delivery of clotting factor VIII to the blood compartment via the oral route (HEMKER et al. 1980) was never followed up.

In vivo targeting of liposomes to cells in the liver has been reported by a number of research groups. Most of this work was initiated to achieve enhanced uptake by the hepatocytes by addressing the hepatocytic galactose receptor first described by ASHWELL and MORELL (1974). Although the incorporation of exposed galactose residues on the liposomal surface invariably led to increased rates of elimination of the liposomes from the circulation with a concomitant increase in hepatic uptake (e.g., SZOKA and MAYHEW 1983; GHOSH et al. 1982; SPANJER and SCHERPHOF 1983), variable results were obtained with respect to the identification of the hepatic cell types involved. From our own work it appeared that SUV containing dimyristoyl PC as their main phospholipid constituent could be directed preferentially to the hepatocytes upon incorporation of a small fraction of lactosylceramide in the liposomal bilayer (SPANJER and SCHERPHOF 1983). However, vesicles based on egg PC were predominantly diverted to the Kupffer cells when they contained lactosylceramide (SPANJER et al. 1984). Also, the incorporation of another galactose-bearing lipid, trisgalactosyl cholesterol (TGC), was shown to direct small liposomes predominantly to the Kupffer cells (SPANJER et al. 1985). These observations were explained by presuming the involvement of the galactose-recognizing binding site on the Kupffer cell surface first described by KOLB-BACHOFEN et al. (1982). This protein factor, which was recently identified as C-reactive protein (KEMPKA et al. 1990), was shown to bind preferentially galactose-bearing particulate material. Increased hepatic uptake of small liposomes carrying digalactosyl diglyceride was reported by DRAGSTEN et al. (1987). From cell separation studies it was concluded that, for positively charged as well as for negatively charged vesicles, the digalactosyl diglyceride led the liposomes to be taken up mainly by the hepatocytes, while inhibition studies suggested that the asialoglycoprotein receptor was involved in this uptake process.

The experiments published by GOSH et al. (1982), who used lactosylceramide as a ligand for galactose receptors, also indicate that uptake by hepatocytes is favored when this galactolipid is incorporated into the liposomal bilayer. It remains difficult to explain, however, how in these experiments the large multilamellar liposomes that were used could have gained access to the parenchymal cells of the liver. The endothelial fenestrations are supposed to be of insufficient diameter to allow passage of such large liposomes across the endothelial lining of the sinusoidal space. Contamination with small vesicles might at least partly account for this observation.

It is interesting to note that strongly preferential uptake of small liposomes by hepatocytes, following intravenous administration, could be achieved readily without the use of any specific ligands. SPANJER et al. (1986) showed that SUV composed of egg PC/cholesterol, although accumulating in the liver rather slowly and only to a relatively small extent, were almost exclusively taken up by the hepatocytes. Incorporation of a negatively charge lipid, phosphatidylserine (PS), caused a several-fold increase in hepatic uptake, without interfering substantially with the intrahepatic distribution favoring the hepatocytes.

Coating of liposomes with polysaccharides has been another approach to achieve organ-specific localization of liposomes after systemic administration. Sunamoto and his colleagues developed, for example, polysaccharides with covalently coupled hydrophobic acyl anchors which could be firmly attached by hydrophobic interaction with liposomal bilayers (SUNAMOTO and IWAMOTO 1986). Such polysaccharide-coated liposomes were shown to localize in the lungs to much higher extents than uncoated liposomes of the same lipid composition (SUNAMOTO et al. 1984). Although not firmly established, it seems likely that these liposomes interacted with the resident intravascular macrophage population in this organ, as suggested by in vitro uptake studies of such liposomes by (alveolar) lung macrophages (TOMONAGA et al. 1985).

G. Intracellular Processing of Liposomes

Once internalized by macrophages or other cells possessing endocytic properties, liposomes are subject to the action of intralysosomal lipolytic enzymes which will degrade the lipid constituents and set free the encapsulated contents. As was pointed out above, the fate of the encapsulated substance will largely depend on its chemical nature. If it is a sufficiently small molecule ($Mr < 400$) it may diffuse out of the lysosomal compartment into the cytosol, unless it is susceptible to any of the lysosomal hydrolases. The use of larger encapsulated molecules will only make sense if they possess hydrolyzable bonds through which the substance can be cleaved to appropriate size. Obviously, such hydrolytic splitting should not interfere with any biological activity which the substance is required to display. As a matter of fact, one might even exploit the hydrolytic potency of the lysosomal compartment by encapsulating an inactive covalent conjugate of the active substance to be delivered, i.e., a prodrug. The larger molecular size has the advantage of diminishing untimely release of the encapsulated material, for example, in the blood-stream. In addition, any material that might still escape from the liposome before it has been internalized by the target cell will not be biologically active.

The rate of release of the biologically active substance obviously depends on the rate of degradation of the liposome. This, in turn, depends on its physical and chemical characteristics. MLV will be degraded more slowly than SUV, as was clearly demonstrated by DERKSEN et al. (1988a) under in vivo conditions in liver and spleen. The parameter in this study was the time-integrated angular perturbation factor calculated from perturbed angular correlation spectroscopy measurements on liposome-encapsulated ^{111}In. This factor provides information on the tumbling rate of the In ion, which in turn is influenced by its direct environment: As long as the In is inside the liposome and bound to a chelator, the factor has a high value; as soon as the ion is released it binds to proteins with a concomitant sharp drop in the perturbation factor (BALDESCHWIELER 1985). By manipulating the liposomal lipid composition the rate of liposome degradation can be further modulated, particularly in the case of MLV. For example, by employing the diether PC analogue dihexadecyl PC as the major phospholipid constituent, in addition to 10% PC and 50% cholesterol, as long as 48 h after intravenous administration nearly half of the In in the liver and spleen is still encapsulated, vs less than 10% with egg PC as the bulk phospholipid. Also the use of disaturated long-chain phospholipid such as dipalmitoyl PC caused the liposomes to display relatively long In retention times in liver and spleen. For SUV little difference in the rate of In release was observed between liposomes of different composition.

By means of an entirely different experimental approach ROERDINK et al. (1989) studied the effect of cholesterol on intracellular processing of liposomes. A combination of ^{3}H-labeled cholesteryl hexadecylether, a non-degradable analogue of cholesterol ester, and cholesteryl-[^{14}C]oleate, the ^{3}H/^{14}C ratio in cells or tissue provides information on the extent of both liposome uptake and degradation; the ^{14}C-labeled oleic acid, set free upon intralysosomal hydrolysis of the cholesterol ester, is in part released from the cells, thus causing an increase in the isotopic ratio. As was predicted, the incorporation of cholesterol resulted in a substantial decrease in the rate at which the isotopic ratio increased. This was found in three different systems:

in the macrophages of the liver following intravenous administration of the liposomes, in these same macrophages (Kupffer cells) following in vitro incubation with liposomes, and in cell-free conditions during incubation of liposomes with lysosomal fractions isolated from liver. In the same study, in vivo data were also collected by means of the perturbed angular correlation spectroscopy method. Both in liver and spleen, a significantly lower rate of liposomal degradation was observed when cholesterol was incorporated in the liposomal bilayer. With the same method DERKSEN et al. (1987, 1988b) observed that the covalent coupling of proteins on the liposomal surface also decreased the susceptibility of liposomes to intracellular degradation. It should be noted that results obtained with the cholesterol ether/ester method tend to present an overestimation of liposome degradation. On the one hand this is due to the fact that not all of the liberated acyl moiety is released from the cell or the tissue, part of it being incorporated into cellular lipids and on the other hand to the ability of the cholesteryl ester to migrate from the inner bilayers of a multilamellar liposome to the surface faster than the liposome is degraded (DERKSEN et al., unpublished). Recently published experiments from our laboratory, in which we compared the rate of release from Kupffer cells in vitro of two radioactive lipid markers of liposomes following their uptake by the cells, confirmed this observation (VAN BORSSUM WAALKES and SCHERPHOF 1990). As a ^{3}H label the lipophilic prodrug 3',5'-dipalmitoyl-5-fluoro-2'-deoxy-[^{3}H]uridine was used and as a ^{14}C label, cholesteryl-[^{14}C]oleate; it was found that the cholesterol ester was degraded substantially more rapidly than the prodrug.

Among the factors responsible for intracellular liposomal disintegration lysosomal phospholipase(s) take a prominent position. Nonetheless other (protein) factors may be of influence as well, as was suggested by DERKSEN et al. (1988a) in an attempt to explain the very rapid and almost composition-independent initial rate of intracellular destabilization of SUV. Nonenzymatic protein factors certainly play a role in extracellular (intravascular) disintegration or destabilization of liposomes. Plasma lipoproteins are the most thoroughly investigated example of this, but complement factors may also be involved.

The variable rates of liposomal degradation, both intra- and extracellularly, and the concomitant variability in solute release from the liposomes, either in the cell or intravascularly, have obvious implications for drug delivery. When the liposome is exploited as an intra- or extracellular drug depot, the rate at which the drug is made available may be of great importance in determining its therapeutic efficacy or its toxicity.

H. Implications for Drug Targeting

In the preceding sections various aspects of the in vivo behavior of liposomes were occasionally considered in view of the drug-targeting concept. In this section I will summarize and extend these considerations.

Stability of liposomes upon exposure to the biological milieu, i.e., body fluids such as lymph, blood, and excreted or interstitial fluids, will determine the rate at which a liposome-associated substance will be released from its carrier and become available to exert its intended biological or pharmacological effect. This stability, measured as the ability to retain an encapsulated or a bilayer-inserted solute, is greatly influenced by the liposomal lipid composition. In addition, the nature of the biological fluid, which is first of all a function of the site of administration, is of great importance in this respect. There are some general rules of thumb for maximization of in vivo liposome stability, such as incorporation of cholesterol and the use of saturated long-chain phospholipids. Nonetheless, for each particular combination of liposome, drug, and route of administration, maximal or rather optimal stability will have to be established experimentally. For some drugs it may be mandatory that drug retention is virtually complete until the (intracellular) target site is reached. In that case maximal stability will be required.

Proper drug action may, however, also require the release of drug, preferably at a premeditated optimal rate, at the site of administration or, in case of intravenous administration, in the circulation. For example, the beneficial effect of encapsulation within liposomes of the cytostatic drug adriamycin on its therapeutic efficacy towards a solid immunocytoma in rats was shown to be based, at least in part, upon its gradual release from the liposomes while still in circulation (STORM et al. 1989). Adriamycin happens to be the most thoroughly investigated cytostatic drug in liposome formulations, including a number of clinical studies (RAHMAN et al. 1980, 1986, 1989b; FICHTNER et al. 1981; FORSSEN and TOKES 1981; GABIZON et al. 1982, 1986, 1989, 1990; OLSON et al. 1982; MAYHEW et al. 1983, 1987; VAN HOESEL et al. 1984; STORM et al. 1987; TREAT et al. 1989; MAYER et al. 1989). It is generally agreed upon that the beneficial effect of liposome encapsulation of this drug can be attributed predominantly to the principle of "site avoidance." The limitations for clinical use of adriamycin reside in its (cumulative) cardio- and nephrotoxicity; encapsulation in liposomes keeps the drug away from these organs and thus diminishes its toxicity. The various investigators do not seem to agree upon the possibility that increased delivery of adriamycin to the tumor tissue may play a role as well (compare for example STORM et al. 1987 and GABIZON et al. 1986). Also, the importance of the liposomal lipid composition is a matter of debate. STORM et al. (1987) observed a less potent antitumor effect with "solid" than with "fluid" liposomes. MAYER et al. (1989) report little influence of the fluidity of the liposomal bilayer on the therapeutic efficacy of liposome-encapsulated adriamycin. In addition to sustained release from circulating liposomes, STORM et al. (1987) point to the role that macrophages, such as the Kupffer cells in the liver, may play in the formation of an intracellular slow-release depot, from which the drug can be released into the circulation upon intralysosomal degradation of the liposome. In this case the liposomal lipid composition is of importance as it will determine the rate of degradation and thus the rate of drug release.

Differences in results between different groups of investigators may be due to the use of differently composed liposomes but also to differences in tumor models. Liposomal adriamycin formulations have been applied in a large number of different tumor models (see references cited above). Furthermore, MAYER et al. (1989) emphasized that the drug-to-lipid ratio can also be an important factor in determining the efficacy of the drug. In addition, they found the size of the vesicles to be of great influence, small size preparations being more effective. This might be a reflection of direct interaction with and uptake of liposomes by tumor cells by means of coated pit endocytosis, which is limited to small liposomes (STRAUBINGER et al. 1983).

    Another area of intensive research on the application of liposomes in antitumor therapy involves the activation of tissue macrophages by liposome-encapsulated biological response modifiers. This approach, which exploits the natural affinity of tissue macrophages for particles such as liposomes, was first employed by POSTE et al. (1979). They showed that encapsulation of lymphokines in liposomes resulted in a large increase in the potency of these substances to activate macrophages to a tumor cytotoxic state and that intravenous injection of liposome-encapsulated lymphokines (FIDLER 1980) and later also muramyl dipeptide (N-acetylmuramyl-L-alanyl-D-isoglutamine, MDP) (FIDLER et al. 1981), caused the efficient eradication of established lung metastases in mice. Others confirmed the validity of this approach, both in different metastatic models, for example liver metastasis (THOMBRE and DEODHAR 1984; DAEMEN et al. 1986a,b; 1990; PHILLIPS et al. 1988; PHILLIPS and TSAO 1989), and with different immunomodulators, such as C-reactive protein (THOMBRE and DEODHAR 1984), synthetic peptides (INAMURA et al. 1985), and interferons (EPPSTEIN et al. 1986; STUKART et al. 1987). The use of lipophilic derivatives of low molecular weight immunomodulators such as MDP should be mentioned here (see also below). It was again FIDLER et al. (1982) who showed for the first time the antitumor activity of liposomal formulations of the lipophilic MDP derivative muramyl tripeptidyl phosphatidylethanolamine (MTP-PE). This was after PABST et al. (1980) had shown that lipophilic MDP derivatives were superior to free MDP in activating macrophages, and GISLER et al. (1982) had reported the synthesis of MTP-PE. PHILLIPS et al. (1985) demonstrated the effectiveness of a diglyceride derivative of MDP in the eradication of experimental metastases, and INAMURA et al. (1985) showed the effectiveness of a synthetic acyltripeptide as a macrophage-mediated antitumor agent. Lipophilic derivatization of an agent such as MDP has two obvious advantages: (1) more efficient incorporation of the drug during liposome preparation and (2) minimal loss of drug from the liposomes while in circulation. MDP released within the vascular compartment is rapidly cleared by the kidneys because of its small size and will never reach concentrations high enough to cause any activation of macrophages.

    With respect to liposome composition, it has been reported by SCHROIT and FIDLER (1982) that incorporation of a negatively charged lipid in the liposomal bilayer, particularly PS, was required for optimal liposome uptake and macrophage activation. In addition, maximal retention in the lung, important for eradication of pulmonary metastases, was also achieved by incorporation of 30 mol-% of PS. These authors also reported a significant influence of the fatty acid composition of the liposomal phospholipid, distearoyl PC being superior to egg PC both with respect to the extent and the duration of the cytotoxic activity of lung alveolar macrophages by liposome-encapsulated MDP. On the other hand, DAEMEN et al. (1989) did not observe any significant influence of the degree of saturation of the liposomal phospholipid on the tumor cytotoxic activity elicited in liver macrophages in monolayer culture. These authors even found liposomes containing a dialkyl PC as the major phospholipid constituent to be not significantly less effective than liposomes containing egg PC, DPPC, or distearoyl phosphatidylcholine (DSPC). Because of the lack of carboxylester bonds the dialkyl PC is not susceptible to phospholipase A activity; these liposomes are degraded relatively slowly (DERKSEN et al. 1988a), presumably by phospholipase C activities. Apparently, the rate at which the MDP is released within the liver macrophages is not a limiting factor in achieving maximal tumor cytotoxicity, as long as substantial liposome degradation is achieved within a period of approximately 48 h, i.e., the time allowed for the macrophages to lyse the tumor cells. It is conceivable that this discrepancy between the results of SCHROIT and FIDLER (1982) and DAEMEN et al. (1989) is caused by the absence of cholesterol from the liposomes used by SCHROIT and FIDLER (1982), while in the liposomes employed by DAEMEN et al. (1989) 50 mol-% cholesterol was always included. As was emphasized by SCHROIT and FIDLER (1982), the incorporation of PS in their liposomes caused considerable leakage of encapsulated solute in serum; it is likely that such leakage is more extensive from egg PC liposomes than from DSPC liposomes and that the latter therefore are more effective as a vehicle to carry the MDP into the macrophages.

Another example of the dramatic influence that incorporation in liposomes may have on the effectiveness of an anticancer drug in vivo is the cytostatic drug 5-fluorodeoxyuridine (FUdR), a derivative, originally designed as a prodrug, of 5-fluorouracil (5FU) (RUSTUM 1983). Following up on the work of SCHWENDENER et al. (1985), we synthesized the dipalmitoyl derivative of FUdR, as the drug itself, once encapsulated, is not retained very tightly in liposomes. The dipalmitoylated derivative can be incorporated up to 15 mol-% in liposomal bilayers, depending on the fluidity of the bilayer-forming lipids (VAN BORSSUM WAALKES and SCHERPHOF 1990). Once taken up by liver macrophages, the cells degrade the liposomes at composition-dependent rates and the lipophilic prodrug is concomitantly released as FUdR (VAN BORSSUM WAALKES and SCHERPHOF, unpublished). Although the rates at which fluid-type and solid-type liposomes are degraded up to five fold, there is hardly any difference in antitumor effect in five widely different tumor models nor in toxicity. Yet, there is a several hundred-fold

(!) increase in antitumor activity as well as in systemic toxicity of the liposomal formulation of the (lipophilized) drug as compared to the free drug, FUdR. Apparently, even the most labile liposome formulation causes a very dramatic extension of the period during which the active (and toxic!) drug becomes available from its intracellular (macrophage) depot, thus causing a sharp increase in its biological effect. Enhanced stabilization of the liposomal membrane, although substantially slowing down the release of active drug, only marginally adds to the antitumor effect and the toxicity. These results, which basically confirm earlier reports by SCHWENDENER et al. (1985), are of interest from the point of view of liposome biology, because they show how dramatic the effects of liposome incorporation of a drug can be. From a therapeutic point of view, however, they are of limited value as therapeutic and toxic dose decrease roughly proportionally upon liposome incorporation.

Cells of MPS have also served as target cells for liposomes carrying antimicrobial agents for the purpose of combatting intracellular parasitic, bacterial, or viral infections in these cells. This topic has been elaborately reviewed recently by ALVING (1988). Well known are the early studies of three groups on the successful use of liposome-encapsulated drugs against the intracellular *Leishmania* parasite (BLACK et al. 1977; ALVING et al. 1978; NEW et al. 1978). Also, the first use of liposome-encapsulated antibiotics dates back to the late 1970s when BONVENTRE and GREGORIADIS (1978) reported on the killing of intracellular *S. aureus* with streptomycin in liposomes. Numerous reports have since then appeared on this subject (see ALVING 1988 for a recent review). Among the most promising results are those on the application of liposomal formulations of the fungicidal drug amphotericin B. Encapsulation of this highly toxic fungicide in liposomes leads to a dramatic reduction in toxicity without substantially influencing the antifungal activity in animal models (GRAYBILL et al. 1982; LOPEZ-BERESTEIN et al. 1983, 1985; MEHTA et al. 1984; TREMBLAY et al. 1984; JULIANO et al. 1987). Successful clinical trials have been carried out with this formulation. LOPEZ-BERESTEIN et al. (1985) treated immune-compromised cancer patients suffering from severe systemic fungal infections and obtained impressive therapeutic effects (LOPEZ-BERESTEIN 1989).

Finally, antimicrobial therapy with liposomes, exploiting the macrophage as a natural target cell for liposome-associated biological response modifiers, has also been reported by a number of investigators. KOFF et al. (1985) showed that liposome-encapsulated MDP protected mice against fatal herpes simplex infection and FRASER-SMITH et al. (1983) demonstrated similarly the protective effect of MDP in liposomes against *Candida* infections in mice. EPPSTEIN et al. (1985) demonstrated that liposome-encapsulated interferon-γ is able to activate macrophages to cytotoxicity against melanoma cells but that this could be attributed entirely to interferon that had leaked from the liposomes. GILBREATH et al. (1985, 1986) provided evidence that liposomal lipids actually inhibit lymphokine-induced macrophage microbicidal activity.

It was suggested that it is the PS constituent, and in particular its metabolite, lyso-PS, that is responsible for this effect (GILBREATH et al. 1986). For interferon-induced microbicidal activity similar phenomena were observed; in addition to the nature of the polar headgroup of the liposomal phospholipids, the fatty acid composition was shown to play an important role in the inhibitory activity of the liposomes as well (GILBREATH et al. 1989).

I. Concluding Remarks

The field of liposome research has experienced a tremendous thrust over the past two decades, culminating in a large number of clinical trials for therapeutic and diagnostic applications currently being carried out (see for example LOPEZ-BERESTEIN and FIDLER 1989). With respect to intravenous application, interactions of liposomes with plasma proteins were shown to affect the solute-retention capacity as well as their fate and destiny in the body. Both were shown to be substantially influenced by the liposomal lipid composition. Also the intracellular degradation of liposomes, which has to precede the release of any liposome-associated drug, was found to be a function of the liposomal composition. In addition to size, composition is therefore a suitable parameter by which important pharmacological parameters can be manipulated. Under in vivo conditions adsorptive or receptor-mediated endocytosis appears to be by far the most common mechanism by which liposome-mediated drug delivery to cells proceeds. This brings along the serious drawback of exposure of the drug to lysosomal conditions. Although, in vitro, convincing evidence of intracellular delivery by means of fusion has been produced, direct fusion with the plasma membrane under in vivo conditions would seem to be a rather remote possibility. However, uptake by endocytosis, immediately followed by acid-induced fusion of the (pH-sensitive) liposomal membrane with the endosomal membrane, may be a feasible approach to deliver a drug to the cytoplasm in the in vivo situation.

A major limitation of the use of liposomes, or any other particulate drug carrier for that matter, is the general tightness of the vascular system which, as a rule, does not allow particles over 10 or 20 nm to escape readily from the circulation. Only in organs lacking a basement membrane and equipped with a fenestrated endothelium, such as liver, spleen, and bone marrow, may small liposomes get easy access to cells outside the circulation. This implies that the most evident target cells for liposomes following intravenous administration are circulating blood cells, vascular endothelial cells, and liver and spleen macrophages, of which the macrophages display by far the highest avidity for liposomes. However, by attenuating the eagerness of the macrophages the rate of elimination from the blood can be slowed down substantially, thus increasing the probability that other cells will participate in liposome uptake. Such attenuation may be achieved either by interfering with the phagocytic function of the macrophages or by manipulating size and composition of the liposomes in such a way that they become less attractive for the macrophage. The latter approach has led to the concept of the "stealth liposome," which goes relatively unnoticed by the liver and spleen macrophages. When the liposomes are small enough such conditions may even be sufficiently favorable to allow for significant extravasation and uptake by cells outside the circulation. Such conditions of reduced competition by macrophages may also be exploited to achieve optimal results with specific targeting devices. All this shows that at the experimental level the liposome undoubtedly deserves the wide attention it receives from large numbers of scientists from many different disciplines. As for the near future, the numerous new conceptual and technical possibilities for in vivo applications of liposomes that have emerged from recent work will require a continuing research effort in order to identify which specific pathological conditions may have the best chance of being successfully challenged by a liposomal approach.

For the time being, it appears that the macrophage-mediated approaches are most promising. The activation of macrophages to tumor cytotoxicity with liposome-associated biological response modifiers, the direct targeting of intracellular parasites or bacteria in macrophages with liposome-encapsulated antibiotics, and the formation of intracellular depots of antimicrobial or cytostatic agents are all examples in which remarkable therapeutic results have been obtained in a variety of animal models. Of the numerous clinical trials which have recently been carried out or are still in progress, the vast majority are based on an approach which either directly or indirectly exploits the resident tissue macrophages in the body as target cells for systemically administered liposomes. Finally, an important result that has emerged from the various trials carried out thus far is that liposomes as such have shown very little toxicity in humans (see for example SCULIER et al. 1986; COUNE et al. 1983). It is to be expected, therefore, that in spite of severe limitations as to the general applicability of liposomes as a systemic drug carrier system, the liposome has a bright future, not merely as an investigational tool but also as the drug carrier of choice in at least a number of specific pharmacological applications.

Acknowledgements. I am grateful to all my former and present coworkers and students for their invaluable contributions to much of the data cited in this chapter. I trust that they will feel satisfactorily acknowledged by the citation density of their work. I thank Rinske Kuperus for her help in preparing the manuscript.

References

Abra RM, Hunt CA (1981) Liposome disposition in vivo. III. Dose and vesicle size effects. Biochim Biophys Acta 666:493–503
Abra RM, Bosworth ME, Hunt CA (1980) Liposome disposition in vivo: effects of predosing with liposomes. Res Commun Chem Pathol Pharmacol 29:349–359.

Abra RM, Hunt CA, Fu KK, Peters JH (1983) Delivery of therapeutic doses of doxorubicin to the mouse lung using lung-accumulating liposomes proves unsuccessful. Cancer Chemother Pharmacol 11:98–101

Abraham W, Downing DT (1990) Interaction between corneocytes and stratum corneum lipid liposomes in vitro. Biochim Biophys Acta 1021:119–125

Abraham W, Wertz PW, Downing DT (1988) Effect of epidermal acylglucosylcer-amides and acylceramides on the morphology of liposomes prepared from stratum corneum lipids. Biochim Biophys Acta 939:403–408

Agarwal K, Bali A, Gupta CM (1986a) Influence of phospholipid structure on the stability of liposomes in serum. Biochim Biophys Acta 856:36–40

Agarwal K, Bali A, Gupta CM (1986b) Effect of phospholipid structure on stability and survival times of liposomes in circulation. Biochim Biophys Acta 883: 468–475

Allen TM (1981) A study of phospholipid interactions between high density lipo-proteins and small unilamellar vesicles. Biochim Biophys Acta 640:385–397

Allen TM (1988) Toxicity of drug carriers to the mononuclear phagocyte system. Adv Drug Delivery Rev 2:55–67

Allen TM (1989) Stealth liposomes: avoiding reticuloendothelial uptake. In: Lopez-Berestein G, Fidler IJ (eds) Liposomes in the therapy of infectious diseases and cancer. Liss, New York, p 405

Allen TM, Chonn A (1987) Large unilamellar liposomes with low uptake into the reticuloendothelial system. FEBS Lett 223:42–46

Allen TM, Cleland LG (1980) Serum-induced leakage of liposome contents. Biochim Biophys Acta 597:418–426

Allen TM, Everest JM (1983) Effect of liposome size and drug release properties on pharmacokinetics of encapsulated drugs in rats. J Pharmacol Exp Ther 226: 539–544

Allen TM, Mehra T (1989) Recent advances in sustained release of antineoplastic drugs using liposomes which avoid uptake into the reticuloendothelial system. Proc West Pharmacol Soc 32:111–114

Allen TM, McAllister L, Mausolf S, Gyorffy E (1981) Liposome-cell interactions. A study of the interactions of liposomes containing entrapped anti-cancer drugs with the EMT 6, S 49 and AE_1 (transport-deficient) cell lines. Biochim Biophys Acta 643:346–362

Allen TM, Ryan JL, Papahadjopoulos D (1985) Gangliosides reduce leakage of aqueous space markers from liposomes in the presence of human plasma. Biochim Biophys Acta 818:205–210

Allen TM, Hansen C, Rutledge J (1989) Liposomes with prolonged circulation times: factors affecting uptake by reticuloendothelial and other tissues. Biochim Biophys Acta 981:27–35

Alving CR (1987) Liposomes as carriers for vaccines In: Ostro MJ (ed) Liposomes from biophysics to therapeutics. Dekker, New York, p 195

Alving CR (1988) Macrophages as targets for delivery of liposome-encapsulated antimicrobial agents. Adv Drug Delivery Rev 2:107–128

Alving CR, Steck EA, Chapman WL Jr, Waits VB, Hendricks LD, Swartz GM Jr, Hanson WL (1978) Therapy of leishmaniasis: superior efficacies of liposome-encapsulated drugs. Proc Natl Acad Sci USA 75:2959–2963

Ashwell G, Morell AG (1974) The role of surface carbohydrates in the hepatic recognition and transport of circulating glycoproteins. Adv Enzymol 41:99–128

Baldeschwieler JD (1985) Phospholipid vesicle targeting using synthetic glycolipid and other determinants. Ann NY Acad Sci 446:349–367

Bali A, Dhawan S, Gupta CM (1983) Stability of liposomes in the circulation is markedly enhanced by structural modification of their phospholipid component. FEBS Lett 154:373–377

Bangham AD, Standish MM, Watkins JC (1965a) Diffusion of univalent ions across the lamellae of swollen phospholipids. J Mol Biol 13:238–252

Bangham AD, Standish MM, Weissmann G (1965b) The action of steroids and streptolysin S on the permeability of phospholipid structures to cations. J Mol Biol 13:253–259

Barber RF, Shek PN (1986) Liposomes and tear fluid. I. Release of vesicle-entrapped carboxyfluorescein. Biochim Biophys Acta 879:157–163

Beaumier PL, Hwang KJ (1983) Effect of liposome size on the degradation of bovine sphingomyelin/cholesterol liposomes in the mouse liver. Biochim Biophys Acta 731:23–30

Bisgaier CL, Siebenkas MV, Williams KJ (1989) Effects of apolipoproteins A-IV and A-I on the uptake of phospholipid liposomes by hepatocytes. J Biol Chem 264:862–866

Black CDV, Gregoriadis G (1976) Interaction of liposomes with blood plasma proteins. Biochem Soc Trans 4:253–256

Black CDV, Watson GJ, Ward RJ (1977) The use of Pentostam liposomes in the chemotherapy of experimental leishmaniasis. Trans R Soc Trop Med Hyg 71: 550–552

Blumenthal R, Ralston E, Dragsten P, Leserman LD, Weinstein JN (1982) Lipid vesicle-cell interactions: analysis of a model for transfer of contents from adsorbed vesicles to cells. Membr Biochem 4:283–303

Bonventre PF, Gregoriadis G (1978) Killing of intraphagocytic *Staphylococcus aureus* by dihydrostreptomycin entrapped within liposomes. Antimocrob Agents Chemother 13:1049–1051

Brown PM, Silvius JR (1990) Hechanisms of delivery of liposome-encapsulated cytosine arabinoside to CV-1 cells in vitro. Fluorescent and cytohoxiciby studies. Biochim Biophys Acta 1023:341–351

Connor J, Huang L (1985) Efficient cytoplasmic delivery of a fluorescent dye by pH-sensitive immunoliposomes. J Cell Biol 101:582–589

Connor J, Huang L (1986) pH-sensitive immunoliposomes as an efficient target-specific carrier for antitumor drugs. Cancer Res 46:3431–3435

Connor J, Yatvin M, Huang L (1984) pH-sensitive liposomes: acid-induced fusion. Proc Natl Acad Sci USA 81:1715–1718

Coune A, Sculier JP, Fruehling J, Stryckmans P, Brassine C, Ghanem G, Laduron C, Atassi G, Ruysschaert JM, Hildebrand J (1983) IV administration of water-insoluble antimitotic compound entrapped in liposomes. Preliminary report on infusion of large volumes of liposomes to man. Cancer Treat Rep 67:1031–1033

Daemen T, Veninga A, Roerdink FH, Scherphof GL (1986a) In vitro activation of rat liver macrophages to tumoricidal activity by free or liposome-encapsulated muramyl dipeptide. Cancer Res 46:4330–4335

Daemen T, Veninga A, Scherphof GL, Roerdink FH (1986b) The activation of Kupffer cells to tumorcytotoxicity with immunomodulators encapsulated in liposomes. In: Kirn A, Knook DL, Wisse E (eds) Cells of the hepatic sinusoid. Kupffer Cell Foundation, Rijswijk, p 379

Daemen T, Veninga A, Roerdink FH, Scherphof GL (1989) Conditions controlling tumor cytotoxicity of rat liver macrophages mediated by liposomal muramyl dipeptide. Biochim Biophys Acta 991:145–151

Daemen T, Dontje BHJ, Veninga A, Scherphof GL, Oosterhuis JW (1990) Therapy of murine liver metastases by administration of MDP encapsulated in liposomes. Select Cancer Ther 6:63–72

Damen J (1982) Interactions of liposomes with plasma lipoproteins. PhD thesis, State University, Groningen, p 80

Damen J, Waite M, Scherphof G (1979) The in vitro transfer of ^{14}C-dimyristoyl phosphatidylcholine from liposomes to subfractions of human HDL as resolved by isoelectric focusing. FEBS Lett 105:115–119

Damen J, Dijkstra J, Regts J, Scherphof G (1980) Effect of lipoprotein-free plasma on the interaction of human plasma high density lipoprotein with egg yolk phosphatidylcholine liposomes. Biochem Biophys Acta 620:336–346

Damen J, Regts J, Scherphof G (1981) Transfer and exchange of phospholipid between small unilamellar liposomes and rat plasma high density lipoproteins: dependence on cholesterol and phospholipid composition. Biochem Biophys Acta 665:538–545

Damen J, Regts J, Scherphof G (1982) Transfer of ^{14}C-phosphatidylcholine between liposomes and human plasma high density lipoprotein: partial purification of a transfer-stimulating plasma factor using a rapid transfer assay. Biochem Biophys Acta 712:444–452

Das PK, Murray GL, Zirzow GC, Brady RO, Barranger JA (1985) Lectin-specific targeting of glucocerebrosidase to different liver cells via glycosylated liposomes. Biochem Med 33:124–131

Dave J, Patel HM (1986) Differentiation in hepatic and splenic phagocytic activity during reticuloendothelial blockade with cholesterol-free and cholesterol-rich liposomes. Biochem Biophys Acta 888:184–190

Derksen JTP, Scherphof GL (1985) An improved method for the covalent coupling of proteins to liposomes. Biochem Biophys Acta 814:151–155

Derksen JTP, Morselt HWM, Scherphof GL (1987) Processing of different liposome markers after in vitro uptake of immunoglobulin-coated liposomes by rat liver macrophages. Biochem Biophys Acta 931:33–40

Derksen JTP, Baldeschwieler JD, Scherphof GL (1988a) In vivo stability of ester- and ether-linked phospholipid-containing liposomes as measured by perturbed angular correlation spectroscopy. Proc Natl Acad Sci USA 85:9768–9772

Derksen JTP, Morselt HWM, Scherphof GL (1988b) Uptake and processing of immunoglobulin-coated liposomes by subpopulations of rat liver macrophages. Biochem Biophys Acta 971:127–136

Desmukh DS, Bear WD, Wisniewsky HM, Brockerhoff H (1978) Long-living liposomes as potential drug carriers. Biochem Biophys Res Commun 82:328–334

Desmukh DS, Bear WD, Brockerhoff H (1981) Can intact liposomes be adsorbed in the gut? Life Sci 28:239–242

Dijkstra J, van Galen WJM, Hulstaert CE, Kalicharan D, Roerdink, FH, Scherphof GL (1984a) Interaction of liposomes with Kupffer cells in vitro. Exp Cell Res 150:161–176

Dijkstra J, van Galen WJM, Scherphof GL (1984b) Effects of ammonium chloride and chloroquine on endocytic uptake of liposomes by Kupffer cells in vitro. Biochem Biophys Acta 804:58–67

Dijkstra J, van Galen WJM, Regts J, Scherphof G (1985a) Uptake and processing of liposomal phospholipids by Kupffer cells in vitro. Eur J Biochem 148:391–397

Dijkstra J, van Galen WJM, Scherphof G (1985b) Influence of liposome charge on the association of liposomes with Kupffer cells in vitro. Effects of divalent cations and competition with latex particles. Biochem Biophys Acta 813:287–297

Dijkstra J, van Galen WJM, Scherphof G (1985c) Effects of (dihydro)cytochalasin B, colchicine, monensin and trifluoperazine on uptake and processing of liposomes by Kupffer cells in culture. Biochem Biophys Acta 845:34–42

Dragsten PR, Mitchell DB, Covert G, Baker T (1987) Drug delivery using vesicles targeted to the hepatic asialoglycoprotein receptor. Biochem Biophys Acta 926:27–279

Duzgunes N, Straubinger RM, Baldwin PA, Friend DS, Papahadjopoulos D (1985) Proton-induced fusion of oleic acid-phosphatidylethanolamine liposomes. Biochemistry 24:3091–3098

Ellens H, Morselt H, Scherphof G (1981) In vivo fate of large unilamellar sphingomyelin/cholesterol liposomes after intraperitoneal and intravenous injection into rats. Biochim Biophys Acta 674:10–18

Ellens H, Mayhew E, Rustum YM (1982) Reversible depression of the reticulo-endothelial system by liposomes. Biochim Biophys Acta 714:479–485

Ellens H, Morselt H, Dontje BHJ, Kalicharan D, Hulstaert CE, Scherphof GL (1983) Effects of liposome dose and the presence of lymphosarcoma cells on blood clearance and tissue distribution of large unilamellar liposomes in mice. Cancer Res 43:2927–2934

Ellens H, Bentz J, Szoka FC (1985) H^+- and Ca^{2+}-induced fusion and destabilization of liposomes. Biochemistry 24:3099–3106

Eppstein DA, Marsh YV, van der Pas MA, Felgner PF, Schreiber AB (1985) Biological activity of liposome-encapsulated murine interferon-gamma is mediated by a cell membrane receptor. Proc Natl Acad Sci USA 82:3688–3692

Eppstein DA, van der Pas MA, Schryver BB, Felgner PL, Gloff CA, Soike KF (1986) Controlled release and localized targeting of interferons. In: Davis SS, Illum L, Tomlinson E (eds) Delivery systems for peptide drugs. Plenum, New York, p 227

Felgner PL, Gadek TR, Holm M, Roman R, Chan HW, Wenz M, Northrop JP, Ringold GM, Danielsen M (1987) Lipofection: a highly efficient, lipid-mediated DNA-transfection procedure. Proc Natl Acad Sci USA 84:7413–7417

Fichtner I, Reszka R, Elbe B, Arndt D (1981) Therapeutic evaluation of liposome-encapsulated daunoblastin in murine tumor models. Neoplasma 28:141–149

Fidler IJ (1980) Therapy of spontaneous metastases by intravenous injection of liposomes containing lymphokines. Science 208:1469–1471

Fidler IJ, Sone J, Fogler WE, Barnes ZL (1981) Eradication of spontaneous metastases and activation of alveolar macrophages by intravenous injection of liposomes containing muramyl dipeptide. Proc Natl Acad Sci USA 78:1680–1684

Fidler IJ, Sone S, Fogler WE, Smith D, Braun DG, Tarcsay L, Gisler RJ, Schroit A (1982) Efficacy of liposomes containing a lipophilic muramyl dipeptide derivative for activating the tumoricidal properties of alveolar macrophages in vivo. J Biol Response Mod 1:43–55

Fogler WE, Fidler IJ (1986) The activation of tumoricidal properties in human blood monocytes by muramyl dipeptide requries specific intracellular interaction. J Immunol 136:2311–2317

Forssen EA, Tokes ZA (1981) Use of anionic liposomes for the reduction of chronic doxorubicin-induced cariotoxicity. Proc Natl Acad Sci USA 78:1873–1877

Fraley R, Subramani S, Papahadjopoulos D (1980) Introduction of liposome-encapsulated SV40 DNA into cells: effect of vesicle composition and incubation conditions. J Biol Chem 255:10431-10435

Fraley R, Straubinger RM, Rule G, Springer E, Papahadjopoulos D (1981) Liposome-mediated delivery of deoxyribonucleic acid to cells: enhanced efficacy of delivery related to lipid composition and incubation conditions. Biochemistry 20:6978–6987

Fraser-Smith EB, Eppstein DA, Larsen MA, Mattews TR (1983) Protective effect of a muramyl dipeptide analog encapsulated in or mixed with liposomes against *Candida albicans* infection. In fect Immun 39:172–178

Freise J, Mueller WH, Broelsch C, Schmidt FW (1980) In vivo distribution of liposomes between parenchymal and non-parenchymal cells in rat liver. Biomedicine 32:118–123

Freise J, Mueller WH, Magerstedt P (1981) Uptake of liposomes and sheep red blood cells by the liver and spleen of rats with normal and decreased function of the reticuloendothelial system. Res Exp Med 178:263–269

Friedman M, Byers SO, Rosenman RH (1957) Resolution of aortic atherosclerotic infiltration in the rabbit by phosphatide infusion. Proc Soc Exp Biol Med 95:586–588

Gabizon A, Papahadjopoulos D (1988) Liposome formulations with prolonged circulation time in blood and enhanced uptake by tumors. Proc Natl Acad Sci USA 85:6949–6953

Gabizon A, Dagan A, Goren D, Barenholz Y, Fuks Z (1982) Liposomes as in vivo carriers of adriamycin: reduced cardiac uptake and preserved antitumor activity in mice. Cancer Res 42:4734–4739

Gabizon A, Meshorer A, Barenholz Y (1986) Comparative long-term study of the toxicities of free and liposome-associated doxorubicin in mice after intravenous administration. JNCI 77:459–469

Gabizon A, Shiota R, Papahadjopoulos D (1989a) Pharmacokinetics and tissue distribution of doxorubicin encapsulated in stable liposomes with long circulation time. JNCI 18:1484–1488

Gabizon A, Sulkes A, Peretz T, Druckmann S, Goren D, Amselem S, Barenholz Y (1989b) Liposome-associated doxorubicin: preclinical pharmacology and exploratory clinical phase. In: Lopez-Berestein G, Fidler IJ (eds) Liposomes in the therapy of infectious diseases and cancer. Liss, New York, p 391

Gabizon A, Peretz T, Sulkes A, Amselem S, Ben-Yosef R, Catane R, Biran S, Barenholz Y (1900) Systemic administration of doxorubicin-containing liposomes in cancer patients: a phase I study. Eur J Cancer Clin Oncol (in press)

Ghosh P, Das PK, Bachhawat BK (1982) Targeting of liposomes towards different cell types of rat liver through the involvement of liposomal surface glycosides. Arch Biochem Biophys 213:266–270

Gilbreath MJ, Nacy CA, Hoover DL, Alving CR, Swartz GM, Meltzer MS (1985) Macrophage activation for microbicidal activity against *Leishmania major*: inhibition of lymphokine activation by phosphatidylcholine-phosphatidylserine liposomes. J Immunol 134:3420–3425

Gilbreath MJ, Hoover DL, Alving CR, Swartz GM, Meltzer MS (1986) Inhibition of lymphokine-induced macrophage microbicidal activity against *Leishmania major* by liposomes: characterization of the physicochemical requirements for liposome inhibiton. J Immunol 137:1681–1687

Gilbreath MJ, Fogler WE, Swartz GM, Alving CR, Meltzer MS (1989) Inhibition of interferon gamma-induced macrophage microbicidal activity agaisnt *Leishmania major* by liposomes: Inhibition is dependent upon composition of phospholipid headgroups and fatty acids. Int J Immunopharmacol 11:103–110

Gisler RH, Schumann G, Sackmann W, Pericin C, Tarcsay L, Dietrich FM (1982) A novel muramyl peptide, MTP-PE: profile of biological activities. In: Yamamura S, Kotani S (eds) Immunomodulation by microbial products and related synthetic compounds. Excerpta Medica, Amsterdam, p 167

Graybill JR, Craven PC, Taylor RL, Williams DM, Magee WE (1982) Treatment of murine cryptococcosis with liposome-associated amphotericin B. J Infect Dis 145:748–752

Green PHR, Glickman RM, Riley JW, Quinet E (1980) Human apolipoprotein A-IV. Intestinal origin and distribution in plasma. J Clin Invest 65:911–919

Gregoriadis G, Neerunjun ED (1975) Homing of liposomes to target cells. Biochem Biophys Res Commun 65:537–544

Gregoriadis G, Ryman BE (1972a) Fate of protein-containing liposomes injected into rats. An approach to the treatment of storage diseases. Dur J Biochem 24: 485–491

Gregoriadis G, Ryman BE (1972b) Lysosomal localization of fructofuranosidase-containing liposomes injected into rats; implications in the treatment of genetic disorders. Biochem J 129:123–133

Gregoriadis G, Senior J (1984) Targeting of small unilamellar liposomes to the galactose receptor in vivo. Biochem Soc Trans 12:337–339

Grosse E, Kieda C, Nicolau C (1984) Flow cytofluorimetric investigations of the uptake by hepatocytes and spleen cells of targeted and untargeted liposomes injected intravenously into mice. Biochim Biophys Acta 805:354–361

Gupta CM, Bali A, Dhawan S (1981) Modification of phospholipid structure results in greater stability of liposomes in serum. Biochim Biophys Acta 648:192–198

Haensler J, Schuber F (1988) Preparation of neo-galactosylated liposomes and their interaction with peritoneal macrophages. Biochim Biophys Acta 946:95–105

Hafeman DG, Lewis JT, McConnell HM (1980) Triggering of the macrophage and neutrophil respiratory burst by antibody bound to a spin-label phospholipid hapten in model lipid bilayer membranes. Biochemistry 19:5387–5393

Heath TD, Fraley RT, Papahadjopoulos D (1980) Antibody targeting of liposomes: cell specificity obtained by conjugation of F(ab')$_2$ to vesicle surface. Science 210:539–541

Heath TD, Bragman K, Matthay K, Lopez NG, Papahadjopoulos D (1985a) Antibody-targeted liposomes: development of a cell-specific drug delivery system. In: Gregoriadis G, Poste G, Senior J, Trouet A (eds) Receptor-mediated targeting of drugs. Plenum, New York, p 407

Heath TD, Lopez NG, Papahadjopoulos D (1985b) The effects of liposome size and surface charge on liposome-mediated delivery of methotrexate-aspartate in vitro. Biochim Biophys Acta 820:74–84

Hemaker HC, Muller AD, Hermens WT, Zwaal RFA (1980) Oral treatment of haemophilia A by gastrointestinal absorption of factor VIII entrapped liposomally. Lancet 1:70–71

Hermetter A, Paltauf P (1983) Interaction between ether glycerophospholipid vesicles and serum proteins in vitro. Biochim Biophys Acta 752:444–450

Ho RJY, Rouse BT, Huang L (1987) Target-sensitive immunoliposomes as an efficient drug carrier for antiviral activity. J Biol Chem 262:13973–13978

Hoekstra D, Tomasini R, Scherphof G (1978) Interaction of phospholipid vesicles with rat hepatocytes in primary monolayer culture. Biochim Biophys Acta 542:456–469

Hoekstra D, Tomasini R, Scherphof G (1980) Interactions of phospholipid vesicles with rat hepatocytes in vitro. Influence of vesicle-incorporated glycolipids. Biochim Biophys Acta 603:336–346

Hoekstra D, van Renswoude J, Tomasini R, Scherphof G (1981) Interaction of phospholipid vesicles with rat hepatocytes. Further characterization of vesicle-cell surface interaction; use of serum as a physiological modulator. Membr Biochem 4:129–147

Howard FD, Petty HR, McConnell HM (1982) Identification of phagocytosis-associated surface proteins of macrophages by two-dimensional gel electrophoresis. J Cell Biol 92:283–288

Huang A, Huang L, Kennel SJ (1980) Monoclonal antibody covalently coupled with fatty acid; a reagent for in vitro liposome targeting. J Biol Chem 255:8015–8018

Hughes BJ, Kennel S, Lee R, Huang L (1989) Monoclonal antibody targeting of liposomes to mouse lung in vivo. Cancer Res 49:6214–6220

Hwang KJ, Luk K-FS, Beaumier PL (1980) Hepatic uptake and degradation of unilamellar sphingomyelin/cholesterol liposomes: a kinetic study. Proc Natal Acad Sci USA 77:4030–4034

Hwang KJ, Luk KF, Beaumier P (1982) Volume of distribution and transcapillary passage of small unilamellar liposomes. Life Sci 31:949–955

Illum L, Davis SS (1984) The organ uptake of intravenously administered colloidal particles can be altered by using a non-ionic surfactant (Poloxamer 338). FEBS Lett 167:79–82

Illum L, Hunneyball IM, Davis SS (1986) The effect of hydrophilic coatings on the uptake of colloidal particles by the liver and by peritoneal macrophages. Int J Parm 29:53–65

Illum L, Davis SS, Mueller RH, Mak E, West P (1987) The organ distribution and circulation time of intravenously injected colloidal carriers sterically stabilized by a block polymer – poloxamine 908. Life Sci 40:367–374

Inamura N, Nakahara K, Kino T, Gotoh T, Kawamura L, Aoki H, Imanaka H, Sone S (1985) Activation of tumoricidal properties in macrophages and inhibition of experimentally induced murine metastases by a new synthetic acyltripeptide, FK-565. J Biol Respanse Mod 4:408–417

Juliano RL, Lin G (1980) The interaction of plasma proteins with liposomes: protein binding and effects on the clotting and complement system. In: Tom BH, Six HR (eds) Liposomes and immunobiology. Elsevier/North-Holland, Amsterdam, p 49

Juliano RL, Stamp D (1975) The effect of particle size and charge on the clearance rates of liposomes and liposome-encapsulated drugs. Biochem Biophys Res Commun 63:651–658

Juliano RL, Grant CW, Barber KR, Kalp MA (1987) Mechanism of the selective toxicity of amphotericin B incorporated into liposomes. Mol Pharmacol 31:1

Kao YJ, Juliano RL (1981) Interactions of liposomes with the reticuloendothelial system. Effects of reticuloendothelial blockade on the clearance of large unilamellar vesicles. Biochim Biophys Acta 677:453–461

Kempka G, Roos PH, Kolb-Bachofen V (1990) A membrane-associated form of C-reactive protein is the galactoside-specific receptor on rat liver Kupffer cells. J Immunol 144:1004–1009

Kimelberg HK, Mayhew EG (1978) Properties and biological effects of liposomes and their uses in pharmacology and toxicology. CRC Crit Rev Toxicol 6:25–79

Kirby C, Gregoriadis G (1980) The effect of cholesterol content of small unilamellar liposomes on the fate of their lipid components in vivo. Life Sci 27:2223–2230

Kirby C, Gregoriadis G (1981) Plasma-induced release of solutes from small unilamellar lipsomes is associated with pore formation in the bilayer. Biochem J 199:251–254

Kirby C, Clarke J, Gregoriadis G (1980a) Effect of cholesterol content of small unilamellar liposomes on their stability in vivo and in vitro. Biochem J 186:591–598

Kirby C, Clarke J, Gregoriadis G (1980b) Cholesterol content of small unilamellar liposomes controls phosphatidylcholine loss to high density lipoproteins in the presence of serum. FEBS Lett 111:324–328

Koff WC, Showalter SD, Hampar B, Fidler IJ (1985) Protection of mice against fatal herpes simplex type 2 infection by liposomes containing muramyl tripeptide. Science 228:495–497

Kolb-Bachofen V, Schlepper-Schaefer J, Vogell W, Kolb H (1982) Electron microscopic evidence for an asialoglycoprotein receptor on Kupffer cells. Cell 21:859–866

Kuipers F, Spanjer HH, Havinga R, Scherphof GL, Vonk RJ (1986) Lipoproteins and liposomes as in vivo cholesterol vehicles in the rat: preferential use of cholesterol carried by small unilamellar liposomes for the formation of muricholic acids. Biochim Biophys Acta 876:559–566

Lasch J, Wohlrab W (1986) Liposome-bound cortisol: a new approach to cutaneous therapy. Biomed Biochim Acta 45:1295–1299

Lazar G, van Galen M, Scherphof GL (1989) Gadoliniumchloride-induced shifts in intrahepatic distributions of liposomes. Biochim Biophys Acta 1011:97–101

Leserman LD, Barbet J, Kourilsky F, Weinstein JN (1980) Targeting to cells of fluorescent liposomes covalently coupled with monoclonal antobody or protein A. Nature 288:602–604

Liu D, Huang L (1989a) Role of cholesterol in the stability of pH-sensitive, large unilamellar liposomes prepared by the detergent-dialysis method. Biochim Biophys Acta 981:254–260

Lu D, Huang L (1989b) Small but not large, unilamellar liposomes composed of dioleoylphosphatidylethanolamine and oleic acid can be stabilized by human plasma. Biochemistry 28:7700–7707

Liu D, Zhou F, Huang L (1989) Characterization of plasma-stabilized liposomes composed of dioleoylphosphatidylethanolamine and oleic acid. Biochem Biophys Res Commun 162:326–333

Lopez-Berestein G (1989) Treatment of systemic fungal infections with liposomal amphotericin B. In: Lopez-Berestein G, Fidler IJ (eds) Liposomes in the therapy of infectious diseases and cancer. Liss, New York, p 317

Lopez-Berestein G, Fidler IJ (1989) Liposomes in the therapy of infectious diseases and cancer. Liss, New York UCLA symposia on molecular cellular biology, new series, vol 89

Lopez-Berestein G, Mehta R, Hopfer RL, Mills K, Kasi L, Mehta K (1983) Treatment and prophylaxis of disseminated infection due to *Candida albicans* in mice with liposome-encapsulated amphotericin B. J Infect Dis 147:939–945

Lopez-Berestein G, Fainstein V, Hopfer R, Mehta K, Sullivan MP, Keating M, Rosenblum MG, Mehta R, Luna M, Hersh EM, Reuben J, Juliano RL, Bodey

GP (1985) Liposomal amphotericin B for the treatment of systemic fungal infections in patients with cancer: a preliminary study. J Infect Dis 151:704–710

Mangat S, Patel HM (1985) Lymph node localization of non-specific antibody-coated liposomes. Life Sci 36:1917–1925

Martin FJ, MacDonald RC (1974) Liposomes can mimic virus membranes. Nature 252:161–163

Martin FJ, Hubbell WL, Papahadjopoulos D, (1981) Immunospecific targeting of liposomes to cells: a novel and efficient method for covalent attachment of Fab' fragments via disulfide bonds. Biochemistry 20:4229–4238

Matthay KK, Abai AM, Cobb S, Hong K, Papahadjopoulos D, Straubinger RM (1989) Role of ligand in antibody-directed endocytosis of liposomes by human T-leukemia cells. Cancer Res 49:4879–4886

Mauk MR, Gamble RC, Baldeschwieler JD (1980) Targeting of lipid vesicles: specificity of carbohydrate receptor analogues for leukocytes in mice. Proc Natl Acad Sci USA 77:4430–4434

Mayer LD, Tai LCL, Ko DSC, Masin D, Ginsberg RS, Cullis PR, Bally MB (1989) Influence of vesicle size, lipid composition and drug-to-lipid ratio on the biological activity of liposomal doxorubicin in mice. Cancer Res 49:5922–5930

Mayhew E, Gotfredsen C, Schneider YJ, Trouet A (1980) Interaction of liposomes with cultured cellsa: effect of serum. Biochem Pharmacol 29:877–886

Mayhew E, Rustum Y, Vail WJ (1983) Inhibition of liver metastase of M5076 tumor by liposome-entrapped adriamycin. Cancer Drug Delivery 1:43–58

Mayhew EG, Goldrosen MH, Vaage J, Rustum YM (1987) Effects of liposome-entrapped doxorubicin on liver metastases of mouse colon carcinomas 26 and 38. 78:707–713

McDougall IR, Dunnick JK, McNamee MG, Kriss JP (1974) Distribution and fate of synthetic lipid vesicles in the mouse. A combined radionuclide and spin label study. Proc Natl Acad Sci USA 71:3487–3491

Mehta K, Lopez-Berestein G, Hersh G, Juliano RL (1982) Uptake of liposomes and liposome-encapsulated muramyl dipeptide by human peripheral blood monocytes. J Reticuloendothel Soc 32:155–164

Mehta R, Lopez-Berestein G, Hopfer RL, Mills K, Juliano RL (1984) Liposomal amphotericin B is toxic to fungal cells but not to mammalian cells. Biochim Biophys Acta 770:230–234

Moghimi SM, Patel HM (1988) Tissue specific opsonins for phagocytic cells and their different affinity for cholesterol-rich liposomes. FEBS Lett 233:143–147

Moghimi SM, Patel HM (1989a) Differential properties of organ-specific serum opsonins for liver and spleen macrophages. Biochim Biophys Acta 984:379–383

Moghimi SM, Patel HM (1989b) Serum opsonins and phagocytosis of saturated and unsaturated phospholipid liposomes. Biochim Biophys Acta 984:384–387

Muller CD, Schuber F (1989) Neo-mannosylated liposomes: synthesis and interaction with mouse Kupffer cells and resident peritoneal macrophages. Biochim Biophys Acta 986:97–105

Munn MW, Parce JW (1982) Antibody-dependent phagocytosis of haptenated liposomes by human neutrophils is dependent on the physical state of the liposomal membrane. Biochim Biophys Acta 692:101–108

Nayar R, Schroit AJ (1985) Generation of pH-sensitive liposomes:use of large unilamellar vesicles containing N-succinyldioleoylphosphatidylethanolamine. Biochemistry 24:5967–5971

New RRC, Chance ML, Thomas SC, Peters W (1978) Antileishmanial activity of antimonials entrapped in liposomes. Nature 272:55–56

New RRC, Black CDV, Parker RJ, Scherphof (1990) Liposomes in biological systems. In: New RRC (ed) Liposomes, a practical approach. IRL, Oxford, p 221

Olson F, Mayhew E, Maslow D, Rustum Y, Szoka FC (1982) Characterization, toxicity and therapeutic efficacy of adriamycin encapsulated in liposomes. Eur J Cancer Clin Oncol 18:167–176

Pabst MJ, Cummings NP, Shiba T, Kusomoto S, Kotani S (1980) Lipophilic deriva-
    tive of muramyldipeptide is more active than muramyl dipeptide in priming
    macrophages to release superoxide anion. Infect Immun 29:617
Pagano RE, Huang L (1975) Interactions of phospholipid vesicles with cultured
    mammalian cells. II. Studies of mechanism. J Cell Biol 67:49–60
Pagano RE, Weinstein JN (1978) Interactions of liposomes with mammalian cells.
    Annu Rev Biophys Bioeng 7:435–468
Papahadjopoulos D, Gabizon A (1987) Targeting of liposomes to tumor cells in vivo.
    Ann NY Acad Sci 507:64–74
Papahadjopoulos D, Poste G, Mayhew E (1974) Cellular uptake of cyclic AMP
    captured within phospholipid vesicles and effect on cell growth behaviour.
    Biochim Biophys Acta 363:404–418
Parker RJ, Sieber SM, Weinstein JN (1981) Effect of encapsulation of a fluorescent
    dye on its uptake by the lymphatics in the rat. Pharmacology 23:128–
    136
Parker RJ, Priester ER, Sieber SM (1982a) Comparison of lymphatic uptake metab-
    olism, excretion and biodistribution of free and liposome-entrapped [^{14}C]
    cytosine-D-arabinofuranoside following intraperitoneal administration to rats.
    Drug Metab Dispos 10:40–45
Parker RJ, Priester ER, Sieber SM (1982b) Effect of route of administration and
    liposome entrapment on the metabolism and disposition of adriamycin in the rat.
    Durg Metab Dispos 10:499–504
Patel HM, Wild AE (1988) Fc receptor-mediated transcytosis of IgG-coated Lipo-
    somes across epithelial barriers. FEBS Lett 234:321–325
Patel HM, Tuzel NS, Ryman BE (1983a) Inhibitory effect of cholesterol on the uptake
    of liposomes by liver and spleen. Biochim Biophys Acta 761:142–151
Patel KR, Li MP, Baldeschwieler JD (1983b) Suppression of liver uptake of liposomes
    by dextran sulfate 500. Proc Natl Acad Sci USA 80:6518–6522
Patel HM, Boodle KM, Vaughan-Jones R (1984) Assessment of the potential use of
    liposomes for lymphoscintigraphy and lymphatic drug delivery. Failure of 99m-
    technetium marker to represent intact liposomes in lymph nodes. Biochim
    Biophys Acta 801:76–86
Patel HM, Tuzel NS, Stevenson WS (1985) Intracellular digestion of saturated and
    unsaturated phospholipid liposomes by mucosal cells. Possible mechanism of
    transport of liposomally entrapped macromolecules across the isolated vascularly
    perfused rabbit ileum. Biochim Biophys Acta 839:40–49
Peeters PAM, Brunink BG, Eling WMC, Crommelin DJA (1989) Therapeutic
    effect of chloroquin (CQ)-containing immunoliposomes in rats infected with
    Plasmodium berghei parasitized mouse red blood cells: comparison with com-
    binations of antibodies and CQ or liposomal CQ. Biochim Biophys Acta 981:
    269–276
Phillips NC, Tsao M-S (1989) Inhibition of murine hepatic tumor growth by liposomes
    containing a lipophilic muramyl dipeptide. Cancer Immunol Immunother 28:
    54–58
Phillips NC, Moras ML, Chedid L, Bernard JM (1985) Activation of alveolar
    macrophage tumoricidal activity and eradication of experimental pulmonary
    metastases by freeze-dried liposomes containing a new lipophilic muramyl
    dipeptide derviative. Cancer Res 45:128–134
Phillips NC, Rioux J, Tsao M-S (1988) Activation of murine Kupffer cell tumoricidal
    activity by liposomes containing lipophilic muramyl dipeptide. Hepatology 8:
    1046–1050
Poste G, Papahadjopoulos D (1976) Lipid vesicles as carriers for introducing materials
    into cultured cells. Influence of vesicle lipid on mechanism(s) of vesicle incorpora-
    tion into cells. Proc Natl Acad Sci USA 73:1603–1607
Poste G, Kirsh R, Fogler WE, Fidler IJ (1979) Activation of tumoricidal properties in
    mouse macrophages by lymphokines encapsulated in liposomes. Cancer Res
    39:881–892

Poste G, Bucana C, Raz A, Bugelski P, Kirsh R, Fidler IJ (1982) Analysis of the fate of systemically administered liposomes and implications for their use in drug delivery. Cancer Res 42:1412–1422

Poste G, Kirsh R, Koestler T (1984) The challenge of liposome targeting in vivo. In: Gregoriadis G (ed) Liposome technology, vol 3. CRC, Boca Raton, p 1

Proffitt RT, Williams LE, Presant CA, Tin GW, Uliana JA Gamble RC, Baldeschwieler JD (1983) Tumor-imaging potential of liposomes loaded with ^{111}In-NTA. Biodistribution in mice. J Nucl Med 24:45–51

Rahman A, Kessler A, More N, Sikic B, Rowden G, Woolley P, Schein P (1980) Liposomal protection of adriamycin-induced cardiotoxicity in mice. Cancer Res 40:1532–1637

Rahman YE, Cerny EA, Patel KR, Lau EH, Wright BJ (1982) Differential uptake of liposomes varying in size and lipid composition by parenchymal and Kupffer cells of mouse liver. Life Sci 31:2061–2071

Rahman A, Carmichael D, Harris M, Roh JK (1986) Comparative pharmacokinetics of free doxorubicin and doxorubicin entrapped in cardiolipin liposomes. Cancer Res 43:2295–2299

Rahman A, Roh JK, Treat J (1989) Preclinical and clinical pharmacology of doxorubicin entrapped in cardiolipin liposomes. In: Lopez-Berestein G, Fidler IJ (eds) Liposomes in the therapy of infectious diseases and cancer. Liss, New York, p 367

Raz A, Bucana C, Fogler WE, Poste G, Fidler IJ (1981) Biochemical, morphological and ultrastructural studies on the uptake of liposomes by murine macrophages. Cancer Res 41:487–494

Richardson EC, Swartz GM, Moe JB, Alving CR (1988/1989) Life-long administration of liposomes and lipid A in mice: effects on longevity, antibodies to liposomes, and terminal histopathological patterns. J Liposome Res 1:93–110

Roerdink FH, Wisse E, Morselt HWM, van der Meulen J, Scherphof GL (1977) Cellular distribution of intravenously injected protein-containing liposomes in the rat liver. In: Wisse E, Knook DL (eds) Kupffer cells and other liver sinusoidal cells. Elsevier/North-Holland, Amsterdam, p 263

Roerdink FH, Dijkstra J, Hartman G, Bolscher B, Scherphof G (1981) The involvement of parenchymal, Kupffer and endothelial liver cells in hepatic uptake of intravenously injected liposomes. Effects of lanthanum and godolinium salts. Biochim Biophys Acta 677:79–89

Roerdink FH, Regts J, van Leeuwen B, Scherphof GL (1984) Intrahepatic uptake and processing of intravenously injected small unilamellar vesicles in rats. Biochim Biophys Acta 770:195–202

Roerdink FH, Regts J, Scherphof G (1986) Effect of lipid composition on the uptake and intracellular degradation of liposomes by Kupffer cells. In: Kirn A, Knook DL, Wisse E (eds) Cell of the hepatic sinusoid. Kupffer Cell Foundation, Rijswijk, p 125

Roerdink FH, Regts J, Handel T, Sullivan SM, Baldeschwieler JD, Scherphof GL (1989) Effect of cholesterol on the uptake and intracellular degradation of liposomes by liver and spleen: a combined biochemical and x-ray perturbed angular correlation study. Biochim Biophys Acta 980:234–240

Rowland RN, Woodley JF (1980) The stability of liposomes in vitro to pH, bile salts and pancreatic lipase. Biochim Biophys Acta 620:400–409

Rowland RN, Woodley JF (1981) The uptake of distearoylphosphatidylcholine/cholesterol liposomes by rat intestinal sacs in vitro. Biochim Biophys Acta 673:217–223

Rudra D, Myant N, Pflug J, Reichl D (1984) The distribution of cholesterol and apolipoprotein A-1 between the lipoproteins in plasma and peripheral lymph from normal human subjects. Atherosclerosis 53:297–308

Rustum YM (1983) Prodrugs: an approach to target-directed chemotherapy. In: Cheng Y-C, et al. (eds) Development of target-oriented anticancer drugs. Raven, New York, p 119

Salord J, Schuber F (1988) In vitro drug delivery mediated by ecto-NAD$^+$-glyco-
hydrolase ligand-targeted liposomes. Biochim Biophys Acta 971:197–206
Salord J, Tarnus C, Muller CD, Schuber F (1986) Targeting of liposomes by covalent
coupling with ecto-NAD$^+$-glycohydrolase ligands. Biochim Biophys Acta 886:
64–75
Scherphof G, Morselt H (1984) On the size dependent disintegration of samll
unilamellar phosphatidylcholine vesicles in rat plasma. Evidence of complete loss
of vesicle structure. Biochem J 221:423–429
Scherphof G, Roerdink F, Waite M, Parks J (1978) Disintegration of phosphatidylcholine liposomes as a result of interaction with high density lipoproteins.
Biochim Biophys Acta 542:296–307
Scherphof G, Morselt H, Regts J, Wilschut J (1979) The involvement of the lipid
phase transition in the plasma-induced dissolution of multilamellar phosphatidylcholine vesicles. Biochim Biophys Acta 556:196–207
Scherphof G, Roerdink F, Hoekstra D, Zborowski J, Wisse E (1980) Stability of
liposomes in presence of blood constituents: consequences for uptake of liposomal lipid and entrapped compounds by rat liver cells. In: Gregoriads G, Allison
AC (eds) Liposomes in biological systems. Wiley, Chichester, p 179
Scherphof G, Roerdink F, Dijkstra J, Ellens H, de Zanger R, Wisse E (1983a) Uptake
of liposomes by rat and mouse hepatocytes and Kupffer cells. Biol Cell 47:
47–58
Scherphof G, van Leeuwen B, Wilschut J, Damen J (1983b) Exchange of phosphatidylcholine between small unilamellar liposomes and human high density
lipoprotein exclusively involves the phospholipid in the outer monolayer of the
liposomal membrane. Biochim Biophys Acta 732:595–599
Schroit AJ, Fidler IJ (1982) Effects of liposome structure and lipid composition on the
activation of the tumoricidal properties of macrophages by liposomes containing
muramyl dipeptide. Cancer Res 42:161–167
Schwendener RA, Lagocki PA, Rahman YE (1984) The effects of charge and size on
the interaction of unilamellar liposomes with macrophages. Biochim Biophys
Acta 772:93–101
Schwendener RA, Superasxo A, Rubas W, Weder HG (1985) 5'-O-Palmitoyl-and
3',5'-O-dipalmitoyl-5-fluoro-2'-deoxyuridine. Novel lipophilic analogues of
5-fluoro-2'-deoxyuridine: synthesis, incorporation into liposomes and preliminary
biolgogical results. Biochem Biophys Res Commun 126:660–666
Sculier JP, Coune A, Brassine C, Laduron C, Atassi G, Ruysschaert JM, Fruehling J
(1986) Intravenous infusion of high doses of liposomes containing NCC 251635, a
water-insoluble cytostatic agent. A pilot study with pharmacokinetic data. J Clin
Oncol 4:789–797
Senior JH (1987) Fate and behaviour of liposomes in vivo: a review of controlling
factors. CRC Crit Rev Ther Drug Carrier Syst 3:123–193
Senior J, Gregoriadis G (1982a) Stability of small unilamellar liposomes in serum and
clearance from the circulation: the effect of the phospholipid and cholesterol
components. Life Sci 30:2133–2136
Senior J, Gregoriadis G (1982b) Is the half-life circulating liposomes determined by
changes in their permeability? FFBS Lett 145:109–114
Senior J, Gregoriadis G (1984) Methodology in assessing liposomal stability in the
presence of blood, clearance from the circulation of injected animals, and uptake
by tissues. In: Gregoriadis G (ed) Liposome technology, vol 3. CRC, Boca
Raton, p 263
Senior J, Gregoriadis G, Mitropoulos KA (1983) Stability and clearance of small
unilamellar liposomes. Studies with normal and lipoprotein-deficient mice.
Biochim Biophys Acta 760:111–118
Senior J, Crawley JCW, Gregoriadis G (1985) Tissue distribution of liposomes
exhibiting long half-lives in the circulation after intravenous injection. Biochim
Biophys Acta 839:1–8

Souhami RL, Patel HM, Ryman BE (1981) The effect of reticuloendothelial blockade on the blood clearance and tissue distribution of liposomes. Biochim Biophys Acta 674:354–371

Spanjer H, Scherphof G (1983) Targeting of lactosylceramide-containing liposomes to hepatocytes in vivo. Biochim Biophs Acta 734:40–47

Spanjer H, Morselt H, Scherphof G (1984) Lactosylceramide-induced stimulation of liposome uptake by Kupffer cells in vivo. Biochim Biophys Acta 774:49–55

Spanjer HH, Scherphof GL, van Berkel TJC, Kempen HJM (1985) The effect of a water-soluble tris-galactoside terminated cholesterol derivative on the in vivo fate of small unilamellar vesicles in rats. Biochim Biophys Acta 816:396–402

Spanjer HH, van Galen M, Roerdink FH, Regts J, Scherphof GL (1986) Intrahepatic distribution os small unilamellar liposomes as a function of liposomal lipid composition. Biochim Biophys Acta 863:224–230

Stein O, Halperin G, Leitersdorf E, Olivecrona T, Stein Y (1984b) Lipoprotein lipase mediated uptake of non-degradable ether analogues of phosphatidylcholine and cholesteryl ester by cultured cells. Biochim Biophys Acta 795:47–59

Stein Y, Halperin G, Leitersdorf E, Dabach Y, Hollander G, Stein O (1984a) Metabolism of liposomes prepared from a labelled ether analog of 1,2-dioleoyl-sn-glycero-3-phosphocholine in the rat. Biochim Biophys Acta 793:354–364

Stevenson RW, Patel HM, Parsons JA, Ryman BE (1982) Prolonged hypoglycemic effect in diabetic dogs due to subcutaneous administration of insulin in liposomes. Diabetes 31:506–511

Storm G, Roerdink FH, Steerenberg PA, de Jong WH, Crommelin DJA (1987) Influence of lipid composition on the antitumor activity exerted by doxorubicin-containing liposomes in a rat solid tumor model. Cancer Res 47:3366–3372

Storm G, Nassander UH, Roerdink FH, Steerenberg PA, de Jong WH, Crommelin DJA (1989) In: Lopez-Berestein G, Fidler IJ (eds) Liposomes in the therapy of infectious diseases and cancer. Liss, New York, p 105

Straubinger RM, Hong K, Friend DS, Papahadjopoulos D (1983) Endocytosis of liposomes and intracellular fate of encapsualted molecules: encounter with a low-pH compartment after internalization in coated vesicles. Cell 43:1069–1079

Straubinger RM, Duzgunes N, Papahadjopoulos D (1985) pH-sensitive liposomes mediate cytoplasmic delivery of encapsulated macromolecules. FEBS Lett 179:148–154

Stukart MJ, Rijnsent A, Roos E (1987) Induction of tumoricidal activity in isolated rat liver macrophages by liposomes containing recombinant rat gamma interferon supplemented with lipopolysaccharide or muramyl dipeptide. Cancer Res 47: 3880–3885

Sunamoto J, Iwamoto K (1986) Protein-coated and polysaccharide-coated liposomes as drug carriers. CRC Crit Rev Ther Drug Carrier Syst 2:117–136

Sunamoto J, Goto M, Iida T, Hara K, Saito A, Tomonaga A (1984) Unexpected tissue distribution of liposomes coated with amylopectin derivatives and successful use in the treatment of experimental legionnaires disease. In: Gregoriadis G, Poste G, Senior J, Trouet (eds) Receptor-mediated targeting of drugs. Plenum, New York, p 359

Szoka FC, Mayhew E (1983) Alteration of liposome disposition in vivo by bilayer situated carbohydrates. Biochem Biophys Res Commun 110:140–146

Szoka FG, Jacobson K, Derzko Z, Papahadjopoulos D (1980) Fluorescence studies on the mechanism of liposome-cell interactions in vitro. Biochim Biophys Acta 600:1–18

Szoka FC, Magnusson K-E, Wojcieszyn J, Hou Y, Derzko Z, Jacobson K (1981) Use of lectins and polyethylene glycol for fusion of glycolipid-containing liposomes with eukaryotic cells. Proc Natal Acad Sci USA 78:1685–1689

Takada M, Yuzuriha T, Katayama K, Iwamoto K, Sunamoto J (1984) Increased lung uptake of liposomes coated with polysaccharides. Biochim Biophys Acta 802: 237–243

Thombre PS, Deodhar SD (1984) Inhibition of liver metastases in murine colon adenocarcinoma by liposomes containing human C-reactive protein or crude lymphokine. Cancer Immunol Immunother 16:145–150

Tomonaga A, Ueda Y, Hirota M, Saito A, Hara K, Goto M, Sunamoto J (1985) The uptake of polysaccharide-coated liposomes by alveolar macrophages. In: Leichard S, Kojima M (eds) Macrophage biology. Liss, New York, p 15

Torchilin VP (1987) Liposomes as targetable drug carriers. CRC Crit Rev Ther Drug Carrier Syst 2:65–115

Torchilin VP, Goldmacher VS, Smirnov VN (1978) Comparative studies on covalent and non-covalent immobilization of protein molecules on the surface of liposomes. Biochem Biophys Res Commun 85:983–990

Torchilin VP, Klibanov AI, Smirnov VN (1982) Phosphatidylinositol may serve as the hydrophobic anchor for immobilization of proteins on liposome surface. FEBS Lett 138:117–120

Treat J, Greenspan AR, Rahman A (1989) Liposome-encapsulated doxorubicin. Preliminary results of phase I and phase II trials. In: Lopez-Berestein G, Fidler IJ (eds) Liposomes in the therapy of infectious diseases and cancer. Liss, New York, p 353

Tremblay C, Barza M, Fiore C, Szoka F (1984) Efficacy of liposome-intercalated amphotericin B in the treatment of systemic candidiasis in mice. Antimicrob Agents Chemother 26:170–173

Tumer A, Kirby C, Senior J, Gregoriadis G (1983) Fate of cholesterol-rich liposomes after subcutaneous injection into rats. Biochim Biophys Acta 760:119–125

Van Borssum Waalkes M, Scherphof GL (1990) Liposome-incorporated 3′,5′-O-dipalmitoyl-5-fluoro-2′-deoxyuridine as a slow-release antitumor drug depot in rat liver macrophages. Select Cancer Ther 6:15–22

Van Hoesel QG, Steerenberg PA, Crommelin DJA, van Dijk A, van Oort W, Klein S, Doux JMC, de Wildt DJ, Hillen FC (1984) Reduced cardiotoxicity and nephrotoxicity with preservation of antitumor activity of doxorubicin entrapped in stable liposomes in the LOU/M Wsi rat. Cancer Res 44:3698–3705

Van Oss CJ, Gillman CF, Bronson PM, Border JR (1974a) Phagocytosis-inhibiting properties of human serum alpha-1 acid glycoprotein. Immunol Commun 3: 321–328

Van Oss CJ, Gillman CF, Bronson PM, Border JR (1974b) Opsonic properties of human serum alpha-2 HS glycoprotein. Immunol Commun 3:329–326

Van Renswoude AJBM, Westenberg P, Scherphof GL (1979) In vitro interaction of Zajdela ascites hepatoma cells with lipid vesicles. Biochim Biophys Acta 558: 22–40

Van Renswoude J, Bridges KR, Harford JB, Klausner RD (1982) Receptor-mediated endocytosis of transferrin and the uptake of Fe in K562 cells: identification of a nonlysosomal acidic compartment. Proc Natl Acad Sci USA 79:6186–6190

Van Rooijen N, van Nieuwmegen R (1984) Elimination of phagocytic cells in the spleen after intravenous injection of liposome-encapsulated dichloromethylene diphosphonate. An enzyme-histochemical study. Cell Tissue Res 238:355–358

Van Rooijen N, van Nieuwmegen R, Kamperdijk EWA (1985) Elimination of phagocytic cells after intravenous injection of liposome-encapsulated dichloromethylene phosphonate. Ultrastructural aspects of elimination of marginal zone macrophages. Virchows Arch [Cell Pathol] 49:375–383

Wang C-Y, Huang L (1987) pH-sensitive immunoliposomes mediate target cell-specific delivery and controlled expression of a foreign gene in mouse. Proc Natl Acad Sci USA 84:7851–7855

Weinstein JN, Leserman LD (1984) Liposomes as drug carriers in cancer chemotherapy. Pharmacol Ther 24:207–233

Weinstein JN, Blumenthal R, Sharrow SO, Henkart P (1978) Antibody-mediated targeting of liposomes: binding to lymphocytes does not ensure incorporation of vesicle contents into the cells. Biochim Biophys Acta 509:272

Weissman G, Korchak H, Finkelstein M, Smolen J, Hoffstein S (1978) Uptake of enzyme-laden liposomes by animal cells in vitro and in vivo. Ann NY Acad Sci 308:235–249

Wisse E, de Zanger R, Jacobs R (1982) Lobular gradients in endothelial fenestrae and sinusoidal diameter favour centrolobular exchange processes: a scanning EM study. In: Knook DL, Wisse E (eds) Sinusoidal liver cells. Elsevier, Amsterdam, p 61

Wisse E, de Zanger RB, Jacobs R, McCuskey RS (1983) Scanning electron microscope observations on the structure of portal veins, sinusoids and central veins in rat liver. Scanning electron Microsc 3:1441–1452

Woodley JF (1986) Liposomes for oral administration of drugs. Crit Rev Ther Drug Carrier Syst 2:1–18

Wright S, Huang L (1989) Antibody-directed liposomes as drug-delivery vehicles. Adv Drug Delivery Rev 3:343–389

Wu MS, Robbins JC, Bugianesi RL, Ponpipom MM, Shen TY (1981) Modified in vivo behaviour of liposomes containing synthetic glycolipids. Biochim Biophys Acta 674:19–29

Yatvin MB, Kreutz W, Horwitz BA, Shinitzky M (1980) pH-sensitive liposomes: possible clinical implications. Science 210:1253

Zborowski J, Roerdink FH, Scherphof GL (1977) Leakage of sucrose from phosphatidylcholine liposomes induced by interaction with serum albumin. Biochim Biophys Acta 497:183–191

CHAPTER 9

Antisense Oligonucleotides as Pharmacological Modulators of Gene Expression

G. DEGOLS, J.-P. LEONETTI, and B. LEBLEU

A. General Principles and Historical Background

Sequence specific interactions between nucleic acids, through Watson-Crick base pairing, or between nucleic acids and proteins, through well defined recognition rules, govern all steps of gene expression.

Specific interference with any such event would in principle provide a way to control the expression of given cellular or viral genes, the long sought target of many therapies. On a theoretical basis, adequate specificity will be attained if oligonucleotidic sequences of sufficient length can be either generated in situ from recombinant vectors or introduced through trans-membrane passage. Although figures vary slightly with the refining of theoretical considerations, it is generally accepted that 12–14-mer and 17-mer sequences, will be represented statistically once in a mRNA population and in the genome of a mammalian cell, respectively (SMITH 1983). This can be achieved through the use of what are now the classic tools of recombinant DNA technology with insertion of a gene fragment in reverse orientation (hence the term "fliped gene") downstream of any constitutively expressed or conditional promoter. Works by IZANT and WEINTRAUB (1984) on eukaryotic cells and by COLEMAN et al. (1984) on prokaryotes have convincingly demonstrated the feasibility of the approach; a large number of publications discussing similar principles have accumulated since then (GREEN et al. 1986; VAN DER KROL et al. 1988b for reviews).

The potential of antisense oligonucleotides has been well demonstrated through the generation of transgenic petunias expressing various patterns of pigmentation (VAN DER KROL et al. 1988a); this was achieved by the expression in flipped orientation of the gene encoding chalcone synthase, an enzyme controlling flavonoid biosynthesis and therefore flower pigmentation. A similar approach has enabled researchers with both academic and industrial affiliations to down-regulate the expression in transgenic tomatoes of polygalacturonase, the enzyme that weakens the structure of fruit cell walls upon ripening (SMITH et al. 1988). The commercial impact of such an achievement will be highly significant if ongoing field trials confirm laboratory experiments. These two examples demonstrate the feasibility of "antisense technology" for generating strains with improved genetic characters. We are evidently still very far from achieving similar goals in mammals for both ethical and technical reasons; somatic genetic diseases will eventually provide applications of antisense in humans. Besides the ethical implications, two major technical difficulties are encountered with this approach: (1) the choice of an efficient target for the antisense RNA and (2) the more classical problems of its expression. We will not dwell more on these aspects; several comprehensive reviews have been published on the subject in the last few years including papers by GREEN et al. (1986) and VAN DER KROL et al. (1988b).

The other method discussed here in more detail consists of introducing pre-formed synthetic oligonucleotides into cells. Although conceptually very simple, as pointed out above, this has proved to be less easy to achieve than initially expected in in vitro studies and has yet to be performed convincingly in vivo. Synthesizing oligonucleotides at the appropriate scale, evaluating their pharmacodynamic properties, promoting their transmembrane passage, and understanding the conditions of their interaction with their intracellular targets are problems which chemists, molecular and cell biologists, and pharmacologists will have to solve before they become part of the therapeutic resources.

Three groups unquestionably deserve the credit for having pioneered this approach. MILLER et al. (1974, 1979), at John Hopkins University (Baltimore, MD, USA) cleverly set out to synthesize neutral oligonucleotide analogues, i.e., phosphotriesters and methylphosphonates, on the assumption that strongly charged unmodified oligonucleotides would not cross cell membranes; their achievements will be discussed in more detail in following sections. ZAMECNIK and STEPHENSON (1978) and ZAMECNIK et al. (1986), at the Worcester Foundation (Shrewsbury, MA, USA) used charged oligonucleotides as a way to down-regulate the expression of retroviruses, e.g., Rous sarcoma virus and more recently human immunodeficiency virus (HIV). Although somewhat "heretical" to some of us initially, their work turned out to be based on solid ground since oligo- and polynucleotides indeed appear to be internalized into intact cells, at least in vitro. Finally, the longstanding efforts of D.G. KNORRE et al. (1985), at the Siberian branch of the USSR Academy of Sciences, have provided us with a collection of invaluable tools in nucleic acid chemistry, some of which will be described in following sections.

The pace of research has accelerated over the last few years; workshops are now regularly held which are devoted totally to antisense technology. They attract an increasing number of participants from academic institutions, governmental agencies, and industry; half a dozen biotechnology companies have appeared to explore possible applications of the technology.

B. Artificial Control of Gene Expression by Synthetic Oligonucleotides: An Overview of Problems and Potential

As pointed out above, the number of publications dealing with the use of antisense oligonucleotides as agents controlling gene expression has increased dramatically in the past 5 years. A list of reviews covering particular aspects of this or relevant related fields in more detail is given at the end of this chapter (see Appendix); the reader should consult them for a more exhaustive coverage.

As expected, most of the published literature deals with the use of antisense oligonucleotides to down-regulate the expression of viral, parasitic, or cellular genes as an alternative to classical genetic analysis. In their excellent review, VAN DER KROL et al. (1988b) list more than one hundred references dealing with the use of antisense synthetic oligonucleotides or antisense RNA; more has been accomplished since then. Although it is obviously difficult to obtain an accurate figure concerning failures, it is clear that difficulties have been frequently encountered.

A recent paper clearly illustrates the problems and limitations arising from the use of antisense oligonucleotides. A 15 base-long unmodified oligonucleotide complementary to BFGF (basic fibroblast growth factor) mRNA specifically inhibits BFGF production in melanoma cells (BECKER et al. 1989). The oligomer concentrations needed, ranging from 5 to 50 µM in in vitro experiments, require efficient and large scale oligonucleotide synthesis. Such high concentrations reflect two of the present drawbacks of this technique: The first concerns the metabolic stability of oligonucleotides in biological fluids or cells; however, cell culture media can easily be manipulated in order to decrease nuclease content using heat inactivated serum (as described in the above mentioned paper) or defined cell culture media. Nothing of this sort can be done for the intracellular stability of oligonucleotides, except for the utilization of analogues of increased resistance towards nucleases. The second concerns the ionic character of oligonucleotides which limits their cellular uptake. Various attempts to ease this problem will be described in a following section. Other frequently encountered problems include the choice of the target, which remains empirical. The most commonly used target is the AUG initiation codon of the mRNA, as was the case for BFGF inhibition. However, the efficiency of a selected target is difficult to predict and can vary with the nature of the oligonucleotide analogues. Moreover, secondary and tertiary target structures, interaction with proteins, and recognition by unwinding activities in intact cells are essentially unknown. Controls are absolutely essential since several cases have been reported of unexpected non-sequence specific effects of synthetic oligonucleotides. For instance in the above mentioned example, hybridization competition by sense oligonucleotide, or exogenous BFGF itself, reversed the growth inhibitory activity of antisense oligonucleotides; omission of the oligonucleotide or use of mismatched oligonucleotides also constitute frequently used negative controls.

C. Oligonucleotide Chemistry and Modifications

The phosphodiester linkage can be hydrolyzed by nucleases, and its anionic charge limits the uptake of the oligonucleotides in cultured cells. Therefore much effort was made to synthesize oligonucleotide analogues with modified internucleotidic linkages (Table 1). An enhanced stability was also obtained by modifying the sugar residue or 3' and /or 5' ends of the oligonucleotide. One of the major concerns in the search for new analogues is to achieve good metabolic stability while maintaining the required specificity for target recognition and antisense action (e.g., recognition of the hybrid by RNase H) and avoiding the occurrence of toxic catabolic products.

I. Modifications of the Phosphodiester Backbone

1. Nonionic Oligonucleotides

The first described modification was the ethylation of the phosphate group leading to an ethyl-phosphotriester nonionic linkage (MILLER et al. 1974), supposedly more favorable for diffusion across cellular membranes. Indeed, these analogues were shown to be taken up by cells where they were deethylated within 24 h and degraded (MILLER et al. 1977). Only a few further reports describe the use of these oligonucleotides.

The methylphosphonate chemistry developed by MILLER et al. (1979) is an alternative to the ethylphosphotriester oligonucleotides previously described. In these analogues, an ionizable oxygen atom of the phosphodiester

Table 1. Backbone modification of antisense oligonucleotides

Phosphodiester bond	R'			References
	$-O-\overset{\overset{\displaystyle \|}{\|}}{\underset{\underset{\displaystyle \|}{\|}}{P}}-O-$			
	R			
Unmodified	R=O	R'=⁻O		STEC et al. (1984)
Phosphorothioate	R=O	R'⁻=S		GRANDAS et al. (1989)
Phosphorodithioates	R=S⁻	R'=S		MILLER et al. (1979)
Methylphosphonate	R=Me	R'=O		MILLER et al. (1974)
Ethylphosphotriester	R=Et	R'=O		MORI et al. (1989)
Phosphoroselenoate	R=O⁻	R'=Se		FROEHLER and MATTEUCCI (1988)
Phosphoramidates	R=NHBU,	—N	NH$_2^+$	AGRAWAL et al. (1988)
	—N	O	R'=O	

linkage was substituted by a methyl group. These analogues are highly resistant towards nuclease degradation and diffuse across the cellular membrane (MARCUS-SEKURA et al. 1987). They have been successfully used in the control of various cellular and viral genes, for instance the *ras* oncogene (YU et al. 1989) and vesicular stomatitis (AGRIS et al. 1986), herpes simplex 1 (SMITH et al. 1986), or human immunodeficiency (SARIN et al. 1988) viral infections. However, the introduction of the methyl group gives rise to diastereoisomers which can be detrimental to hybridization (QUARTIN and WETMUR 1989). This could explain the high concentrations $(50-200\,\mu M)$ generally needed for an effective antisense inhibition. The introduction of stereoselective synthesis of P-homochiral oligonucleotide methylphosphonate could resolve this drawback (LESNIKOWSKI et al. 1988). Moreover, RNase H, which is believed to be involved (see below) in the potentiation of some antisense effects through cleavage of the target mRNA, does not recognize the target RNA-methylphosphonate hybrids (MAHER and DOLNICK 1988). FURDON et al. (1989) have synthesized hybrid oligonucleotides containing only a few methylphosphonate residues; the stability of these hybrid molecules was markedly increased and RNase H recognition was restored.

2. Isoelectric Oligonucleotides

Another modification of the phosphate linkage consists in the substitution of an ionizable oxygen by a sulfur atom (STEC et al. 1984). As with methylphosphonates, these phosphorothioates analogues are resistant to nuclease degradation and are synthesized as a mixture of diastereoisomers; however, the melting points of the hybrids formed with complementary targets are not as severely affected as those of unmodified oligonucleotides. Phosphorothioate analogues as inhibitors of HIV multiplication have in particular been studied; they are active in a $5-50\,\mu M$ concentration range. In vitro, the phosphorothioate oligonucleotide-RNA hybrids were shown to be recognized by RNase H (STEIN et al. 1988). They seem to act by two different mechanisms: a non-sequence dependent effect, through non-specific interactions most probably with proteins, (MATSUKURA et al. 1987) and sequence specific effects though base pairing with target sequences (MATSUKURA et al. 1989). The relative efficiency of different analogues were compared in the specific inhibition of CAT gene expression in transfected cells (MARCUS-SEKURA et al. 1987). Phosphorothioate oligonucleotides were twice as potent as methylphosphonates and four times more potent than unmodified oligonucleotides.

Interesting prospects are provided by the recent synthesis of achiral phophorodithioates oligonucleotides (GRANDAS et al. 1989). Preliminary results obtained in cell-free experiments show that these analogues inhibit HIV and avian myeloblastosis virus (AMV) reverse transcriptase at concentrations lower than phosphorothioates (CARUTHERS, personal communication); however, no hybridization data have been reported.

The substitution of the ionizable oxygen atom by selenium gives phosphoroselenoate analogues. These compounds are isoelectric and closely isostructural with the normal phosphodiester oligonucleotides. They have, unfortunately, decreased hybridization properties, are less active than phosphorothioates in the nonspecific inhibition of HIV, and are more cytotoxic to cultured cells (MORI et al. 1989).

3. Phosphoramidate Oligonucleotides

The replacement of the ionizable oxygen of the phosphodiester linkage by primary and secondary amines was facilitated by the introduction of H phosphonate chemistry (FROEHLER and MATTEUCCI 1988). While resistant to nuclease degradation, these oligonucleotides form unstable duplexes. However, they have been used successfully, within the same concentration range as phosphorothioates, in the nonspecific inhibition of HIV multiplication (AGRAWAL et al. 1988).

The phosphate backbone-modified oligonucleotides described in this section are diastereoisomeric mixtures and form less stable hybrids than normal phosphodiester oligonucleotides. However, the contribution of the P atom chirality to the overall destabilization of the hybrids may be less than expected and a distortion of the backbone due to stereoelectric factors has to be considered as well (FROEHLER and MATTEUCCI 1988; IMBACH, personal communication).

II. Modifications of the Sugar Moiety

1. Sugar-Modified Oligonucleotides

Another approach to modifying an oligonucleotide involves the alteration of the sugar moieties (Table 2). The reversion of the configuration of the 1' carbon atom of the sugar residue results in α-oligonucleotides analogues (MORVAN et al. 1986). These analogues are resistant to nucleases (BACON et al. 1988) and form stable duplexes in parallel orientation with RNA (GAGNOR et al. 1987). In vitro the hybrids between α-oligonucleotide and RNA are not recognized by RNase H (GAGNOR et al. 1989). This could explain their poor efficiency in translation arrest: no inhibition of interleukin-6 mRNA translation was observed in a reticulocyte lysate with an α-oligonucleotide directed against the initiation codon region (GAGNOR et al. 1987). However, at the same concentration, an α-oligonucleotide targeted against the cap region of the rabbit β-globin mRNA specifically inhibited its translation (BERTRAND et al. 1989). In this case interferences with the binding of translation initiation factors could explain the inhibitory effect. The poor efficiency of α-analogues was confirmed in intact cells, since an α-oligonucleotide directed against a vesicular stomatitis virus (VSV) mRNA did not exhibit antiviral activity compared to the unmodified oligonucleotide (LEONETTI et al. 1988). Recently, phosphorothioate analogues of α-oligonucleotides were tested for their anti-

Table 2. Sugar modified oligonucleotides

Sugar modifications		References
Deoxyribose	HO — Base / O / O H	
Alpha-deoxyribose	HO / O / Base / O H	MORVAN et al. 1986
Ribose	HO — Base / O / O O / H H	
2'-O-Methyl	HO — Base / O / O O / H Me	SPROAT et al. 1989

HIV activity; the homopolymeric dC$_{28}$ and the anti-rev α-phosphorothioate sequences appear to be as active as phosphorothioate in the regular β configuration (RAYNER et al. 1990).

2. Oligoribonucleotide Analogues

Since the availability of automated RNA synthesis, a few examples of oligoribonucleotide analogues have been reported. (2'-O-methyl)ribonucleotides present interesting properties: less susceptibility to RNase and nucleolytic enzymes, stabilization to alkaline treatment, and stable formation of heteroduplexes with RNA (SPROAT et al. 1989). This analogue has been efficiently utilized in the form of chimeric molecules with interspersed ribo- and deoxyribonucleotides to cleave RNA with RNase H (SHIBAHARA et al. 1987); it was also used to study snRNP structure and to inhibit splicing (LAMOND et al. 1989). Recently, the synthesis of phosphorothioate analogues of (2'-O-methyl)ribonucleotides has been described and the relative efficiency of these ribonucleotide analogues was tested in the inhibition of HIV;

only the phosphorothioate or the partially phosphorothioate form of the analogue exhibited antiviral effects (SHIBAHARA et al. 1989).

III. Functionalization of Oligonucleotide Ends

Progress in oligonucleotide chemistry has been used to synthesize analogues, circumventing some of the problems listed above; much is still under way and we will focus mainly on derivatives already shown to be active in intact cells. The covalent linkage of reagents to the end of the oligonucleotide can increase its affinity for the nucleic acid target and also protect it from exonucleases; some cause an irreversible alteration of the target. Different approaches were investigated (Table 3), but only a few have been shown to be

Table 3. Antisense oligonucleotide functionalizations

Functionalizations	References
Trimethylpsoralen	KULKA et al. (1989)
N-2-chloroethyl-N-methylaminobenzylamine	KNORRE et al. (1987)
2-Methoxy-6-chloro-9-amino-acidine	VERSPIEREN et al. (1987) ZERIAL et al. (1987)

Photoactivable (covalent linkage)

$R'—O—P—O—NH—(CH_2)_2—NH—CH_2$

Alkylation of DNA (covalent linkage)

Intercalation in DNA (stabilization of hybridization)

usable in vivo in their present form. For example, oligonucleotides linked to free radical generating groups, i.e., EDTA Fe (BOUTORIN et al. 1984), phenanthroline Cu (CHEN and SIGMAN 1986), etc., are of interest in cell-free experiments to generate sequence specific damage to mRNA, or single- or double-stranded DNA. However, target degradation by free radicals is slow, and limits their utilization in cells.

Vlassov and co-workers have developed oligonucleotides linked to alkylating reagents (V. KNORRE et al. 1985). They were shown to react spontaneously with bases after hybridization with their nucleic acid target. Successful inhibition of the tick-borne encephalitis virus was reported even in vivo after intrathecal inoculation of mice (KNORRE et al. 1989). However, alkylating reagents may react before reaching their expected target, creating a potential source of nonspecific effects and toxicity.

Cell uptake was supposed to decrease with increasing oligonucleotide length. Since less stable hybrids are formed with short oligonucleotides, they were linked to intercalating agents in order to stabilize them (HELENE et al. 1985). One of the most commonly used intercalating agents is acridine. A 12-mer oligonucleotide directed to the 5' end of the mini-exon of *Trypanosoma brucei* mRNA inhibits cell-free translation more efficiently when linked to acridine (VERSPIEREN et al. 1987); such intercalating agent conjugated oligonucleotides kill cultured trypanosomes at high concentration $(80\,\mu M)$. Sequence specific antiviral effects were also observed on type A influenza virus in cell cultures (ZERIAL et al. 1987).

The intercalating properties and photoreactivity with pyrimidine bases of UV activatable reagents, such as psoralen (SHI and HEARST 1986), offer interesting prospects. Methylphosphonate oligonucleotides linked to psoralen induce 80% photoadduct formation on their that nucleic acid targets (LEE et al. 1988). This potentiates the biological activity of antisense oligonucleotides: indeed, a dodecamer methylphosphonate linked to psoralen inhibits 98% of herpes simplex virus multiplication at $5\,\mu M$, compared to $100\,\mu M$ with a methylphosphonate oligonucleotide (KULKA et al. 1989).

D. Internalization Pathway of Antisense Oligonucleotides and Alternative Methods to Increased Cellular Uptake

I. Mechanism of Uptake of Oligonucleotides in Cells

As mentioned previously, the prevailing view is that polyanionic molecules such as oligonucleotides can only permeate poorly through cellular membranes. Nonetheless, biological effects are obtained with unmodified antisense oligonucleotides, generally at high concentrations; this implies the delivery of functional oligonucleotides into the cytoplasmic compartment.

LOKE et al. (1989) demonstrated that fluorescently labelled oligonucleotides are actively transported across cellular membranes in a temperature dependant way. In a similar approach YAKUBOV et al. (1989) reported two internalization pathways. At high concentration a fluid phase endocytosis seems to be predominant, while at low concentration, when a substantial part of the oligonucleotide is adsorbed at the cell surface, uptake is mediated by an adsorbtive process involving the acidic compartments of endocytosis. This second internalization pathway suggests the presence of (specific) cell surface binding proteins involved in transport. Indeed, the two groups identified an 80 kD a membrance protein which can be affinity labelled with oligonucleotides. The biological role of this protein, and the mechanisms by which oligonucleotides are released in the cytosol remain to be ascertained. A better knowledge of this mechanism will eventually be helpful in the design of new analogues with improved uptake properties.

II. Modifications of Oligonucleotides to Increase Cell Uptake

In order to increase the uptake of oligonucleotides into cells, different alternatives were investigated (Fig. 1). The pioneer work of Ts'o, Miller, and their co-workers demonstrate the value of nonionic methylphosphonate oligonucleotides. As mentioned above, these analogues were designed to diffuse passively across cellular membranes (MARCUS-SEKURA et al. 1987) and have been used successfully to inhibit the expression of several viral and cellular genes. Their uptake is clearly different from anionic oligonucleotides: in competition experiments LOKE et al. (1989) demonstrated that methylphosphonate oligonucleotides do not block the uptake of fluorescently tagged phosphorothioate or phosphodiester oligonucleotides. Prospects and limitations of these analogues have been discussed in the preceding section.

The modification of oligonucleotides with cholesterol moieties was shown to enhance the uptake of oligonucleotides linked to an alkylating agent by about two orders of magnitude in L929 cells; this can be attributed to an increased interaction of the oligonucleotide with the cell membrane (BOUTORIN et al. 1989). In the same way, LETSINGER et al. (1989) reported an increased antiviral efficiency of phosphorothiates or unmodified oligonucleotides linked to cholesterol; only nonspecific anti-HIV activity of homopolymers was tested.

Linkage of oligonucleotides to poly-L-lysine (PLL), a well known polycationic carrier, significantly decreases both the concentration required for the inhibition of VSV multiplication (LEMAITRE et al. 1987) and HIV cytopathogenicity (STEVENSON and IVERSEN 1989) as compared to unmodified oligonucleotides (unpublished results) or to methylphosphonates (AGRIS et al. 1986). PLL is taken up by the cell through a nonspecific adsorbtive endocytosis which concentrates the transported molecules into the acidic compartments (SHEN and RYSER 1978; LEONETTI et al. 1990a). The efficiency of PLL as a carrier differs greatly between cell lines. Moreover, it is

Methylphosphonates (diffusion across cellular membranes)
Miller et al. 1979

Linkage to cholesterol (unknown mechanism)
Boutorin et al. 1989

Linkage to poly-L-lysine (nonspecific adsorbtive endocytosis)
Lemaitre et al. 1987

Fusion liposomes (fusion with cellular membranes)
Loke et al. 1989

Targeted liposomes (endocytosis through specific receptor interactions)
Leonetti et al. 1990

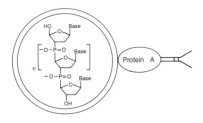

Fig.1. Modifications improving oligonucleotide uptake. The proposed mechanism of internalization is indicated in *parentheses*

not yet understood how a sufficient amount of oligonucleotide can escape from the acidic compartments without being degraded and go on to reach its cytoplasmic or nuclear target. Thus, passage from the acidic compartments to the cytoplasm is a common limitation to the delivery of unmodified oligonucleotides or PLL conjugates.

To bypass the cellular uptake machinery and introduce oligonucleotides directly into the cytoplasm, unmodified and phosphorothioate oligonucleotides were encapsulated into fusion liposomes. An inhibition of c-*myc* oncogene expression was observed in HL 60 cells with an encapsulated phosphorothioate oligonucleotide directed to the c-*myc* mRNA translation initiation site, while in the same conditions unencapsulated oligonucleotides were inefficient (LOKE et al. 1988); unfortunately, cells had to be exposed to polyethylene glycol. Fusogenic liposomes (ARAD et al. 1986) or pH-sensitive immunoliposomes (CONNORS et al. 1984) have been used efficiently to deliver plasmid DNA into cells and could offer interesting prospects for the delivery of oligonucleotides. More recently we encapsulated an antisense oligonucleotide directed to the VSV N protein mRNA into antibody targeted liposomes (LEONETTI et al. 1990b). With this technique, oligonucleotides are active in amounts one to two orders of magnitude lower than those reported for unencapsulated oligonucleotides. The major interest of such a liposome approach is to allow a double specificity: (1) a particular cell selected with the targeting antibody on the liposome and (2) a particular mRNA in the cell selected by complementarity with the oligonucleotide. However, the targeted liposomes are taken up through the endocytic compartments (STRAUBINGER et al. 1983) and the problems of intracellular distribution raised above are not overcome. Fusogenic liposomes targeted with antibodies would, in theory, represent a more efficient alternative, since they combine the advantages of the two techniques, direct passage across the cellular membrane and specificity for a cell surface determinant.

In the same way, the microinjection of oligonucleotides should allow their specific delivery into the nucleus or cytoplasm. This offers interesting prospects for studies of intracellular oligonucleotide metabolism, distribution, etc.; however, no published data are available except for *Xenopus laevis* oocytes (DASH et al. 1987). Interesting results in mammalian cells were obtained with double-stranded oligonucleotides corresponding to the consensus cAMP response element (BERKOWITZ et al. 1989). The response has to be very sensitive since only a small amount of cells can be microinjected. Electropermeabilization (for a review see KNIGHT and SCRUTTON 1986) can be potentially employed to affect a larger number of cells but is limited by the small amount of material introduced into cells; preliminary results have reported uptake but not yet any biological activity (BASILE et al. 1989).

E. Mechanism of Action of Antisense Oligonucleotides

Among all the utilizations of synthetic oligonucleotides as modulators of gene expression (Fig. 2), the antisense strategy generally appears to be the most frequently used. The oligonucleotides are designed to hybridize to a selected complementary sequence on the target mRNA or its precursors, such as the 5′ end, the translation initiation site, or the acceptor or donor splicing sites.

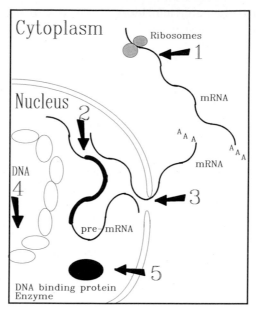

Fig.2. Possible intracellular targets of synthetic oligonucleotides. Synthetic oligonucleotides have been designed to interfere with cytoplasmic mRNA expression (*1*) or with pre-mRNA nuclear processing (*2*); possible interferences with nucleocytoplasmic transport (*3*) should be considered, as documented for antisense RNA (KIM and WOLD 1985). Direct interference with DNA (*4*) for instance, through triple helix formation, or with DNA binding proteins (*5*) represents an interesting alternative prospect

As an example, antiviral effects were obtained with an oligonucleotide directed to the splice acceptor junction of herpes simplex virus I immediate early mRNA 4; this was consequent to an inhibition of splicing since the unspliced form of this RNA accumulated in oligonucleotide treated cells (KULKA et al. 1989).

The mechanisms of action of antisense oligonucleotides may differ with the target site and the choice of the oligonucleotide analogue. In addition, no accurate picture of mRNA or pre-mRNA secondary and tertiary structure can be provided using existing algorithms (EHRESMANN et al. 1987) and the various structural protein binding sites (mRNPs, hnRNPs, snRNPs) are almost completely ignored. Several reports have shown that translation inhibition by antisense oligonucleotides is drastically dependent upon the target of the oligonucleotide. As an example, the translation of Sendai virus nucleocapsid protein and phosphoprotein mRNAs in rabbit reticulocyte lysate is blocked by an oligonucleotide complementary to a site adjacent to the cap site (GUPTA 1987).The inhibitory effect decreases with an oligonucleotide complementary to the translation initiation site and is abolished with an oligonucleotide complementary to the coding region. The inhibiting capacity of an oligonucleotide directed to the 5′ noncoding region can be explained by secondary structures generated by the oligonucleotide hybridization, which prevent the binding of the translation initiation factors (LAWSON et al. 1986). This dependence on the target site is less pronounced in in vitro translation experiments with wheat germ lysate (MINSHULL and HUNT 1987) and in *Xenopus laevis* oocytes. DASH et al. (1987) demonstrated that the microinjection of short oligonucleotides in *Xenopus* oocytes leads to a degradation of the complementary mRNA by means of an RNAse H-like activity. Furthermore, complementation of reticulocyte lysates with RNase H significantly improves the translation arrest by complementary oligonucleotides (MINSHULL and HUNT 1987). This enzyme is generally detected in the nuclei of mammalian cells and is able to hydrolyze the RNA strand of an RNA-DNA hybrid; it was thus suggested that an endogenous RNAse H-like activity may be largely responsible for the specific inhibiting properties of antisense oligonucleotides observed in cultured cells. In line with this assumption, treatment of normal human T lymphocytes with an oligonucleotide directed to c-*myb* mRNA indeed leads to a decrease of c-*myb* protein level correlated with a decrease of c-*myb*. mRNA (GEWIRTZ et al. 1989); this suggests an oligonucleotide-mediated degradation of the mRNA target. The exact implication of an RNAse H activity in intact cells remains to be ascertained since oligonucleotide analogues unrecognized by RNAse H, such as methylphosphonates (WALDER 1988) or α-oligonucleotides (BERTRAND et al. 1989), are efficient at least in cell-free experiments on certain targets.

Additional difficulties might result from the melting of antisense-target hybrids by helix unwinding activities. The point has been raised by the recent work of BASS and WEINTRAUB (1987) and REBAGLIATI and MELTON (1987) as an explanation for the inefficiency in *Xenopus laevis* eggs of antisense RNA sequences previously tested for their ability to down-regulate various gene products in *Xenopus laevis* oocytes. More troubling still, this developmentally regulated helicase turned out to be an RNA modifying enzymatic activity converting adenosine to inosine (BASS and WEINTRAUB 1988). Unwinding activities might be of more general occurrence as WAGNER and NISHIKURA (1988) reported a mammalian unwinding activity co-regulated with the cell cycle. This is no surprise since DNA and RNA bear intramolecular secondary structures which have to be melted for gene expression to take place. Knowledge of the regulation of such activities and of their mode of action might be of importance to devise more efficient antisense oligonucleotides.

F. Biological Potential of Synthetic Oligonucleotides

The antisense approach is generally based on the inhibition of mRNA expression, but additional targets have to be considered in some specific situations. For instance in our own studies (DEGOLS et al. 1989) on the antiviral activity of oligonucleotides directed against (VSV), it was found that oligonucleotides complementary to the so-called intergenic sequence (a largely conserved genomic sequence critical to both viral mRNA polyadenylation and transcription re-initiation on the polycistronic genomic RNA) was indeed a very effective target. On the other hand, the "leader" sequence (the polymerase primary binding site on the viral genome) could not be used as a target for oligonucleotides in the same experimental system. Such observations illustrate the difficulty of predicting effective targets.

Antisense technology relies on the well known interaction properties of double-stranded nucleic acids. More recently, homopolypurines and homopolypyrimidines were shown to hybridize in a triple helix on double-stranded nucleic acids via the formation of Hoogsteen hydrogen bondings (HOOGSTEEN 1959). This property allows interaction of interfering oligonucleotide with double-stranded DNA, a less abundant target than mRNA (HELENE and TOOLME 1990 for a recent review). Promising results were obtained with an oligonucleotide designed to bind to DNA at the 5′ end of the human c-*myc* gene (COONEY et al. 1988); cell-free transcription experiments show a correlation between triplex formation and the repression of c-*myc* mRNA synthesis. Interestingly the target sequence on the c-*myc* gene is a binding site for transcription initiation factors. Interference between triple helix formation and the binding of the transcription factor Sp I on DNA has also been described in *Escherichia coli* cellular extracts (MAHER et al. 1989). At first, physicochemical analyses were focused on triple helix hybridization between polypurine and polypyrimidine sequences; however, alternative possibilities may exist since this new code has not yet been broken down completely. Indeed, heterologous sequences have recently been shown to hybridize successfully in triple helixes (GRIFFIN and DERVAN 1989), which enlarges the application field to various sequences. Moreover, some base modifications (5-methylcytosine) can increase the stability of the hybrid under physiological conditions (MAHER et al. 1989).

Inhibition of protein binding on DNA is an interesting way to modulating gene expression; it is flexible since it allows potentially either the inhibition of gene expression through competition with transcriptional activating factors or the activation through competition with inhibiting factors. Beyond the formation of triple helixes, it is possible to interfere with DNA binding proteins by titrating these factors with double-stranded oligonucleotides carrying their recognition sequence. Gel retardation and southwestern blot experiments have widely demonstrated the usefulness of double-stranded oligonucleotides for this purpose. Recently, microinjected double-stranded oligonucleotides carrying the consensus cAMP response element (CRE) have been shown to abolish the induction of endogenous c-*fos* gene by cAMP (BERKOWITZ et al. 1989).

Numerous studies on HIV have pointed out the possibility of inhibiting virus multiplication with non-sequence specific oligonucleotides; an approach somewhat different from the preceding ones. Phosphorothioates oligonucleotides (dC_{28}) were the most potent (MATSUKURA et al. 1987) and the antiviral effects are presumably due to the interaction of the oligonucleotide with viral reverse transcriptase (MAJUMDAR et al. 1989). Cell-free experiments indicate that dC_{28} is a linear competitive inhibitor of HIV reverse transcriptase. Not only lentivirus reverse transcriptases are sensitive to dC_{28} as initially thought, since similar results were obtained with HSV2 induced DNA polymerase. In contrast, this compound showed less inhibition of human DNA polymerases α, β, and λ as well as HSV1 and Epstein-Barr virus induced DNA polymerase.

The use of synthetic oligoribonucleotides offers a number of possible alternatives to the existing strategies for gene expression modulation. Indeed, short oligoribonucleotides could conceivably be useful to mimicking protein binding sites, for instance viral polymerase binding sites, pre-mRNA processing sites, or translational repressors, thereby interfering with specific events in viral or cellular gene expression. Their use as mere substitutes to oligodeoxyribonucleotides as antisense moieties could be envisaged as well, although no predictions can be made as far as relative efficiencies are concerned. Indeed, RNA-RNA hybrids have a greater stability than RNA-DNA ones; on the other hand RNAs are usually metabolically less stable than DNAs and no amplification of the antisense effect through RNase H processing of the hybrids will occur in this case. Another interesting prospect is the now well established catalytic activities associated with RNAs, recognition of which resulted from original studies of the sequence specific endoribonuclease activities of *Tetrahymena* ribozyme (MCSWIGGEN and CECH 1989) or RNase P associated H_1 RNA (BARTKIEWICZ et al. 1989). Synthetic ribozymes have been constructed and shown to be active both in cell-free extracts (HASELOFF and GERLACH 1988; UHLENBECK 1987) and in intact cells (CAMERON and JENNINGS 1989); whether the down-regulation of the reporter gene, CAT in the latter example, directly results from RNA cleavage remains, however, to be established. The relative efficiencies of ribozyme, antisense RNA and antisense DNA as specific inhibitors of U7 snRNP–dependent histone pre-mRNA processing have been compared in nuclear extracts. Antisense DNA is less active than antisense RNA but inhibits the processing reaction in an irreversible manner; ribozymes have not proven very efficient in this particular study (COTTEN et al. 1989). It is thus obviously too early to evaluate the relative potentials of these approaches.

Selective cleavage of RNA or DNA can be obtained with hybrid molecules consisting of an oligonucleotide fused to a nuclease; the oligonucleotide ensures the sequence specificity of the cleavage. Interesting results were obtained using hybrid molecules with staphylococcal nuclease (ZUCKERMANN and SCHULTZ 1989) and with the class II restriction endonuclease *Fok* I (KIM et al. 1988). This particular approach will benefit from progresses in the synthesis of oligonucleotide-peptide conjugates and more generally from the design of peptide targeted oligonucleotides.

G. Prospectives of In Vivo Utilization of Antisense Oligonucleotides

Whatever their potential as demonstrated by in vitro or cell-free experiments, the in vivo use of antisense oligonucleotides is still untested. There are essentially two types of basic problems to be faced (i) synthesis of the oligonucleotides at the adequate degree of purity and scale and (ii) determination of their pharmacological properties in terms of toxicity and bio-availability. The available information is still very scarce as expected for such a novel and still expensive approach. It is the authors' feeling that the use of (targeted-specific) transporters will be required to eventually turn oligonucleotides into useful clinical products; similar issues have been raised for peptide drugs as well (EPPSTEIN and LONGENECKER 1988).

The widespread use of synthetic oligonucleotides as molecular biology tools is due to the availability of efficient and automated methods for their synthesis. Most of the oligonucleotide analogue chemistry reviewed in the preceding section has been adapted to solid phase synthesis with good yields on commercial automatic DNA synthesizers. However, the amounts and cost of material required even for in vitro studies somewhat limits experimentation. As an example, the synthesis of material required for liposome entrapment at the present efficiency of encapsulation requires two to three rounds of synthesis with a 1 μmole reaction and costs around US 1000.

A significant scale-up has already been achieved, by Applied Biosystem and Gilead Sciences for instance, and animal toxicity studies have been started. No acute toxicity has been found in the few studies reported so far on unmodified phosphodiesters (GOODCHILD et al. 1988), methylphosphonates (SARIN et al. 1988), or phosphorothioates (AGRAWAL et al. 1988). A preliminary study (reviewed in ZON 1989) indicates that unmodified and phosphorothioate oligonucleotides were slightly mutagenic, and, interestingly, no significant differences in mutagenicity were observed with the relative intracellular availability. A high clearance rate ($t^{1/2}$ in plasma of around 10 min) with elimination in the urine has been reported with unmodified oligonucleotides injected in mice (BABKIN et al. 1988).

A dramatic decrease in manufacturing costs, the use of more potent analogues, and/or a better control of their administration will be required, as reviewed at the recent NCI-NIAID sponsored workshop on "Oligodeoxynucleotides as antisense inhibitors of gene expression: therapeutic implications" (ROTHENBERG et al. 1989).

A wide range of drug delivery systems has been developed and some show interesting prospects for clinical application. They belong essentially to two classes, synthetic or natural polymers (polypeptides for instance) and particulate materials lipid vesicles and nanospheres for instance). This very active field has been reviewed many times (see for example TOMLINSON 1987; JULIANO 1987). The credibility of using such tools for the delivery of antisense oligonucleotides to intact cells relies on the following considerations: (a) Whatever the progress in oligonucleotide chemistry, the cost will probably remain high unless a real breakthrough is made. (b) Although prospects for their use as catalytic moieties exist (see preceding section), oligonucleotides generally have to be used at a relatively high effector to target ratio; direct interference with gene expression at the chromatin level might change this situation but represents an even more remote prospect. (c) Oligonucleotides are rapidly eliminated from body fluids through nuclease degradation (this can be partly overcome by the use of suitable analogues as reviewed in previous sections) and rapid clearance (see above). (d) Antisense oligonucleotides should by definition be specific for their intracellular target(s), at variance with many more conventional drugs; thus, blocking the expression of a gene (for instance, the overexpression of an oncogene) in a given tissue or cell type might be advantageous. However, the catabolism of oligonucleotide analogues or conjugates will inevitably liberate degradation products with their own potential nonspecific toxicity (e.g., the intercalating agent of acridine oligonucleotide derivatives or the alkylating moiety of the corresponding conjugates). Even unmodified oligonucleotides might turn out to be deleterious if they accumulate in certain cell types. (e) The in vivo administration of oligonucleotides implies their efficient transport specific barriers (for instance the mucosal epithelium following nonparenteral administration), in addition to the cellular one.

As described above, PLL has successfully been used to internalize unmodified oligonucleotides with antiviral or antiproliferative activity in vitro; immunogenicity and toxicity delay their in vivo utilization. Polysulfated polyanions have been shown to enhance the specific biological activity of oligonucleotide – PLL conjugates and to diminish their nonspecific toxicity (LEONETTI et al. unpublished results). Since the in vitro tolerance of cultured cells to PLL conjugates has been shown to be enhanced by polyanions, further studies including in vivo ones might be worth pursuing. Such tools obviously lack targeting properties; more sophisticated PLL-based delivery systems might be constructed and tested for oligonucleotide delivery, for instance neoglycoproteins with various lectin-recognition properties (WU and WU 1988). Alternatively, direct coupling of oligonucleotides to cell surface specific determinants (for instance, tumor specific antigens, transferrin receptors) might be conceived. It has to be recalled, however, that antisense modulation of gene expression requires the functional internalization of a relatively large number of molecules into target cells, at variance with the agents studied so far. The abundance of the surface determinant, its rate of recycling, and its mode of internalization will be critical factors in this respect. Coupling of several oligonucleotide moieties to an inert carrier might be a solution to both the amount of carried drug and to a full maintenance of cell surface recognition properties. The difficulties experienced in the use of polypeptide conjugates such as bioavailability and intracellular trafficking of the carried drug are not expected to be particularly different for oligonucleotides (ARNOLD 1985; NEVILLE 1987; FIUME et al. 1988 for reviews on the PLL, immunotoxin, and asialoglycoprotein fields, respectively).

Lipid vesicles represent an interesting alternative prospect for the in vivo delivery of antisense oligonucleotides. Liposomes of various sorts (GREGORIADIS 1988) as well as reconstituted paramyxovirus particles (HELENIUS et al. 1987), erythrocytes (KANEDA et al. 1989) or low density lipoproteins (VAN BERKEL et al. 1985) have been used by several groups to deliver various drugs and macromolecules to intact cells. This type of approach presents a number of theoretical advantages; indeed, the encapsulation of oligonucleotides within the aqueous internal compartment protects them from degradation by nucleases in biological fluids or from immune reactions. Moreover, liposomes have been successfully designed to release encapsulated drugs in a controlled manner, which might be of critical importance in the antisense oligonucleotides field (WRIGHT and HUANG 1989).

As pointed out in previous sections, lipid vesicles can be associated with targeting moieties such as antibodies or lectins. However, serious practical difficulties have generally been encountered upon in vivo extrapolation of the in vitro data. They deal with physical stability of the lipid vesicles within biological fluids (BONTE and JULIANO 1986), targeting out of the vascular compartment, and escape from capture by the reticuloendothelial system (GREGORIADIS 1988). Similar problems are expected to be encountered with lipid vesicles carrying antisense oligonucleotides but no experimental data have yet been disclosed. It is encouraging that significant progress has been made recently in the targeting of various liposomes outside of the reticuloendothelial system. Highly significant in this respect is the recent achievement by the group of L. Huang (HUGUES et al. 1989) in successfully targeting intravenously inoculated immunoliposomes to mouse lungs through monoclonal antibodies specific for lung capillary endothelial cells.

In conclusion, antisense oligonucleotides have already proven to be efficient for the in vitro modulation of various cellular and viral genes thus providing invaluable tools for assessing their individual role in intact cells.

In vivo experimentation and eventual clinical application are probably still far ahead at variance with the provocative editorial of a *Wall Street Journal* issue on the "Promise seen in anti-sense medicine – an approach aiming at neutralizing harmful genes."

Local administration, for instance in the treatment of skin diseases, might well represent a first practical goal, since Ts'o and colleagues already report preliminary data on the local treatment of mouse herpes simplex type I ear infection by methylphosphonates (MILLER and Ts'o 1987).

References

Agrawal S, Goodchild J, Civeira MP, Thornton AH, Sarin PS, Zamecnik PC (1988) Oligodeoxynucleoside phosphoramidates and phosphorothioates as inhibitors of human immunodeficiency virus. Proc Natl Acad Sci USA 85:7079–7083

Agris CH, Blake K, Miller P, Reddy M, Ts'o POP (1986) Inhibition of vesicular stomatitis virus protein synthesis and infection by sequence-specific oligodeoxyribonucleoside methylphosphonates. Biochemistry 25:6268–6275

Arad G, Hershkovitz M, Panet A, Loyter A (1986) Use of reconstituted Sendai virus envelopes for fusion-mediated microinjection of double-stranded RNA: inhibition of protein synthesis in interferon-treated cells. Biochim Biophys Acta 859:88–94

Arnold LJ (1985) Polylysine drug conjugates. Methods Enzymol 112:270–285

Babkin IV, Boutorin AS, Ivanova EM, Ryte AF (1988) Study of chemical conversion of radioactive (N-2-chloroethyl-N-methylamino)benzyl 5'—^{32}P—phosphamide of oligodeoxyribonucleotides in vivo. Biokhemiia 53:384–393

Bacon TA, Morvan F, Rayner B, Imbach JL, Wicksrom E (1988) α-Oligodeoxynucleotide stability in serum, subcellular extracts and culture media. J Biochem Biophys Methods 16:311–318

Bartkiewicz M, Gold HA, Altman S (1989) Identification and characterization of an RNA molecule that copurifies with RNase P activity from HeLa cells. Genes Dev 3:488–499

Basile D, Mir LM, Paoletti C (1989) Voltage-dependent introduction of [alpha] octothymidylate into electropermeabilized cells. Biochem Biophys Res Commun 159:633–639

Bass BL, Weintraub H (1987) A developmentally regulated activity that unwinds RNA duplexes. Cell 48:607–613

Bass BL, Weintraub H (1988) An unwinding activity that covalently modifies its double-stranded RNA substrate. Cell 55:1089–1098

Becker D, Meier CB, Herlyn M (1989) Proliferation of human malignant melanomas is inhibited by antisense oligodeoxynucleotides targeted against basic fibroblast growth factor. EMBO J 8:3685–3691

Berkowitz LA, Riabowol KT, Gilman MZ (1989) Multiple sequence elements of a single functional class are required for cyclic AMP responsiveness of the mouse c-fos promoter. Mol Cell Biol 9:4272–4281

Bertrand JR, Imbach JL, Paoletti C, Malvy C (1989) Comparative activity of α- and β-anomeric oligonucleotides on rabbit β globin synthesis: inhibitory effect of CAP targeted α-oligonucleotides. Bioch Biophys Res Commun 164:311–318

Bonte F, Juliano RL (1986) Interaction of liposomes with serum proteins. Chem Phys Lipids 40:359–371

Boutorin AS, Vlassov VV, Kazakov SA, Kutiavin IV, Podymnogin MA (1984) Complementary addressed reagents carrying EDTA-Fe(II) groups for directed cleavage of single-stranded nucleic acids. FEBS Lett 172:43–46

Boutorin AS, Gusvkova LV, Ivanova EM, Kobetz ND, Zarytova VF, Ryte AS, Yurchenko LV, Vlassov VV (1989) Synthesis of alkylating oligonucleotide derivatives containing cholesterol or phenazinium residues at their 3'-terminus and their interaction within mammalian cells. FEBS Lett 254:129–132

Cameron H, Jennings PA (1989) Specific gene suppression by engineered ribozymes in monkey cells. Proc Natl Acad Sci USA 86:9139–9143

Chen CHB, Sigman DS (1986) Nuclease activity of 1.10-phenantroline-copper: sequence-specific targetting. Proc Natl Acad Sci USA 83:7147–7151

Coleman J, Green PJ, Inouye M (1984) The use of RNAs complementary to specific mRNAs to regulate the expression of individual bacterial gene. Cell 37:429–436

Connors J, Yatvin MB, Huang L (1984) pH-sensitive liposomes: acid-induced liposome fusion. Proc Natl Acad Sci USA 81:1715–1718

Cooney M, Czernuszewicz G, Postel EH, Flint SJ, Hogan ME (1988) Site-specific oligonucleotide binding represses transcription of the human c-*myc* gene in vitro. Science 241:456–459

Cotten M, Schaffner G, Birnstiel ML (1989) Ribozyme, antisense RNA, and antisense DNA inhibition of U7 small nuclear ribonucleoprotein-mediated histone pre-mRNA processing in vitro. Mol Cell Biol 9:4479–4487

Dash P, Lotan I, Knapp M, Kandel ER, Goelet P (1987) Selective elimination of mRNAs in vivo: Complementary oligodeoxynucleotides promote RNA degradation by an RNAse H-like activity. Proc Natl Acad Sci USA 84:7896–7900

Degols G, Leonetti JP, Gagnor C, Lemaitre M, Lebleu B (1989) Antiviral activity and possible mechanisms of action of oligonucleotides-poly(L-lysine) conjugates targeted to vesicular stomatitis virus mRNA and genomic RNA. Nucleic Acids Res 17:9341–9350

Dervan PB (1989) oligonucleotide recognition of double-helical DNA by triple helix formation. In: Cohen JS (ed) Oligodeoxynucleotides antisense Inhibitors of gene expression. pp 197–210

Ehresmann C, Baudin F, Mougel M, Romby P, Ebel JP, Ehresmann B (1987) Probing the structure of RNAs in solution. Nucleic Acids Res 15:9109–9128

Eppstein DA, Longenecker JP (1988) Alternative delivery systems for peptides and proteins as drugs. CRC Crit Rev Ther Drug Carrier Sys 5:99–139

Fiume L, Busi C, Mattioli A, Spinosa G (1988) Targeting of antiviral drugs bound to protein carriers. CRC Crit Rev Ther Drug Carrier Syst 4:265–284

Froehler B, Ng P, Matteucci M (1988) Phosphoramidate analogues of DNA: synthesis and thermal stability of heteroduplexes. Nucleic Acids Res 16:4831–4839

Furdon PJ, Dominski Z, Kole R (1989) RNase H cleavage of RNA hybridized to oligonucleotides containing methylphosphonate, phosphorothioate and phosphodiester bonds. Nucleic Acids Res 17:9193–9204

Gagnor C, Bertrand JR, Thenet S, Lemaitre M, Morvan F, Rayner B, Malvy C, Lebleu B, Imbach JL, Paoletti C (1987) Alpha-DNA VI: comparitive study of alpha- and beta-anomeric oligonucleotides in hybridization to mRNA and in cell-free translation inhibition. Nucleic Acids Res 15:1049–10436

Gagnor C, Rayner B, Leonetti JP, Imbach JL, Lebleu B (1989) Parallel annealing of alpha anomeric oligodeoxyribonucleotides to natural mRNA is required for interference in RNase H mediated hydrolysis and reverse transcription. Nucleic Acids Res 17:5107–5113

Gewirtz AM, Anfossi G, Venturelli D, Valpreda S, Sims R, Calabretta B (1989) G_1/S transition in normal human T-lymphocytes requires the nuclear protein encoded by c-*myb*. Science 24:180–183

Goodchild J, Agrawal S, Civeira MP, Sarin PS, Sun D, Zamecnik PC (1988) Inhibition of human immunodeficiency virus replication by antisense oligodeoxynucleotides. Proc Natl Acad Sci USA 85:5507–5511

Grandas A, Marshall WS, Nielsen J, Caruthers MH (1989) Synthesis of deoxycytidine oligomers containing phosphorodithioate linkages. Tetrahedron Lett 30:543–546

Green PJ, Pines O, Inouye M (1986) The role of antisense RNA in gene regulation. Annu Rev Biochem 55:569–597

Gregoriadis G (ed) (1988) Liposomes as drug carriers. Recent trends and progress. Wiley, Chichester

Griffin LC, Dervan PB (1989) Recognition of thymine adenine base pairs by guanine in a pyrimidine triple helix motif. Science 245:967–970

Gupta KC (1987) Antisense oligodeoxynucleotides provide insight into mechanism of translation initiation of two Sendai virus mRNAs. J Biol Chem 262:7492–7496

Haseloff J, Gerlach WL (1988) Simple RNA enzymes with new and highly specific endoribonuclease activities. Nature 334:585–591

Hélène C, Montenay-Garestier T, Saison I, Takasugi M, Toulme JJ, Asseline U, Lancelot G, Maurizot JC, Toulme F, Thuong NT (1985) Oligodeoxynucleotides covalently linked to intercalating agents: a new class of gene regulatory substances. Biochimie 67:777–783

Helenius A, Doxsey S, Hellman I (1987) Viruses as tools in drug delivery. In: Biological approaches to the controlled delivery of drugs. Ann NY Acad Sci 507:1–6

Hoogsteen K (1959) The stucture of crystals containing a hydrogen-bonded complex of 1-methylthymine and 9-methyladenine. Acta Cristallogr 12:822–823

Hugues BJ, Kennel S, Lee R, Huang L (1989) Monoclonal antibody targeting of liposomes to mouse lung in vivo. Cancer Res 49:6124–6220

Izant JG, Weintraub H (1984) Inhibition of thymidine kinase gene expression by antisense RNA: a molecular approach to genetic analyses. Cell 36:1007–1015

Juliano RL (ed) (1987) Biological approaches to the controlled delivery of drugs. Ann NY Acad Sci 507

Kaneda Y, Iwai K, Uchida T (1989) Increased expression of DNA cointroduced with nuclear protein in adult rat liver. Science 243:375–378

Kim SK, Wold B (1985) Stable reduction of thymidine kinase activity in cells expressing high levels of antisense RNA. Cell 42:129–138

Kim SC, Podhajska Aj, Szybalski W (1988) Cleaving DNA at any predetermined site with adapter-primers and class-IIS restriction enzymes. Science 240:504–506

Knight DE, Scrutton MC (1986) Gaining access to the cytosol: the technique and some applications of electropermeabilization. Biochem J 234:497–506

Knorre DG, Vlassov VV, Zarytova VF, Karpova GG (1985) Nucleotide and oligonucleotide derivatives as enzyme and nucleic acid targeted irreversible inhibitors. Chemical aspects. Adv Enzyme Regul 24:277–300

Knorre V, Vlassov VV, Zarytova VF (1985) Reactive oligonucleotide derivatives and sequence-specific modification of nucleic acids. Biochimie 67:785–789

Knorre V, Vlassov VV, Zarytova VF (1989) Oligonucleotides linked to reactive groups. In: Cohen JS (ed) Oligodeoxynucleotides: antisense inhibitors of gene expression. Macmillan, London, p 173

Kulka M, Smith CC, Aurelian L, Fishelevich R, Meade K, Ts'o POP (1989) Site specificity of the inhibitory effects of oligo(nucleoside methylphosphonate)s complementary to the acceptor splic junction of herpes simplex virus type 1 immediate early mRNA 4. Proc Natl Acad Sci USA 86:6868–6872

Lamond AI, Sproat B, Ryder U, Hamm J (1989) Probing the structure and function of U2 snRNP with antisense oligonucleotides made of 2'-O-Me-RNA. Cell 58: 383–390

Lawson TG, Ray BK, Dodds JT, Grifo JA, Abramson RD, Merrick WC, Betsch DF, Veith HL, Thach RE (1986) Influence of 5' proximal secondary structure on the translation efficiency of eukaryotic mRNAs and on their interaction with initiation factors. J Biol Chem 261:13979–13989

Lee BL, Murakami A, Blake KR, Lin SB, Miller PS (1988) Interaction of psoralen-derivatized oligodeoxyribonucleoside methylphosphonates. Biochemistry 27: 3197–3203

Lemaitre M, Bayard B, Lebleu B (1987) Specific antiviral activity of a poly(L-lysine)-conjugated oligodeoxyribonucleotide sequence complementary to vesicular stomatitis virus N protein mRNA initiation site. Proc Natl Acad Sci USA 84:648–652

Leonetti JP, Rayner B, Lemaitre M, Gagnor C, Milhaud PG, Imbach JL, Lebleu B (1988) Antiviral activity of conjugates between poly(L-lysine) and synthetic oligodeoxyribonucleotides. Gene 72:323–332

Leonetti JP, Machy P, Degols G, Lebleu B, Leserman L' (1990b) Antibody-targeted liposomes containing oligodeoxyribonucleotide sequences complementary to viral RNA selectively inhibit viral replication. Proc Natl Acad Sci USA 87:2448–2451

Leonetti JP, Degols G, Lebleu B (1990a) Biological activity of oligonucleotide-poly(L-lysine) conjugates: mechanism of cell uptake. Bioconjugate Chem 1:149–153

Lesnikowski ZJ, Jaworska M, Stec WJ (1988) Stereoselective synthesis of P-homochiral oligo(thymidine methanephosphonates). Nucleic Acids Res 16: 11675–11689

Letsinger RL, Zhang G, Sun DK, Ikeuchi T, Sarin P (1989) Cholesteryl conjugated oligonucleotides: synthesis, properties, and activity as inhibitors of replication of human immunodeficiency virus in cell culture. Proc Natl Acad Sci USA 86: 6553–6556

Loke SL, Stein C, Zhang X, Avigan M, Cohen J, Neckers LM (1988) Delivery of c-*myc* antisense phosphorothioate oligodeoxynucleotide to hematopoietic cells in culture by liposome fusion: specific reduction in c-*myc* protein expression correlates with inhibition of cell growth and DNA synthesis. Curr Top Microbiol Immunol 141:282–289

Loke SL, Stein CA, Zhang XH, Mori K, Nakanishi M, Subasinghe C, Cohen JS, Neckers LM (1989) Characterization of oligonucleotide transport into living cells. Proc Natl Acad Sci USA 86:38474–3478

Maher LJ, III Dolnick BJ (1988) Comparative hybrid arrest by tandem antisense oligodeoxyribonucleotides or oligodeoxyribonucleoside methylphosphonates in a cell-free system. Nucleic Acids Res 16:3341–3357

Maher LJ, III Wold B, Dervan PB (1989) Inhibition of DNA binding proteins by oligonucleotide-directed triple helix formation. Science 245:725–730

Majumdar C, Stein CA, Cohen JS, Broder S, Wilson SH (1989) Stepwise mechanism of HIV reverse transcriptase: primer function of phosphorothioate oligodeoxy-nucleotide. Biochemistry 28:1340–1346

Marcus-Sekura CJ, Woerner AM, Shinozuka K, Zon G, Quinnan GV (1987) Comparative inhibition of chloramphenicol acetyltransferase gene expression by antisense oligonucleotide analogues having alkyl phosphotriester, methylphosphonate and phosphorothioate linkage. Nucleic Acids Res 15: 5749–5763

Matsukura M, Shinozuka K, Zon G, Mitsuya H, Reitz M, Cohen JS, Broder S (1987) Phosphorothioate analogs of oligodeoxynucleotides: inhibitors of replication and cytopathic effects of human immunodeficiency virus. Proc Natl Acad Sci USA 84:7706–7710

Matsukura M, Zon G, Shinozuka K, Robert-Guroff M, Shimada T, Stein CA, Mitsuya H, Wong-Sthall F, Cohen JS, Broder S (1989) Regulation of viral expression of human immunodeficiency virus in vitro by an antisense phos-phorothioate oligodeoxynucleotide against rev (art/trs) in chronically infected cells. Proc Natl Acad Sci USA 86:4244–4248

McSwiggen JA, Cech TR (1989) Stereochemistry of RNA cleavage by the Tetrahymena ribozyme and evidence that the chemical step is not rate-limiting. Science 244:679–683

Miller PS, Ts'o POP (1987) A new approach to chemotherapy based on molecular biology and nucleic acid chemistry: matagen (masking tape for gene expression). Anticancer Drug Design 2:117–128

Miller PS, Barret JC, Ts'o POP (1974) Synthesis of oligodeoxyribonucleotide ethylphosphorodiesters and their specific complex formation with transfer ribonucleic acid. Biochemistry 13:4887–4896

Miller PS, Braiterman LT, Ts'o POP (1977) Effects of a trinucleotide ethyl phos-photriester, $G^mp(ET)G^mp(ET)U$, on mammalian cells in culture. Biochemistry 16:1977–1996

Miller PS, Yano J, Yano E, Caroll C, Jayaraman K, Ts'o POP (1979) Non ionic nucleic acid analogues synthesis and characterization of dideoxyribonucleotide methylphosphonates. Biochemistry 18:5134–5143

Minshull J, Hunt T (1987) The use of single-stranded DNA and RNAse H to promote quantitative "hybrid arrest of translation" of mRNA/DNA hybrids in reticulocyte lysate cell-free translation. Nucleic Acids Res 16:6433–6451

Mori K, Boiziau C, Cazenave C, Matsukura M, Subasunghe C, Cohen JS, Broder S, Toulme JJ, Stein CA (1989) Phosphoroselenoate oligodeoxynucleotides:

synthesis, physico-chemical characterization, anti-sense inhibitory properties and anti HIV activity. Nucleic Acids Res 17:8207–8219

Morvan F, Rayner B, Imbach JL, Chang DK, Lown JW (1986) a-DNA I. Synthesis, characterization by high field ^{1}H-NMR, and base-pairing properties of the unnatural hexadeoxyribonucleotide α- d(CpCpTpTpCpC) with its complement β-d(GpGpApApGpG). Nucleic Acids Res 14:5019–5035

Neville DM Jr (1987) Immunotoxins for in vivo therapy: where are we? In: Biological approaches to the controlled delivery of drugs. Ann NY Acad Sci 507: 155

Quartin RS, Wetmur JG (1989) Effect of ionic strength on the hybridation of oligonucleotides with reduced charge due to methylphosphonate linkages to unmodified oligodeoxynucleotides containing the complementary sequence. Biochemistry 28:1040–1047

Rayner B, Matsukura M, Morvan F, Cohen JS, Imbach JL (1990) Activité anti-VIH in vitro d'oligonucléotides a-phosphorothioates d'anomeried. C R Acad Sci Paris 310[III]:61–65

Rebagliati MR, Melton DA (1987) Antisense RNA injections in fertilized frog eggs reveal an RNA duplex unwinding activity. Cell 48:599–605

Rothenberg M, Jonhson G, Laughlin C, Green I, Cradock J, Sarver N, Cohen JS (1989) Oligodeoxynucleotides as anti-sense inhibitors of gene expression: therapeutic implications. JNCI 81:1539–1544

Sarin PS, Agrawal S, Civeira MP, Goodchild J, Ikeuchi T, Zamecnik PC (1988) Inhibition of acquired immunodeficiency syndrome virus by oligodeoxynucleotide methylphosphonates. Proc Natl Acad Sci USA 85:7448–7451

Shen WC, Ryser H-P (1978) Conjugation of poly-L-lysine to albumin and horseradish peroxidase: a novel method of enhancing the cellular uptake of proteins. Proc Natl Acad Sci USA 75:1872–1876

Shi YB, Hearst JE (1986) Thermostability of double-stranded deoxyribonucleic acids: effects of covalent additions of a psoralen. Biochemistry 25:5895–5902

Shibahara S, Mukai S, Nishiara T, Inouye H, Ohtska E, Morisawa H (1987) Site-directed cleavage of RNA. Nucleic Acids Res 15:4403–4415

Shibahara S, Mukai S, Morisawa H, Nakashima H, Kobayashy S, Yamamoto N (1989) Inhibition of human immunodeficiency virus (HIV-1) replication by synthetic oligo-RNA derivatives. Nucleic Acids Res 17:239–252

Smith CC, Aurelian L, Reddy MP, Miller PS, Ts'o POP (1986) Antiviral effect of an oligo(nucleoside methylphosphonate) complementary to the splice junction of herpes simplex virus type 1 immediate early pre-mRNA 4 and 5. Proc Natl Acad Sci USA 80:3232–3236

Smith CJS, Watson CF, Ray J, Bird CR, Morris PC, Schuch W, Grierson D (1988) Antisense RNA inhibition of polygalacturonase gene expression in tomatoes. Nature 334:724–726

Sproat BS, Lamond AI, Beijer B, Neuner P, Ryder U (1989) Highly efficient chemical synthesis of 2'-O-methyloligoribonucleotides and tetrabiotinylated derivative; novel probes that are resistant to degradation by RNA or DNA specific nucleases. Nucleic Acids Res 17:3373–3386

Stec WJ, Zon G, Egan W, Stec B (1984) Automated solid phase synthesis, separation, and stereochemistry of phosphorothioate analogues of oligodeoxyribonucleotides. J Am Chem Soc ●: 6077–6079

Stein CA, Subasinghe C, Shinozuka K, Cohen JS (1988) Physicochemical properties of phosphorothioate oligodeoxynucleotides. Nucleic Acids Res 16:3209–3221

Stevenson M, Iversen PL (1989) Inhibition of human immunodeficiency virus type 1-mediated cytopathic effects by poly(L-lysine)-conjugated synthetic antisense oligodeoxyribonucleotides. J Gen Virol 70:673–682

Straubinger RM, Hong K, Friend K, Papahadjopoulos P (1983) Endocytosis of liposomes and intracellular fate of encapsulated molecules: encounter with a low pH compartment after internalization in coated vesicles. Cell 32:1069–1079

Tomlinson E (1987) Theory and practice of site-specific drug delivery. Adv Drug Delivery Rev 1:87–198

Uhlenbeck OC (1987) A small catalytic oligoribonucleotide. Nature 328:596–600

Van Berkel TJC, Kruijt JK, Spanjer MH, Nagelkerke JF, Harkes L, Kempen HJM
(1985) The effect of a water-soluble trls-galactoside-terminated cholesterol
derlvatlve on the fate of low density lipoproteins and liposomes. J Biol Chem
260:2694–2699

Van der Krol AR, Lenting PE, Veenstra J, van der Meer IM, Koes RE, Gerats AGM,
Mol JNM, Stuitje AR (1988a) An antisense chalcone synthase gene in transgenic
plants inhibits flower pigmentation. Nature 333:866–869

Van der Krol AR, Mol JNM, Stuitje AR (1988b) Modulation of eukaryotic gene
expression by complementary RNA or DNA sequences. Biotechniques 6:
958–975

Verspieren P, Cornelissen AWCA, Thuong NT, Hélène C, Toulmé C (1987) An
acridine-linked oligodeoxynucleotide targeted to the common 5' end of
trypanosome mRNAs kills cultured parasites. Gene 61:307–315

Wagner RW, Nishikura K (1988) Cell cycle expression of RNA duplex unwindase
activity by mammalian cells. Mol Cell Biol 8:770–777

Walder J (1988) Antisense DNA and RNA: progress and prospects. Genes Dev
2:502–504

Wright S, Huang L (1989) Antibody-directed liposomes as drug-delivery vehicles. Adv
Drug Delivery Rev 3:343–389

Wu JY, Wu CH (1988) Evidence for targeted gene delivery to HEPG$_2$ hepatoma cells
in vitro. Biochemistry 27:887–892

Yakubov LA, Deeva EA, Zarytova VF, Ivanova EM, Ryte AS, Yurchenko LV,
Vlassov VV (1989) Mechanism of oligonucleotide uptake by cells: involvement of
specific receptors? Proc Natl Acad Sci USA 86:6454–6458

Yu Z, Chen D, Black RJ, Blake K, Ts'o POP, Miller P, Chang EH (1989) Sequence
specific inhibition of in vitro translation of mutated or normal ras p21. J Exp
Pathol 4:97–108

Zamecnik PC, Stephenson M (1978) Inhibition of Rous sarcoma virus replication and
cell transformation by a specific oligodeoxynucleotide. Proc Natl Acad Sci USA
75:280–284

Zamecnik PC, Goodchild J, Taguchi Y, Sarin PS (1986) Inhibition of replication and
expression of human T-cell lymphotropic virus type II in cultured cells by
exogenous synthetic oligonucleotides complementary to viral RNA. Proc Natl
Acad Sci USA 83:4143–4146

Zerial A, Thuong NT, Hélène C (1987) Selective inhibition of the cytopathic effect of
type A influenza viruses by oligodeoxynucleotides covalently linked to an intercalating agent. Nucleic Acids Res 15:9909–9919

Zon G (1989) Pharmaceutical considerations. In: Cohen JS (ed) Oligodeoxynucleotides: antisense inhibitors of gene expression. Macmillan, London, p 233

Zuckermann RN, Schultz PG (1989) Site-selective of structured RNA by a
staphylococcal nuclease-DNA hybrid. Biochemistry 86:1766–1770

Further Reading

Cohen J (ed) (1989) Oligonucleotides: antisense inhibitors of gene expression.
Macmillan, London Topics in molecular and structural biology, vol 12. The first
book completely devoted to the field of oligonucleotides synthesis, biological
properties, and prospect of clinical utilization.

Gene (1988) 72:1–378. An entire issue of Gene reporting the EMBO/INSERM
workshop on "Regulation of gene expression by RNA structure and anti-
messengers," held at Les Arcs (France) in March 1988. The entire field of
synthetic oligonucleotides was covered, as well as regulation of gene expression
by naturally occurring antisense RNAs. Aspects of post-transcriptional regulation
of gene expression which might be useful to conceive synthetic oligonucleotides of
increased efficiency were also examined.

Green PJ, Pines O, Inouye M (1986) The role of antisense RNA in gene regulation. Annu Rev Biochem 55:569–597. One of the first and still valid comprehensive reviews of the antisense field with particular emphasis on bacterial systems.

Van der Krol AR, Mol JNM, Stuitje AR (1988) Modulation of eukaryotic gene expression by complementary RNA or DNA sequences. Biotechniques 6: 958–975. One of the most recent reviews covering both the "flipped" gene and the synthetic oligonucleotide approaches; tables illustrating the variety of genes artificially regulated by antisense RNAs or synthetic oligonucleotides might be useful.

Stein CA, Cohen J (1988) Oligodeoxynucleotides as inhibitors of gene expression: a review. Cancer Res 48:2659–2668. A short review on synthetic oligonucleotide analogues and their potential, with particular emphasis on phosphorothioates.

Zon G (1988) Oligonucleotide analogues as potential chemotherapeutic agents. Pharm Res 5:539–549. A recent review covering synthetic oligonucleotides chemistry and prospects for their scaled up synthesis and pharmacological utilization.

Miller PS, Agris CH, Aurelian L, Blake KR, Glave SA, Smith SB, Murakami A, Reddy MP, Smith CC, Spitz SA, Ts'o POP (1986) Matagen (masking tape for gene expression): a family of oligonucleoside methylphosphonates. In: Chagas C, Pullman B (eds) Molecular mechanisms of carcinogenic and antitumor activity. Pontificia Academia Scientiarum, Vatican City, p 169. A review devoted to the use of methylphosphonates as regulators of gene expression.

Juliano RL (ed) (1987) Biological approaches to the controlled delivery of drugs. Ann NY Acad Sci 507. A complete issue covering the general problems of drug delivery.

Tomlinson E (1987) Theory and practice of site-specific drug delivery. Adv Drug Delivery Rev 1:87–198. A comprehensive review on the problems and prospects of drug delivery.

Subject Index

Handbook of Experimental Pharmacology

Editorial Board: G. V. R. Born, P. Cuatrecasas, H. Herken

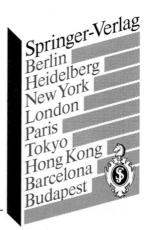

Springer-Verlag
Berlin
Heidelberg
New York
London
Paris
Tokyo
Hong Kong
Barcelona
Budapest

Handbook of Experimental Pharmacology

Editorial Board: G. V. R. Born, P. Cuatrecasas, H. Herken

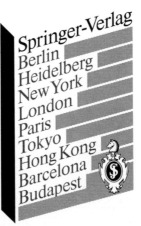

Springer-Verlag
Berlin
Heidelberg
New York
London
Paris
Tokyo
Hong Kong
Barcelona
Budapest